No Time to Teach?

A NURSE'S GUIDE TO PATIENT AND FAMILY EDUCATION

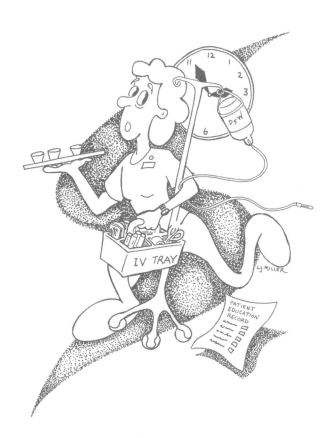

No Time to Teach?

A NURSE'S GUIDE
TO PATIENT AND
FAMILY EDUCATION

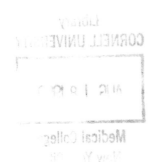
Fran London, RN, MS

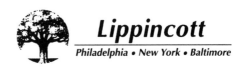

Lippincott

Philadelphia • New York • Baltimore

Acquisitions Editor: Susan M. Glover, RN, MSN
Coordinating Editorial Assistant: Bridget Blatteau
Project Editor: Nicole Walz
Senior Production Manager: Helen Ewan
Production Coordinator: Pat McCloskey

Design Coordinator: Carolyn O'Brien
Indexer: Ellen Murray
Compositor: The PRD Group, Inc.
Printer: R.R. Donnelley & Sons—Crawfordsville

9 8 7 6 5 4 3 2 1

Library of Congress Cataloging in Publications Data

London, Fran.
 No time to teach? : a nurse's guide to patient and family
education / Fran London.
  p. cm.
 Includes bibliographical references and index.
 ISBN 0-7817-1644-6 (alk. paper)
 1. Patient education. 2. Nurse and patient. 3. Nursing.
I. Title. II. Title: Nurse's guide to patient and family education.
 [DNLM: 1. Patient Education Nurses' Instruction. 2. Teaching methods Nurses' Instruction. W 85 L847n 1998]
RT90.L66 1999
615.5′071—dc21
DNLM/DLC
for Library of Congress
                     99-14488
                       CIP

Dedication

"You should never be afraid.
Acting boldly if you must
To fulfill your sacred trust
And be faithful to the promises you made."

—lyrics from *Just While We're Here*

This book is dedicated to my friends:
Doug Fletcher, RN
Bob Diskin, BSN, BFA, RN
Diane Rumsey, RN
Georgia Moss, RN

They came together from Arizona, New York, Pennsylvania, and Florida to creatively promote patient care we could be proud of and to improve nurses' quality of life. They came together through the *Journal of Nursing Jocularity,* to put on another performance of the first musical-comedy about the essence of nursing, *Who's Got the Keys?*

On May 1, 1998, in one instant, they died together in a motor vehicle accident. They taught me, with a shared goal, planning, and collaboration, nurses could accomplish that which seems absolutely impossible. I now see how we are only limited by the walls we create with our minds. We've got the keys.

I will miss them.

"We were only passing through
I wonder if you only knew
How much you gave,
How much we took for granted . . .
Some of us with broken dreams
Disillusioned by the things we've seen,
Some of us with broken bones
You soothe us and give us a home . . .
Because of all the things you do
We're living now with hope renewed.
You offer us your love just while we're here."

—lyrics from *Just While We're Here*

If you want to hear more:

Diskin, B. (1997). *Just While We're Here*. Lyrics from the musical-comedy, *Who's Got The Keys?* Canaan, NY: Muse-Med, Inc.

For information about the musical, *Who's Got the Keys?*

(cassettes, CDs, performances) and other products, contact Ted Fiebke, BSN, RN at:
   Nur–Sing Media, Inc.
   P.O. Box 42
   10 Footbridge Road
   Columbiaville, New York 12050-0042
   Phone: (518)828-3271
   E-mail: efiebke@berk.com

Thanks

We and all the events of our lives are connected. Everyone who ever touched my life made this book possible. My sister, Joan, the creative one. My husband, Jay, who listened to my tales of the process of book writing, offered his unique insights, and encouraged me to keep working ("Are you done yet?"). The list is endless. I'll limit my list of thanks to those who had a direct impact on the creation of this book.

To Bean Cromwell, MS, RN, my preceptor, mentor, and friend. She set high standards, expected me to meet them, and showed me how. When Bean moved beyond inpatient staff nursing, I wondered, "Who'll be my role model, now that my role model's gone?" I didn't realize how strongly I had internalized her lessons.

To all the nurses on the 4-1400 unit of Strong Memorial Hospital, where I grew into the nurse I am today. That was an immersion experience in quality nursing and teamwork.

To Patricia Hryzak Lind, MS, RNC, who taught me how to use the SMOG readability test to make medication teaching sheets more understandable, and for telling me about a humor conference down-state, where I discovered the very first issue of the *Journal of Nursing Jocularity*.

To Kathy Werner, PhD, RN, who started The Emily Center, shared her vision, and gave me the opportunity to build the Patient/Family Education Program at Phoenix Children's Hospital.

To frustration. Without it, the existing books on patient education would have been enough. I can't sit around quietly when something needs to be said.

To those who provided resources, expertise, experiences, or took the time to review my drafts and hone this work:
Yvonne Brookes, RN
Ruth Brooks, MS, RN
Candice Brown, MLIS
Leslie Cole
Beth Cooksey
Sandy Cornett, RN
Marla Cushman, RN
Kim Dent
Jane Diaz, MS, RN
Douglas Fletcher, RN
Nina Gaby, MS, RN
Fran Hoekstra, RN
Mary Holtschneider, BSN, RN
Irene Jacobs
Melani Jaskowiak, MS, RN

Susan Cort Johnson
Suzanne Hall Johnson, MN, RNC, CNS
Dori London
Cathy Miller, RN
Eileen Mitchell, MS, RN
Sally Moffat, MS, RN
Lisa Jane Moore, RN
Esther Muñoz, BS, RN
Joyce Nieiemic, RN
Florence Nightingale
Judy O'Haver, MS, RN
Susan Ohton, RN
Chris Oless, RN
Penny Overgaard, RN
Lori Parker-Hartigan, RN
Genevieve Panzella
Paula Pastore, RN
Rodney Pease, MD
Debbie Perry, MSN, RN
Charlene Pope, CNM, MPH
Vicki Provo
Barbara Rayes
Carol Robinson, MS, RN
Steven Schnall
Julie Schneider, MS, RN
Ele Shnier
Debra Skidmore, BSN, RN
Robin Smith, DO
Jane Snyder
Keith Stefanczyk
Dennis Swain
A. Kim Sweet, RN
Lisa Vanatta, MS, RD
March Warn, RN, CNOR
Kathleen Tripp Werner, PhD, RN
A. White, MS, RN
Patty Wooten, BS, RN
Jillian Wright
Philip Yarbrough, RN
To Susan M. Glover, RN, MSN, my editor, who had faith and offered
me both roots and wings on this writing journey—and extended my
deadline. To Bridget Blatteau, her assistant, who understood, cared,
and implemented.

Thank you.

Preface

What brought me to write this book on patient and family education? In many ways, popular culture.

As a child, my favorite movie was *Dark Victory*. In 1939, *Dark Victory* won academy awards for Best Picture and Best Score, and Bette Davis won Best Actress. In it, rich, strong, beautiful Bette Davis gets a brain tumor, falls in love, and dies. I was too young to understand it was a tale of tragic romance. I missed the point completely. Instead, to me it was a movie about the importance of telling patients the truth. (Bette's doctor didn't tell her she had a tumor; she found out by accident and got angry.) I thought the moral of the story was that doctors should explain to patients what they are experiencing, and give them the ability to make informed choices. I missed the point, but gained a life mission. Because of this movie, I have been a patient advocate since childhood. (My experience also demonstrates that when teaching is not developmentally appropriate for the learner, the message may not be understood as intended.)

Then, as I got older, I found a new favorite movie, *Harold and Maude*. The message there: experience and celebrate life. Control your destiny. Do the right thing. Question authority. Enjoy. Just do it. (It also contains a message I know many nurses share: there are worse things in life than death.) This movie struck a chord in me. It resonated. It was my song.

Most people get their movie reviews from their local newspapers. Not me. My favorite movie reviewer is a psychiatrist, Frank Pittman. His insightful columns in *The Family Therapy Networker* put movies into perspective. He looks at the messages popular films send, and the big picture of the relationship between culture, art, and life. (Well, what do you expect? He's a psychiatrist.) Dr. Pittman has said the key to mental health is to see your life as a comedy, and not as a tragedy. Bad things happen to main characters in both, but the quality of life is better in comedies. Tragic heroes strive for ideals in an ugly, mean world. The main characters of tragedies are heroes, bigger than life, who despair the human condition. On the other hand, the main characters in comedies are human, just like everyone else. Their world can be crazy or bizarre. They learn from their goofs and experiences, and, in response, change and grow. Main characters in comedies don't fight reality, they accept and work within it. The theme of tragedies is "it's not our fault," and comedies, "we asked for it." Attitude makes all the difference in outcome. The key to mental health is to see your life, not as a tragedy, but as a comedy. We choose, with our attitudes, between misery and healthful coping.

What does this have to do with patient education? We nurses can let the state of health care today frustrate us. We can blame the system, say it's not our fault we have no time to teach, despair the human condition, and be miserable. Or we can accept reality and responsibility, change perspective, turn tragedy into comedy and figure out how to teach in this crazy world. Same situation, healthier attitude, better outcomes.

Now it sounds like all I did while I was growing up was watch movies. Not true. My favorite book was Robert Pirsig's *Zen and the Art of Motorcycle Maintenance*. It was timed perfectly; it was published when I was in my pensive period. Don't let the title mislead you. It's a book about the quest for truth. It talks about what's really important. It's a book about Quality. The message: if you're not aiming for Quality, why bother?

So that's the story of the making of *No Time to Teach?* I grew up, like most other people, watching movies and reading books. I learned lessons, integrated them, transformed them, and applied them to today's problems.

To be explicit, the message of this book is: give your patients and families the information they need. Do what you know is right and keep that light attitude. You'll survive, they'll learn, and Quality will prevail.

We know teaching patients and families is important because it's the only way to quality care. Research that tells us how to teach effectively. Now we just have to get out there, apply what we know, get creative, have fun, and do it.

And enjoy the process, because the process is life!

Fran London, MS, RN
flondon@phxchildrens.com

 ## If you want to know more:

Higgins, C. (1971). *Harold and Maude.* Hollywood, CA: Paramount Pictures Corporation.

Pirsig, R. M. (1974). *Zen and the art of motorcycle maintenance.* New York, NY: Bantam Books.

Pittman, F. (1995). Turning tragedy into comedy. *The Family Therapy Networker,* 19(6), 36-40.

Robinson, C. (1939, 1967). *Dark Victory.* Culver City, CA: MGM/UA Home Video, Inc.

Contents

Why Bother Teaching?

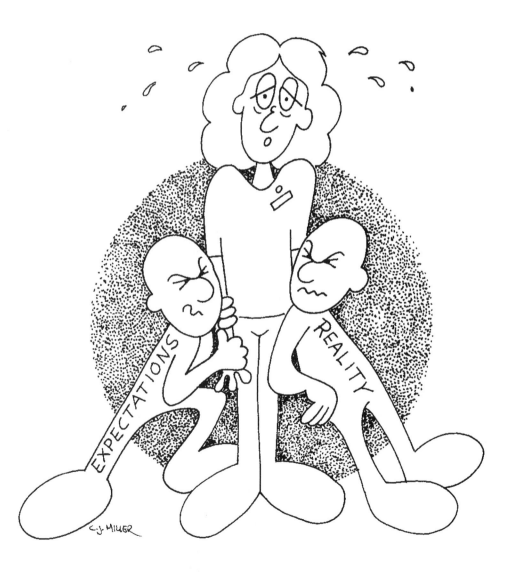

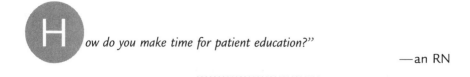

ow do you make time for patient education?"

—an RN

. . . .

Think about nursing school. How did you learn about patient education?

One of your assignments involved teaching a patient or family member. You had several weeks to plan and complete this assignment. You prepared your teaching materials, methods, and ways to evaluate learning. You were anxious, afraid the learner would ask questions you could not answer. When it was time, you sat down with your learner and had a teaching session. When you were done, you asked, "Do you have any questions?" There were some tough moments, but you got through them. You survived teaching. You documented the session in detail.

The assignment taught you a lot about planning, assessment, intervention, evaluation, and teaching. After the experience, talking with patients and families became a little more comfortable.

Then you work as a nurse, and the situation changes.

> *"Nurses have been taught in their basic education how to teach patients—to set objectives, develop plans and to meet those objectives, develop educational materials, set aside teaching time, and sit down and teach. When they get into the real world and are faced with harsh realities, they quickly find this approach impossible.*
>
> *More often than not, they 'throw out the baby with bath water,' hoping someone else will do the teaching they know is necessary. The textbook approach no longer is possible."*
>
> —Ruzicki, 1989, p. 629

Have you given up because you have no time to teach?

Why Bother?

If you continue to define patient teaching in this old textbook approach, in this old paradigm, frustration could overwhelm you. You might throw up your hands and think, "Why bother trying to teach?"

If you work in a hospital, as soon as your patients are well enough to hear your teaching, they are discharged. If you work in home care or in an outpatient setting, the situation is no better. You have too many patients and too little time to teach.

Furthermore, unless you are a diabetes educator, teaching time is rarely reimbursed by third-party payers. Most of the time teaching falls under the package of nursing care activities. Even if you can demonstrate that you need more time to teach, it is difficult to get payment for your time and efforts.

However, teaching is expected. It's in your job description, the Nurse Practice Act, your organization's policies and procedures, and Joint Commission on Accreditation of Health Care Organizations' (JCAHO) standards. Even patients and families expect to get information from you.

Do you feel you're getting mixed messages? Do you feel caught between expectations and reality?

"I Don't Teach. I Save Lives."

One way to avoid the dissonance between expectations and reality is to deny that you teach, but this can only be accurate if you have absolutely no contact with patients or family members who can perceive your presence.

Some nurses say, "I don't teach. I save lives." What does saving lives mean? Most health care professionals rescue patients from physiological events. Physicians, emergency medical technicians, and respiratory therapists all save lives. How are nurses different?

Some define nursing as the discipline that treats human response. Humans respond on many levels. They respond to trauma with bleeding. They respond to germs with fevers. They respond to crises with questions, such as, "What caused this?" and "What do I do now?"

Nurses are liaisons between people and their experiences of change. A liaison connects two or more separate entities so they can work together effectively. This change could be an illness, injury, or life transition. Experiences need to be integrated into patients' lives physically, emotionally, and spiritually. Nurses facilitate that process. Nurses encourage growth and independence. They help patients identify their abilities and coach them toward optimizing self-care.

One way this integration can be facilitated is through information sharing: patient and family teaching.

Can You Avoid Teaching?

Imagine these scenes:

- A nurse walks up to a patient and, without any explanation, gives a shot.
- A patient exclaims, "I could never do that at home!" and the nurse responds, "Oh, OK."
- A mom asks, "What do I do if this happens again?" and the nurse says, "Just bring him back here."
- At discharge, a nurse hands a patient three new prescriptions and says, "You may leave now."
- A family member asks, "What caused this?" and the nurse replies curtly, "Who knows?"

If you were the patient or family member in these situations, would you feel good about the care you received? Can a nurse really avoid teaching? Put another way, is patient and family education a nursing state or a nursing trait?

What's the difference? A *state* is temporary. It comes and goes. An example of a state would be laughter. A *trait* is an intrinsic part of a person. It's always there, whether or not it shows. A trait would be a sense of humor.

Patient education may look like a state when a nurse is assessing understanding of a diagnosis, demonstrating a dressing change, or evaluating knowledge of medication side effects. However, education is intrinsic to nursing.

You cannot avoid teaching. You educate every time you are in view or hearing of patients and families. A patient or family member may see you wash your hands before a procedure, hear you explain to a child how it will feel to have an intravenous (IV) line placed, or watch you operate the feeding pump. Whether or not you are aware of it, your every action teaches something. Educating patients and families is a trait of nursing.

Did you ever have a patient who readjusted his own IV pump or monitor? No nurse intentionally taught that patient to adjust the settings, right? This is evidence that education is a nursing trait.

Reframing Patient and Family Education

Here's another way to look at it. Do we need the nursing diagnosis of Knowledge Deficit?

Some nurses (Dennison & Keeling, 1989) have stated that Knowledge Deficit doesn't even meet the clinical criteria of a nursing diagnosis. One of the criteria for a legitimate nursing diagnosis is clinical utility. By calling Knowledge Deficit a nursing diagnosis, we define the patient's problem as a lack of information.

This implies that providing information will change behavior and outcomes, which is rarely true. If this were true, the warnings on cigarette packages and alcohol bottles would have eliminated smoking and drinking by now. Instead, patient and family education goes beyond information giving to a teaching or coaching role. A nurse helps a patient interpret an illness and integrate that experience and its implications into his or her life.

With this reframing, teaching becomes a tool, not a goal. A diagnosis of Knowledge Deficit ends with knowledge acquisition. This is nice but not very useful. Other nursing diagnoses focus on promoting changes in behavior that can directly improve health outcomes. These may be related to body, mind, or spirit. By eliminating the diagnosis of Knowledge Deficit, teaching becomes reframed from a nursing state into a nursing trait.

For example, consider the nursing diagnosis of Altered Nutrition. Many people know about calories and fats but need help applying that knowledge in ways that can improve their health. The nursing diagnosis Knowledge Deficit related to cardiac disease presents the same problem. It does not guide nursing practice as clearly as Impaired Health Maintenance related to inadequate risk factor reduction or Altered Nutrition: More than body requirements. To improve risk factor reduction, teach what the risk factors are and coach behavioral changes.

How Does This Save Time?

If you view patient and family education as a task, you separate it from other nursing activities. A task requires effort and time. You can perform a task and check it off your list. You may delegate a task to another member of the health care team.

If you view teaching as a task, how do you prioritize it amongst your other tasks? Are you trained as a nurse or as a teacher? Wouldn't you tend to put other nursing tasks first?

If you view teaching as a nursing trait, it becomes one of the factors that defines nursing care. Teaching becomes part of the essence of nursing. You become aware of the informal teaching you do incidentally while you are providing nursing care. You answer a patient's question, prepare a patient for a procedure, explain the purpose of a piece of medical equipment.

If you recognize these informal moments as educational, claim them as nursing care, and document them, you do not need "time to teach." If you view teaching as a tool that nurses use to accomplish therapeutic goals, you will use it in the context of other nursing tasks. You will teach while you give medication or provide emotional support. You will integrate it into nursing care and take a little extra time. The first step is to acknowledge the teaching you are doing.

How do you make time for patient and family education? Integrate it. Don't task it out.

Is Teaching Cost-Effective?

Yes. A review of studies that looked at the cost benefits of patient education concluded the following:

> *"On the average, for every dollar invested in patient education, $3 to $4 were saved. . . . None of the studies reported that education cost more than it saved."*
> —Bartlett, E. E., 1995, p. 89

Patient and family education is good for the bottom line. When calculating staffing needs, it is a good investment to consider the time needed to teach.

Giving Fish Versus Teaching Fishing

The trademarked slogan for Time Life Medical states that *no prescription is more valuable than knowledge*. It's a quotation from our former Surgeon General, C. Everett Koop.

That's a powerful statement.

Prescriptions are written by licensed, educated professionals for specific treatments that are unavailable without prescriptions. By definition, a prescription is very valuable. It is not easy to get.

Knowledge is even more valuable than a prescription. This doesn't mean *information*, which is just data, but *knowledge*, information that is understood and known. No prescription is more valuable than knowledge.

You know why you teach. Medical care consumers want knowledge. The goals of education are to enable the learner:

- To make informed decisions
- To develop basic self-care skills to survive
- To recognize problems and know what to do in response
- To get questions answered, find resources for answers

This knowledge is much more powerful than any prescription. After all,

"Give a man a fish and he will eat for a day. Teach a man to fish, he will eat for a lifetime."

—Confucius

This can be paraphrased:
Give a patient a treatment and address current symptoms.
Teach a patient to treat himself, and he controls his health behaviors for a lifetime.

In Summary: Why Bother Teaching?

Teaching is not a bother. You can't avoid it. Teaching is part of the essence of nursing. You can't give a treatment or comfort a patient without assessing for or providing information. You shouldn't give a medication without informing the patient about its purpose and potential side effects. You can't optimize self-care without discussing signs and symptoms that need follow-up care.

Therefore, if you must teach, choose to do it well. The good news is that if you integrate teaching into nursing care, you do not need a lot of time to teach. Every moment with the patient is teaching time.

It's unrealistic to expect to hold teaching sessions like you learned in school, yet patient and family education is valuable, essential and unavoidable. What now?

If we focus on needing blocks of time to teach and we cannot get those blocks of time, we may not teach. The essence of nursing is not task accomplishment but therapeutic intervention. Anyone can do tasks. Nurses integrate tasks into nursing care.

"Nurses who utilize their expertise for educational purposes can establish themselves as specialists in the health profession and make a marked difference in the lives of patients, family, and their community."
—Fetter, 1997, p. 119

Patient and family education is not negotiable. Explaining to patients what is happening to them and teaching them to take care of themselves must be done. Education is the ultimate cost-containment tool. Knowledge is the ultimate therapeutic intervention.

"All truths wait in all things."

—Walt Whitman

To go with the flow of managed care, we need to look at patient and family education as a holistic intervention. *Holistic* means dealing with wholes or integrated systems rather than with parts. Patient teaching needs to be integrated into health care at every level: the environment, our relationships with other health care providers, our systems, our supplies, our measures of success.

At any point in the continuum of health care, knowledge is integrated. Education is always present.

This is something like a hologram. Recall the three-dimensional projection at the beginning of the movie Star Wars when Princess Leia asked for help? That was a hologram, which is made with film and laser lights. If the film of a hologram is broken or cut up, each small portion contains information about the whole object. Every point is coded into a large area of the hologram (Outwater & Hamersveld, 1995). If you take a hole-puncher to hologram film, the dot of film you cut out will literally hold the whole picture.

In the same way, with every interaction we have with patients and families, the whole of what they need to know is present. Information permeates the environment in people and things. Everyone has information about how to make informed decisions, perform basic self-care, respond to problems, and find resources for answers. Every piece contains the whole. Our human interaction is to help learners transform this information into personal, relevant knowledge. We evaluate their needs and readiness and manage the flow so that learners can best use what they get.

It is no longer a question of having time to teach. Change the nature of teaching from episodic to omnipresent, and time is no longer an issue.

The next chapter discusses how to teach well. As you refine your teaching skills, you will learn to hone in on the essentials and spend your teaching efforts in the areas where they do the most good.

If you want to learn more:

Bartlett, E.E. (1995). Cost-benefit analysis of patient education. *Patient Education and Counseling, 26*, 87–91.

Dennison, P.D., & Keeling, A.W. (1989). Clinical support for eliminating the nursing diagnosis of knowledge deficit. *Image: Journal of Nursing Scholarship, 21*(1), 142–144.

Fetter, M.S. (1997). Patient-family-community education: No longer frills. *MedSurg Nursing, 6*(3), 119–120.

Outwater, C., & Hamersveld, V. (1995). Practical holography. http://www.holo.com/holo/book/book1.html: Dimensional Arts Inc.

American Hospital Association. (1996). *The joint commission's 1996 accreditation manual for hospitals: The new care of the patient.* Washington, DC: AHA.

Rankin, S.H., & Stallings, K.D. (1996). *Patient education: Issues, principles, practices* (3rd ed.). Philadelphia: Lippincott-Raven.

Ruzicki, D.A. (1989). Realistically meeting the educational needs of hospitalized acute and short-stay patients. *Nursing Clinics of North America, 24*(3).

No Time to Teach Well?

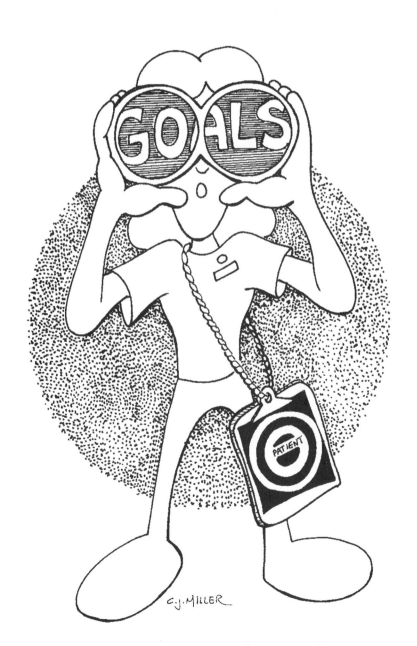

t's difficult to get patient education going, especially in a busy clinic. How do other people make time?"

"How do you cover a vast amount of information in a limited amount of time?"

"How do you make time for patient education?"

—questions from RNs

....

It's not easy to provide quality patient and family education. Box 2-1 lists the challenges identified by nurses in a variety of practice settings. Check the ones you share.

BOX 2-1 Teaching Challenges Checklist

- ☐ Other nursing tasks, like giving medications and physical assessments, are a higher priority than teaching.
- ☐ Night shift: Patients are asleep.
- ☐ Day shift: Patients are getting tests or treatments and are unavailable to teach.
- ☐ Pediatrics: Parents are not there to teach.
- ☐ Don't know what to teach.
- ☐ Don't know how to teach.
- ☐ Don't know the answers to patients' questions.
- ☐ Don't know what the patient has.
- ☐ Don't know in what condition the patient will leave.
- ☐ Don't know if the patient will survive.
- ☐ Don't know what the doctor told the patient and family.
- ☐ Don't know where the patient will be discharged.
- ☐ Don't know what will happen in home care.
- ☐ Don't know what happened in the hospital.
- ☐ The doctor didn't write an order for teaching.
- ☐ Patients and family members are too anxious/angry/medicated/ distracted to learn.
- ☐ Just as they are able to participate in learning, patients are discharged.
- ☐ Patients and family members are not motivated to learn.
- ☐ Don't know how to identify teaching needs for discharge on admission.
- ☐ Too busy keeping patient alive.
- ☐ No one is accountable to continue or complete teaching.
- ☐ No one follows up if I don't do teaching.

Box 2-1 *(Continued)*

☐ No quiet place to teach.
☐ Don't know what resources are available with which to teach.
☐ Don't know where to get supplies.
☐ Teaching supplies are not stocked.
☐ Teaching materials are at too high a reading level.
☐ Teaching materials are not in the patient's language.
☐ Videotapes are missing.
☐ Hard to get foreign language interpreters.
☐ No time to document teaching.
☐ Documentation form is hard to use.
☐ Forms don't have enough space to support quality documentation.
☐ Forms require double documentation.
☐ Others don't document the teaching they've done, so I don't know where they left off.
☐ No one else on the health care team reads my documentation on teaching.
☐ There is no form for documenting follow-up phone calls.
☐ Easier not to start teaching; I feel like I failed if I don't do all the teaching that needs to be done.
☐ Others are better at teaching than I am.
☐ Procrastinate teaching.
☐ Waiting for the perfect time to teach.
☐ Unable to schedule time with patient to teach.
☐ Teaching gets interrupted with other tasks.

and the most popular concern:

☐ No time to teach.

Which duties do you drop from your busy day so that you can spend more time teaching? All are essential. Nothing can be dropped. How do you add more hours to your day? You can't. How do you solve the problem of no time to teach? Take advantage of the time you do have, and use your time and resources well.

Financial pressures force us to delegate more care to the patient and family. Orem's theory of optimizing self-care is more relevant than ever, whether we work in a hospital, office, clinic, school, or home care. Those same financial pressures mean we have precious little time in which to prepare patients and families for their new responsibilities. Is it even possible to do the teaching we need to do in the time we have?

Teaching is a big contributor to the quality of our professional practice. When our teaching is successful, we feel good. We know the learner will do well on his or her own. On the other hand, we're frustrated when teaching is less than a success. If only we had enough time to teach . . .

Time is a limited resource, and we have little control over it. The only logical response to the cry, "no time to teach!" is to get more time. If we can't get more time, we are hopeless. If we stay focused on the lack of time, we are powerless to improve the quality of the education we provide. This cry keeps us from moving forward.

Over what variables of patient and family education do we have control? Everything else: our skills, our methods, our tools, our team efforts toward a shared goal. If we optimize the variables we can control, we will be able to teach more effectively in the time we have. The beautiful side effect is that if we demonstrate that teaching improves outcomes, we can advocate for more teaching time.

Time-Saving Teaching Tips

"Patient education activities often seem to be caught in a vicious cycle in which lack of understanding for the role of patient education in health care and health maintenance, and lack of education and training in patient education, combined with insufficient support and resource allocation, lead to a lack of success, which in turn further weakens any attempts to improve patient education efforts."

—Grueninger, 1995, pages 47–48

Top Time-Saving Teaching Tips

Keep focused on the goals of patient and family education.

Partner with the learner to establish learning objectives.

Assess knowledge and ability before you teach.

Don't make assumptions.

Focus on teaching behaviors and skills.

Get the learner actively involved.

Take advantage of teachable moments.

Individualize your teaching.

Help the learner believe.

Evaluate learning.

Share your teaching with the rest of the health care team.

Does this sound familiar? How can we teach more effectively? Research in education tells us how. The top time-saving teaching tips are summarized in Box 2-2. These teaching tips are the first step to breaking out of this vicious cycle. They are behavioral. They don't require fancy multimedia presentations, expensive equipment, or special spaces for teaching. You can apply them as part of your professional practice, without permission or commitment from your employing organization.

If you follow these tips, then without an increased budget, the quality of your patient and family education will improve. As your teaching improves, you can advocate for increased support and resource allocation, which will increase your success. Turn that cycle into a growth spiral. In the following sections, each tip is described and introduced with real-life situations nurses have identified.

Keep Focused on the Goals of Patient and Family Education

Her kid was going home from the hospital that afternoon with a new diagnosis of asthma. The patient's mom said she was a high school graduate, but she couldn't grasp the concept of lungs and oxygen exchange at all. He needed meds and monitoring, but the mom couldn't even understand what asthma was! Inflammatory response and involuntary muscles were beyond her.

The goals of patient and family education are action focused. They all answer the learner's question, "what can I do?" The short-term goals are to help the learner:

- Make informed decisions
- Develop basic self-care skills to survive
- Recognize problems and know what to do in response
- Get questions answered and find resources for answers

"If you neglect to ask what is the purpose of the project your choices of how to solve it become arbitrary and you will suffer the nagging feeling of that arbitrariness."

— Wurman, 1989, page 82

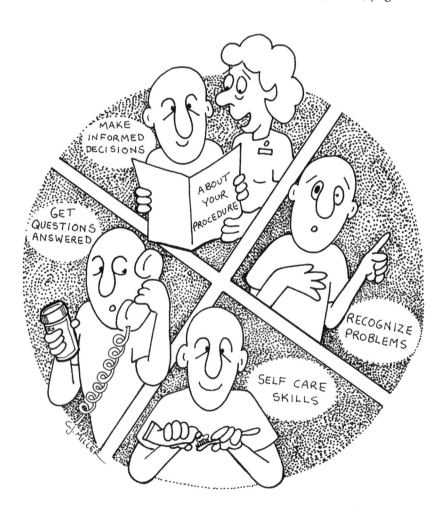

The long-term goal of patient education is to help learners develop positive health-related attitudes and adopt and maintain behaviors conducive to health. Meeting the short-term goals moves patients toward this.

If you keep these goals in mind, you'll spend less time on side issues. Did the mom in the anecdote really have to understand anatomy and physiology to learn how to take care of her son?

Partner With the Learner to Establish Learning Objectives

The patient, in her late 40s, cried inconsolably. She came into the ED for heavy menstrual bleeding, but she wasn't even soaking two pads an hour. "I have cancer, don't I?" she kept asking. "It's OK, you can tell me the truth. It's cancer, isn't it?"

I tried to teach her about normal menstruation, perimenopause, and how the large doses of aspirin she was taking might be related to her bleeding, but she just wanted to talk about cancer. She wouldn't listen to me!

If your goal for patient and family education is compliance, your teaching is only successful if the learner complies with instructions and obeys directives.

". . . but if the patient is not included in deciding how learning will be applied, and the goals of patient education are not mutually agreed on between the teacher and the learner, behavioral changes will not occur."
—Rankin and Stallings, 1996, page 101

Partnering with the learner to establish learning objectives accomplishes several things:

- It informs the learner that patient and family education is part of the treatment plan.
- It involves the learner in the process.
- It establishes mutuality; you and the learner agree from the start.

If you and the learner have different agendas, your educational efforts will not be effective. What does the learner want to know?

If what the learner is asking doesn't make sense to you in the context, ask questions to find out why that is important to the learner. Why was the patient in the emergency department sure she had cancer?

What else was going on in her life, and why was she in the emergency department? Use that information to make your teaching relevant to the learner. Then, set realistic objectives. Use documentation forms to record and share with other members of the health care team key points to be covered.

Assess Knowledge and Ability Before You Teach

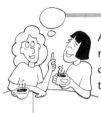

A woman called the emergency room complaining of diarrhea. I told her "For your diarrhea, take Mylanta or Immodium." Her response was "I'll have to take Mylanta. I can't take Immodium because it's a pill. I'm pregnant and my doctor told me not to take any pills."

Assessing knowledge and ability before teaching accomplishes several things:

- Find out what the learner knows so you can reinforce appropriate behaviors and skills and correct misperceptions.
- Find out what the learner believes so you can individualize teaching.
- Find out what the learner doesn't know.
- Find out the learner's ability to learn at this time.
- Do not make assumptions.
- Assess, and you won't waste time teaching things the learner knows.

The learner in this anecdote seems to think in concrete terms. Her physician probably intended to communicate that she needed to avoid unnecessary medications to protect her unborn child. She heard, "don't take pills."

Most health care professionals don't appreciate how much more they know about health and illness than the average person. What is obvious to you may not be obvious to the learner. For example, you know why a tetanus shot (tetanus toxoid or ATT) is given. A study in an accident and emergency unit investigating 500 patients' understanding of the use of ATT found that 50.4% thought that ATT is an antibiotic, 81% thought it protected against wound infection, and 35.6% thought it meant they didn't need antibiotics (Davies, Luke, & Burdett-Smith, 1996). Unless we ask, we don't know what the learner believes.

It is tempting to cut teaching time by doing less assessment. However, the less you know about the learner's understanding, the more off-target your teaching could be. You can waste a lot of precious time teaching the wrong information or the wrong way. Your impact on health outcomes is dependent on individualized teaching based on your assessment.

In other words,

"There are two parts to solving any problem: what you want to accomplish and how you want to do it. . . You must always ask the question 'What is?' before you ask the question 'How to?'"

—Wurman, 1989, page 81

Don't Make Assumptions

In the women's clinic where I work as a nurse practitioner, I was assessing a 33-year-old patient. The woman reported she was not married but sexually active and not using any contraceptives. I warned the woman that she may have been safe so far, but she was putting herself at risk, and I jumped into a lecture about the importance of protection. The more I talked, the more the patient's eyes glazed over. I tried repeating myself and talked with even more enthusiasm.

Finally, I paused and asked the patient why she wanted to risk unmarried pregnancy and STDs and the patient said, "I don't need contraception. I have sex with a woman."

Assumptions can be insidious time wasters. Assumptions are not all bad. They help us function in a complex world. We would be unable to accomplish much if we didn't generalize what we know. Each of us takes certain things for granted, assuming they are true for everyone. However, assumptions can also get in the way of seeing things as they are.

One way to uncover your assumptions is to pay attention to the process of teaching. The following three situations may indicate you have made an assumption:

- You are lecturing and not having an interactive discussion with the learner.
- You repeat the same information several times because you are not getting through.
- The learner is not accepting your teaching, either passively, through politeness, or actively, through argument or rejection.

To avoid making assumptions, you should interact with the learner. Ask questions. Listen to the responses. Explore the learner's understandings and point of view. Then, adapt your teaching to work with the learner's point of view. If your teaching is not working, find out why.

This anecdote illustrates how our assumptions come out of our experiences and expectations. Most of the patients at the women's clinic are probably heterosexual. However, 10% of the population is not. The nurse practitioner not only made an incorrect assumption, she did not notice the cues that told her to stop and reassess. She wasted teaching time.

Focus on Teaching Behaviors and Skills

Several years ago, before the advent of the multiservices lab, we did endoscopies in the OR. Our scheduling staff would tell patients, "Don't eat breakfast the morning of your endoscopy exam."

We had one older gentleman—a farmer from a rural county—under a local-with-sedation anesthetic for an esophigoscopy. The surgeon irrigated and pumped, irrigated and pumped, and irrigated and pumped some more but still couldn't see anything. Exasperated, the surgeon aborted the procedure, and said, rather crossly, to the patient, "I thought we told you not to eat any breakfast this morning!"

"Honest, Doc" the patient replied (rather hoarsely), "I didn't eat no breakfast. All I had was a banana and a cup of coffee."

Make sure terms are clearly defined. Then, evaluate understanding of what to do and when. Share only enough anatomy and physiology to support your teaching. Some learners are turned off with too much technical talk. Other learners want enough science to understand why they need to do things a certain way. Others thrive on medical details. Use your understanding of the learner to individualize your teaching.

In this anecdote, the health care team's definition of breakfast was not the same as the farmer's definition. The behavior the team wanted was no food intake. They didn't say that. If they had taken a moment to evaluate their teaching, they would have identified the problem.

Get the Learner Actively Involved

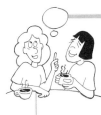

She just sat there, smiled, and nodded as I taught her about warfarin, signs of bleeding, and what medicines to avoid. At the end, I asked her if she had any questions, and she said no. But how do I really know she understood me? How do I know she will use this medicine safely?

Talking, writing, and doing help the learner process new information and learn it through many sensory pathways. Listening to the health care provider, watching a video, or reading a handout are passive methods and much less effective. Follow up each passive method with active involvement. Ask the learner to tell you how the information will be applied or to do an activity that demonstrates understanding.

Some people are intimidated by health care professionals. The patient in the example may have been a quiet person, not easily engaged in conversation. Often, patients don't understand that you are teaching; they see it as a casual conversation. Many patients expect treatments that treat or cure the problem, not information on how to care for themselves. Avoid this problem by making your teaching overt. Tell patients and family members the treatment includes teaching about procedures, choices, and self-care. Tell them they will be taught by health care providers all the time, and their job is to understand and ask questions if they don't.

Give learners paper and pencil to write questions as they arise so that they can ask the appropriate member of the health care team. Explain the roles of the members of the health care team so they know who to talk to about what.

"Asking questions provides adults with a means of controlling the amount, timing, and type of information they will obtain. By asking questions, an individual can seek more information or limit the amount of cognitive input they receive."

—Tripp, 1987, page 173

By getting the learner actively involved, we are also promoting partnership. This partnership helps minimize inequality, often a barrier to learning. When this sense of partnership is missing,

> *"At some level what we're communicating is the feeling that we know, others don't, and we've got to Change Minds. Changing Minds is a tricky game, especially when it's being fed with urgency and self-righteousness. There's often an air of superiority in what we say. People instinctively back off. They feel like they're being told, being 'should' upon."*
> —Dass & Gorman, 1985, page 158

When teaching flows out of an interaction, the conversation moves toward a dialogue and away from an "I know what's best for you" lecture. Consequently, we build an alliance that can support healthy behaviors.

Take Advantage of Teachable Moments

I just ran in to hang the IV bag and he looked up at me and said, "Have you ever seen anybody else have these problems, or is it just me?"

Even though I had a million things to do, I took a moment and asked what he meant. I listened, reassured him that he's not alone and told him I could get him information on a support group. Then I asked if he wanted me to get one of their members to come to visit him in the hospital. He was such a private person, I didn't expect him to be interested, but he said yes!

The best time to teach is when the learner asks a question or a skill is being performed. During a teachable moment, you have a defined topic and a motivated learner primed for active involvement.

One study concluded that, "the information provided to patients is distributed unevenly over time . . . patients received too much information on the day of admission, while they received little information at discharge" (Breemhaar, van den Borne, & Mullen, 1996, page 42). We can more evenly distribute information if we attend to teachable moments in each of our interactions with patients and families. Spreading out our teaching would also lessen our own pressures, because teaching won't all be done at the last minute. Our teaching would also be more effective, because a motivated learner learns best.

The teachable moment in this anecdote started with a vague comment. It could have been easily whisked away with an equally vague, "Oh, I've seen lots of patients who were much worse off than you! You'll be fine!" However, the nurse explored the situation and found an opportunity to intervene, teach, and actively help an otherwise reticent patient.

> *"It may be that by utilizing people's natural learning processes, patient education could be done more efficiently and effectively. Instead of patient education being a separate component of patient care, it would become an integral part of all phases of patient care."*
>
> —Tripp, 1987, page 176

The time to teach is in the moment. Take advantage of natural learning processes, and integrate informal teaching into your patient care.

Individualize Your Teaching

One fine day I erred significantly. I assumed the patient was being discharged with a Foley in place and taught the fine art of leg bag usage and gravity drainage bags. She was extremely attentive and had no questions. No questions until I finished, the she asked me, "Now why would I want a catheter? It sounds like a royal pain in the ass, and all I did was get my bone spurs took care of. What do my feet have to do with my bladder?"

Uh oh, wrong patient, wrong teaching.

What does this learner know now? What does this learner need to know? How does this learner best learn? You will save teaching time if you adapt to the learner.

This anecdote is an example of how not individualizing teaching can cost you time and credibility. The easiest way to individualize teaching is to shift focus from your need to teach to the learner's need to learn.

This involves taking a risk. When you individualize teaching, the learner may ask a question you can't answer or may reveal some emotional conflict you feel unprepared to face. The goal of teaching is not to keep you comfortable and safe, but to help learners care for themselves. Practice. Develop the skills to face these challenging situations, and learn what resources you can access for support.

Help the Learner Believe

My favorite scene from the movie *Star Wars* reminds me of the importance of teaching patients to believe in themselves.

Luke Skywalker was confused and frustrated. Yoda told him to pick up that huge Xwing class starfighter using his mind. Luke could not do it.

Luke Skywalker: "I don't believe it."

Yoda: "That is why you fail."

Then, using the power of the Force, Yoda raised the space ship out of the muck.

—Lucas, 1980

Does the learner believe he or she can do the skill or behavior? A person who does not believe he or she can perform a skill is less likely to be able to do it.

This example may be from fiction, but it very clearly illustrates the need to believe. Luke Skywalker was unable to lift the space ship out of the swamp, because, given his experience and understanding of physics, he did not believe it was possible. Yoda, on the other hand, had a better understanding of the Force, and knew Luke could channel that energy and perform the task. Then, as Luke acquired belief, he was able to accomplish tasks he previously thought were impossible.

A person with self-efficacy believes he or she can do it. There is one important thing to remember about self-efficacy: It is specific to a task. A person may be professionally competent and have a healthy self-esteem but have low self-efficacy about a task like losing weight or quitting smoking.

This means self-efficacy is not always obvious. You need to assess for it. It also means that because self-efficacy is not global, but specific, your interventions can make a difference.

How? If your learner does not believe he or she can do it, address the lack of belief first. If you do not address it, you will waste teaching time moving on to details the learner cannot apply. Help the learner build confidence before facing the task. Break up the skill into small steps the learner can master. It may help to introduce the learner to another of the same socioeconomic or ethnic group who succeeded at the task. This will show the learner that he or she, too, can do it.

Evaluate Learning

I remember teaching Broviac care to the parents of a 6-year-old, Troy. We spent many teaching sessions with discussion, demonstration, hands-on practice, printed instructions, and questions and answers. Mom was always very attentive.

Next summer, while doing a dressing change at camp, Troy insisted that I simply wipe off the exit site with tap water and apply a Band-Aid. When I asked him about our routine of alcohol/Betadine cleansing followed by an occlusive dressing, he firmly protested, 'but that's not the way you taught my mom to do it!' (I might add this child had no complications of line site infections!)

Remember, what we teach does not equal what patients put into practice. What you say may not be what the learner hears. What the learner hears may not be what the learner does. What the learner does while you're watching may not be what the learner does when you're not around. Improvements in health outcomes are dependent on behaviors and skills that are applied day to day.

The purpose of evaluation is not to have something to document to make JCAHO reviewers happy. The long-term goal of patient and family education is to improve health outcomes. Short-term evaluation of learning tells us if the information was transferred. Long-term evaluation of learning tells us if it was applied consistently over time, and if it was enough to improve health outcomes.

Evaluating learning gives us feedback on how we are teaching. Was our message clear? Did our assumptions interfere? To be sure, we need to evaluate learning at the time of teaching and periodically over time.

Short-term evaluation of teaching is direct. Present the learner with situations that may occur, and ask how the learner will respond. Have the learner demonstrate the skill at least three times. Something may go wrong (sterile field may be broken, step may be skipped), and the learner can practice problem-solving skills. Present these activities not as threatening tests or pop quizzes, but as supported practice for competent self-care.

Asking, "Do you have any questions?" is not the most effective way to evaluate learning. Learners may feel they should have understood or may feel their questions are silly or insignificant, so they may choose not to ask them. If you feel the learner has an unasked question, you may say, "Is there anything I could have explained better?" This puts the responsibility on your explanation, rather than emphasizing the learner's inability to grasp information.

Long-term evaluation of your teaching is best done with interactive conversation. How is the information being applied? Is it being applied consistently? What sorts of challenges have come up? Have outcomes changed? Evaluation also reinforces teaching and helps the learner see the connection between behaviors and outcomes.

In this anecdote, the nurse evaluated short-term learning. When Troy got the Broviac, his mom demonstrated that she learned good technique. However, follow-up visits showed that long-term evaluation did not occur. Did Mom not remember what she learned, or did she understand the teaching clearly but decide all those supplies were a waste of money, and a Band-Aid was just as effective? Did she not have the money or insurance to pay for supplies, settling instead for what she could afford? Evaluating teaching in follow-up visits might have revealed the truth sooner.

Share Your Teaching With the Rest of the Health Care Team

We recently performed a combined procedure on an infant just under a year old. One of our ENT docs put in PE ventilating tubes for chronic serous otitis media, and then a urologist came in and corrected a hypospadius condition on the same patient. As we were prepping for the hypospadius, following the PE tube, the patient's mother called in to the OR suite (who gave her the direct number, and why, I'll never know) in an obvious state of panic. What had gone wrong, she wanted to know. We assured her that everything was fine and that her son was doing well. She, however, insisted that something must be wrong because someone told her that the procedure would only take 20 minutes. We informed her that the first part of the procedure, anesthetic induction and PE tube placement, would take 20 minutes. The rest of the procedure would take at least 2 hours. After we had promised to call her with progress reports, she calmed down and hung up.

Someone probably gave the mother the wrong information about the length of time the surgery would take. When you are performing patient/family instruction, you must be certain of all of the information you give them.

The other possibility is that the mother was given the correct information, but in an agitated state, she misunderstood what she had been told. This underlines the importance of having your patients and families repeat back to you the information you gave them so you can evaluate the degree to which the teaching has been successful.

If you don't document your assessments, teaching, or evaluation, other team members may waste time by repeating what you have done. Hold other team members accountable for sharing their teaching progress with you. Build on one another's efforts by working together.

This example emphasizes the need for coordination of teaching. Provide correct information. Provide information in writing, when possible. Provide resources to be accessed, and avoid panic calls into the operating room. You can't anticipate every problem, but you can create an environment that supports patients and family members through stressful times.

Interactive Teaching

Does your current style of teaching patients differ from the interactive, informal style described here? Most nurses teach informally, in the moment, but do not recognize this integrated teaching as official patient education worthy of documentation. Notice when you teach informally now. Acknowledge your own self-efficacy. You can do it. You do have time to teach!

Are you still unclear on how emphasizing an interactive style will decrease teaching time? If you follow these tips, you may take a few more moments to ask questions and listen to the learner, but this will also minimize your frustration with time-wasting ineffective education. You will understand the situation better. In the past, if the learner wasn't understanding the information, your best option may have been to repeat yourself in a slightly different way. Now, you have other responses. Ask yourself if your goals are the learner's goals, if you're making assumptions, if the learner believes he or she can do it, and what the learner needs to succeed. Now you have more options.

You may be using some of these skills already. If so, use them with awareness, knowing they actively save you teaching time. You may need to add some of these skills to your repertoire. If so, there will be some transition time while you are learning to apply these skills. Be patient with yourself and your coworkers. Those frustrating, last-minute crisis teaching situations will still come up. Be ready for them. Before they do, read Box 2-3 on page 28.

We can break out of the vicious cycle of unsuccessful patient and family education efforts. For details on what you can do to gain skills in patient and family education and to increase support and resource allocation, read on.

BOX 2-3

Your Patient's Going Home and You Haven't Done Teaching Yet?

Let's say you get the order for discharge from the hospital, and there's no documentation that any teaching has been done. Here's what to do next:

1. Identify essential knowledge. What does the patient and family absolutely, positively have to know to be safe and promote healing at home? When will the learner next encounter a health care provider who can evaluate, review, and continue your teaching?
2. Identify the learner's concerns. What does the learner want to know to feel safe and comfortable at discharge?
3. Evaluate essential knowledge. What does the patient and family know already? Present a problem that may arise at home, and ask how the learner would deal with it. Whenever possible, have the learner show you. Actions reinforce learning and overcome language barriers.
4. Use your resources. A last-minute lecture won't stick. Get out the pamphlets, videos, audiotapes, models, crayons, and flash cards. Teach whatever the learner needs to know before discharge. Active involvement in the material speeds learning.
5. Refer the learner to resources. Provide a written list of phone numbers and contacts, such as doctors, clinical nurse specialists, rehabilitation services, emergency numbers, hotlines, consumer health libraries, and support groups. Call the social worker if you need help with this.
6. Communicate with other health care team members. Document what the learner knows and what still needs to be taught at future encounters with health care providers. Make sure copies go to those who will be doing follow-up teaching.
7. If the situation isn't safe, advocate. As a registered nurse, you are licensed and required by law to exercise your professional judgment when doing your job. "I was just following orders" will not hold up in court. Nurses are accountable as patient advocates. If you have concerns, pull the facts together and call a team meeting. What will it take for a safe discharge? Does the patient need a visit from a home health nurse tonight, a clinic appointment for the next morning, or one more day in the hospital?
8. Support patients' rights. Without placing blame, inform patients and family members of their rights. Encourage them to expect that their rights will be maintained and to speak up when they feel they are not. Provide appropriate phone numbers, as necessary.

Box 2-3 *(Continued)*

9. Do what you can to avoid crisis teaching in the future. Most topics don't need an hour of sit-down time with the patient and family to teach. In every nurse–patient interaction, you assess knowledge or teach. Document at least one bit of teaching on every patient every shift, and encourage your colleagues to do so. Advocate for patient and family education on task forces, at meetings, and in political forums. Patient and family education is an essential nursing responsibility. JCAHO expects it and patients deserve it.

If you want to learn more:

Breemhaar, B., van den Borne, H.W., & Mullen, P.D. (1996). Inadequacies of surgical patient education. *Patient Education and Counseling, 28*(1), 31–44.

Dass, R., & Gorman, P. (1985). How can I help? *Stories and Reflections on Service.* New York: Alfred A. Knopf.

Davies, F., Luke, L.C., & Burdett-Smith, P. (1996). Patients' understanding of tetanus immunization. *Journal of Accident and Emergency Medicine, 13*(4), 272–273.

Grueninger, U.J. (1995). Arterial hypertension: Lessons from patient education. *Patient Education and Counseling, 26*(1–3), 37–55.

Lucas, G. (1980). *The Empire Strikes Back.* Beverly Hills, CA: 20th Century Fox.

Rankin, S.H., & Stallings, K.D. (1996). *Patient education: Issues, principles, practices* (3rd ed.). Philadelphia: Lippincott-Raven.

Stallings, K.D. (1996). *Integrating patient education in your nursing practice.* Horizon Video Productions, distributed by Glaxo Wellcome Inc.

Tripp, K.R. (1987) *Perspectives on adult learning: Maternal coping with a monitored child in the home.* Unpublished doctoral dissertation, Arizona State University.

Wurman, R.S. (1989). *Information anxiety: What to do when information doesn't tell you what you need to know.* New York: Bantam Books.

Create a Learning Environment

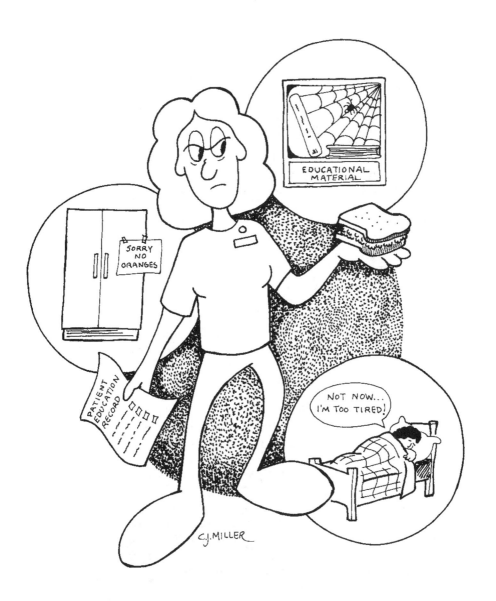

We know that if nurses have materials available at their fingertips, it helps save some time."

—Reid, 1998, page 101

• •

"Don't fix problems. Design them out."

—Leland Kaiser (1997)

• •

Ele Brown was scheduled to be discharged the next day. I checked her education record to see what teaching had been done. The patient's name and number were on top of the form, but the record was blank.

Because Ms. Brown would need to give herself hormone injections at home, I checked the cabinet for the video that teaches the technique. The video wasn't there. I asked the unit secretary. The secretary said she hadn't seen it and couldn't remember who last used it.

I wished I had a handout with the steps written out. Too late now. So I grabbed a blank piece of progress note paper to create a handout while teaching.

I went to the med room for the syringe, needle, alcohol, and saline. I checked the refrigerator for an orange for the patient to practice on, but all I found was a tuna fish sandwich. That wouldn't work.

Ms. Brown has the bed by the window, and her curtains were pulled shut. She was trying to sleep, but the woman in the next bed had a game show blaring on the television. The curtain between them provides only visual privacy, and not even that. The panels don't meet, and you can peek between them.

I entered, announcing my intention to teach. Ms. Brown said she had been up all night in pain, and the medicine she got that morning was finally working and she'd rather sleep, thank you.

I was frustrated, but relieved, because I hadn't even checked my orders yet. The shift got so busy that I never got back to Ms. Brown to do the teaching. Instead, I passed in a report that, "Discharge teaching still needs to be done."

Does this sound familiar? Clearly, this environment does not promote teaching and learning. Written records offered no evidence that any teaching was done. The video was gone. There was no orange, or anything else, on which to practice giving injections. There was no quiet teaching spot, no privacy, and no time.

Improve the Teaching Environment

When nurses discuss barriers to patient and family education, we often focus on details over which we have little control, like patients being discharged too soon or brief office visits. We may jump to solutions before we thoroughly analyze barriers to our teaching. We choose time savers, like teaching groups instead of individuals, before we find out where our time is wasted. Consequently, we overlook aspects of the environment we can easily improve.

This is unfortunate, because improvements in the environment can make a big difference. Even one adjustment to your work space can facilitate every future teaching effort. If you control the design of a space, you can influence the consciousness elicited by that space. A true learning environment encourages learners to seek information and create time to learn and encourages teachers to be ready and able to teach.

> *"You may have more power to affect your work environment than you realize. Some people have great freedom in outfitting their immediate work area . . ."*
>
> —Venolia, C. (1988), page 154

No matter what your place in the hierarchy, you can take action to improve your work environment. Start by changing one thing you can control. A single success will enhance your belief that you can be effective. This is called *self-efficacy*. If you want, recruit an enthusiastic colleague to work with you. Demonstrate to others the value of investing in creating a learning environment, then harness their enthusiasm to promote system changes.

What changes in your environment can effectively optimize teaching time? Leland Kaiser (1997) says a good space supports people, lets them do what they can do, and challenges them to reach out and grow. He says the space compensates, facilitates, potentiates, provides choices, induces people to try choices, and offers high rewards or reinforcements. Is your workspace designed to offer these qualities? If not, what, specifically, can you do to create a learning environment?

Here are some suggestions. Some you can do independently, and some call for a team effort. Others demand cooperation across departments or organizations. Some you may implement as written; others need to be modified to apply to your workplace. Some may just stimulate your own creativity.

Organize Your Teaching Tools

How do you identify obstacles in your environment? Analyze each part of the problem. The nurse in the previous situation asked, "Where is the video?" The nurse knew the video existed but did not know where or how to find it. What is the solution?

Keep teaching tools in an order every user understands so they are accessible when needed.

- ☐ Develop a list of available teaching tools. Organize the list by topic, alphabet, or both.
    - ☐ Make the list accessible to team members so they know what is available.
    - ☐ Make the list available to learners so they may initiate learning when they are motivated.
- ☐ Organize teaching tools in one place so they can be found when needed.
    - ☐ File handouts in a box or cabinet.
    - ☐ Keep models on a shelf.
    - ☐ Store videos on a locked cart, with the video cassette recorder (VCR) and monitor.
- ☐ Create a system for maintaining teaching tools. This system should:
    - ☐ Replace consumables.
    - ☐ Keep track of items in use.
    - ☐ Clean reusables.

Acquire Needed Teaching Tools

After you organize your current teaching tools, you will know what you have and can identify gaps in the collection. The nurse in the beginning of this chapter wished she had a handout with the steps written out. What do you need?

- ☐ Identify what teaching tools are needed.
    - ☐ Survey staff. What are they creating at the bedside? What teaching materials do they want?
    - ☐ Review education records. What topics are taught most? Do you need additional resources to teach those topics better?
    - ☐ Survey learners. What do they wish they had in writing, in pictures, and on video?
    - ☐ Prioritize your needs. What topics do you need most often or carry the greatest risk if not taught well?

☐ Write or call for free teaching tools. Many government agencies, not-for-profit groups, and pharmaceutical companies offer posters, handouts, and videos.
☐ Create a teaching tool that is needed.
    ☐ Write that handout.
    ☐ Make a notebook of pictures showing steps of a skill.
    ☐ Create a poster that uses photos to illustrate a skill that is frequently taught.
☐ Prepare a wish list of teaching supplies. Identify the person or committee responsible for or invested in effective patient and family education, and propose that money be budgeted for these teaching supplies.
☐ Because people learn differently, have tools that allow you to teach the same information in several different ways (handouts, audiotapes, and videotapes).

Create a Physical Environment That Facilitates Learning

An environment that does not support teaching wastes much valuable teaching time. The environment includes everything outside you. Environment is the place, temperature, sounds, lighting, furniture, supplies, and people.

The space needs to be conducive to learning. What alternatives are available if Ms. Brown's roommate won't turn down her television? Is there another, private place where teaching can occur?

The space in which you work can promote learning or hinder it.

☐ Identify environmental barriers to learning.
    ☐ What interferes with your patients' and families' learning?
    ☐ What makes it hard for them to pay attention?
☐ Directional and informational signs should be written in languages of your learners.
☐ Identify quiet, private spaces for teaching.
☐ Ensure that teaching spaces are well lit.
☐ Arrange seating to promote conversation.
☐ Manage distracting sights, sounds, and smells.
☐ Identify spaces that can be reserved for teaching, when necessary.
☐ Create a cart with teaching materials and practice supplies that can be brought to the learner.
☐ Identify spaces for diversionary activities. Nonlearners need someplace to go so they won't distract learners.

Create an Environment That Inspires Learning

The environment needs to prepare and inspire the learner to participate in learning. For example, one hospital has touch screen computers by the elevators. The graphics are colorful and directions easy to follow. Any literate patient or visitor can use these computers to print out general information on illnesses, diagnostic tests, treatments, first aid, health promotion, roles of health care team members, and directions to services on campus. These computers offer information in English and Spanish.

- ☐ Inform patients and families that learning will occur during interactions with health care providers. Encourage them to participate.
- ☐ Write a poster or handout for patients and families: *How to Make the Most of Your Hospital Stay* or *How to Make the Most of Your Office Visit or Home Visit.* Let the learner know what resources are available for self-learning:
  - ☐ Roles of health care team members
  - ☐ Classes offered
  - ☐ Videos
  - ☐ Pamphlets
  - ☐ Computer programs and self-learning modules available
  - ☐ Stress management and diversionary activities available, such as a humor cart or basket
- ☐ Give every patient a paper and pencil to write down questions as they arise. This promotes active participation in learning.
- ☐ Do you have enough time with families to teach? If not, why not? Do visiting hours limit their time to learn? Do they know their roles include learning? Do they understand what they need to learn and why?
- ☐ Post information attractively in the halls and waiting rooms. Focus on general information that applies to many of your patients, such as good handwashing technique, how to take medicine, milestones of growth and development, nutrition, exercise, or stress management tips. These may be in the following forms:
  - ☐ Posters
  - ☐ Pamphlets
  - ☐ Notebooks
  - ☐ Bulletin board with changing postings
- ☐ Do the magazines in your waiting room promote health?
  - ☐ Choose periodicals that emphasize good nutrition, fitness, and mental health.
  - ☐ Add books supporting health promotion, too. Consider investing in a lending library based on the honor system.

☐ Written materials should be available in the languages your learners speak.

☐ Obtain directories of self-help groups. Keep them in a place where patients and families can access them.

☐ Provide handouts or inservices for patients and family members on topics like *how to find and use community resources.*

☐ Post opportunities to learn in the community (presentations, workshops, classes) to encourage self-motivated learning.

One controlled study (Mead, Rhyne, Wiese, Lambert, & Skipper, 1995) concluded that patient education materials available in a waiting room were not effective in increasing the number of preventive services performed by physicians. Although the pamphlets encouraged patients to ask their physicians about cholesterol testing, Pap smears, tetanus boosters, and mammograms, the experimental group did not have more tests than the control group. More studies are needed on educational materials in the environment to clarify this issue. However, this study does reinforce that a learning environment alone is not enough to change behaviors and that interactions between learners and educating caregivers are essential.

The Bigger Picture

Systems are also part of the environment. Systems need to support communications between health care team members. What have others taught Ms. Brown? Has she seen the video yet? Where should this be documented? Who had the video last, and where is it now? What system is in place to communicate this information? Does the system encourage teaching throughout the hospitalization, or is discharge the only trigger for evaluation of learning?

Systems need to support patient and family education. Education documentation forms need to be user-friendly. Teaching tools need to be available and accessible. Responsibilities need to be assigned. Who's in charge of stocking, obtaining, or creating teaching tools? Who orders supplies and manages the budget? Team members need to be held accountable for their responsibilities.

Promote Communication Between Team Members

Efficient teaching depends on team work. Each team member builds on the teaching of others. Teaching goes quicker when insights on individualizing teaching are shared.

☐ Document your teaching.
☐ When you're getting report, ask what teaching was done, where it was documented, and what needs to be covered next.
☐ Promote continuity of care. Communicate to the next health care provider what teaching still needs to be done or reinforced.
☐ Post articles in the staff lounge that promote patient and family education on topics like how to teach with a video.
☐ When you precept orientees, talk about how to promote an educational environment.
☐ Join a committee that is working on patient and family educational issues.
☐ Gather a team to optimize the educational environment. Identify environmental barriers to education.
    ☐ Are documentation forms user-friendly?
    ☐ Are teaching materials readily available?
    ☐ Is equipment, like a VCR or audiotape player, available?

Then work together to create a better system.

Create Systems That Promote a Learning Environment

This environment includes the systems that support your teaching, such as documentation forms, family visiting hours, and a workload that provides you with time to teach. Environment also encompasses the atmosphere and tone of the workplace. Policies, procedures, forms, and communications can undermine or support learning.

☐ Identify barriers to learning and evaluation of learning in existing systems. Question why it has to be done that way.
    For example, Planetree Hospital (Gilpin, 1993) has a program in which patients who are interested, alert, and able can take responsibility for their own medications while hospitalized. A physician writes an order to initiate the three-stage self-medication program. In the first stage, the patient learns about the medication. In the second stage, the patient asks for the medication at the right time, every time it is due. In the third stage, the patient keeps an 8-hour supply of medications at the bedside to take as prescribed. This transitions the patient toward self-medication at home. This system helps health care providers identify problems before discharge.
☐ Evaluate the focus of your systems.
    ☐ Are they based on provider convenience or the convenience of the patient and family?
    ☐ Are nurses available to teach when families are visiting?

☐ If families or friends will be caring for the patient at home, are they able to learn and practice this in the hospital? Planetree Hospital (Gilpin, 1993) has a Care Partner Program that formalizes this process.

☐ Do systems encourage and support assessment and evaluation of learning throughout the hospitalization or only on discharge?

☐ Refocus systems to serve patients and families, and to support learning.

For example, are language interpretation services available when needed? If not, gather data that demonstrate the need for interpreters, and present your proposal through appropriate channels.

Promote Consistency and Continuity of Teaching

Learning occurs over time, during interactions with every health care provider. Enhance learning by working together across systems.

☐ Primary care providers, clinics, specialists, and home care providers need to collaborate. For example, each should teach the same technique for dressing changes. Each should use the same procedures and teaching materials. If this is difficult, look at recent research together and negotiate an acceptable compromise. This will minimize confusion in the learner, facilitate learning through reinforcement, and promote alliance and compliance.

☐ Ask other health care providers their assessments of your patient's learning needs and the status of teaching. Read their notes.

☐ Communicate your evaluation of teaching with the other health care providers your patient sees. Tell them your concerns.

Hold the Gains

You can do a lot to create a learning environment. However, though you may act independently to initiate environmental change, it requires a team activity to maintain that improvement. Even simple changes, like organizing teaching tools, need to be maintained, or they will become disorganized over time.

Ultimately, the environmental change that matters most is in the attitudes of your colleagues. Change is superficial until health care team members become a part of the process. Attitude change occurs internally, as each team member understands how barriers in the environment can interfere with teaching and how improvements to the environment can facilitate teaching. Team members will readily support change when they appreciate how a learning environment promotes quality care. This process can effectively start at any level of the organizational hierarchy. Whatever your official role, it can begin with you.

Think of yourself as a catalyst for creating an environment that supports teaching and learning. You may work alone to initiate change. Then, to ensure their use and the continuation of improvements, promote awareness within the health care team. Inform them of the changes you made and how they facilitate teaching. Periodically ask team members how the changes are working, and modify them as needed. Nourish team members' enthusiasm for creating a learning environment. Organize team efforts to maintain and continue environmental changes.

An enthusiastic health care team will work to hold the gains made in creating a learning environment. For every change made, the team must identify and implement the following:

☐ A system to maintain the change. Who is accountable?
☐ A system to monitor the change. Is it consistently implemented? If not, why not? If so, is it producing the results you expected?

For example, let's say pamphlets from the American Lung Association will now be stocked in a file cabinet. The manager and the unit secretary agree this is an appropriate duty to be added to the unit secretary's role. The unit secretary is now accountable. She places an index card with reorder information five pamphlets from the bottom of the pile. It instructs the person about to teach to give the card to the unit secretary. She will then order more before they run out. Users are informed about this reorder system and their role. This is a system to maintain the change of stocking pamphlets.

This change can be monitored in several ways. Users inform the unit secretary when stock is out. No stock may mean the pamphlet is used more often than anticipated, and the index card needs to be moved higher in the pile. No stock may also mean the unit secretary did not order the pamphlets when he or she received the card from a user. The unit secretary needs to be held accountable to fulfill his or her role. A user who did not give the card to the unit secretary, but left it on the pile of pamphlets, needs to be held accountable as well.

On the other hand, no stock may mean the source did not supply the pamphlets. Is it a rare occurrence, is it an unreliable source, or is the pamphlet out of print? Perhaps a similar pamphlet from another source needs to be considered.

Where Improvements Can Lead

So how would teaching go if the nurse in the opening story worked in an environment that supported learning? Here's the tale again, after changes in the environment:

Ele Brown was to be discharged the next day and would need to give herself hormone injections at home. I checked her education record to see what teaching had been done. The form has been updated daily since admission, filled in by nurses, a physician, and a social worker. It indicated that Ms. Brown had and understood teaching handouts and had viewed the video on self-injection. Ms. Brown had not yet demonstrated the technique.

I asked the charge nurse to cover my patients while I was teaching, and I gave her a brief update on each. The charge nurse replied, "No problem."

I went to the teaching cart and checked out supplies for self-injection: the model abdomen, syringe, needle, alcohol, and saline. I also checked out the self-injection steps in photos. First, I would ask Ms. Brown to put the photos in order and describe the process. This will help Ms. Brown review and enhance her confidence and help me evaluate her readiness to move on.

Ms. Brown had the bed by the window, and her curtains were pulled shut. The woman in the next bed was in the patient lounge, watching television.

I entered, announcing my intention to teach. Ms. Brown responded with a smile. She complimented the effectiveness of the teaching she received on pain management before admission, and the staff's responses to her medication needs. She said she slept comfortably though the night. I acknowledged the compliment and began teaching.

Create an Environment to Enhance Patient and Family Education

How could your patient care area enhance patient and family education? Draw the ideal environment here.

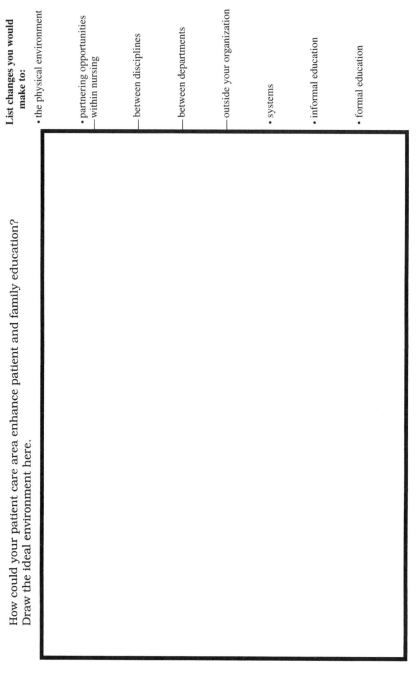

List changes you would make to:

• the physical environment

• partnering opportunities
  within nursing

  between disciplines

  between departments

  outside your organization

• systems

• informal education

• formal education

From: No Time To Teach? A Nurse's Guide to Patient and Family Education   Permission granted to photocopy for individual use by Lippincott Williams & Wilkins

Figure 2.1

Take the First Step

Creating a learning environment is work, but it is a good investment. An environment that supports patient and family education will save you time in teaching preparation and ensure the supplies you need are available. All this will help minimize frustration. Most of all, it will let you teach when your learner is ready.

Here is an exercise to get you started on your path to change. Get out your crayons or colored pencils. (If you don't have any, buy some. They are a great teaching resource.) Draw in this book or make one copy of the exercise (Fig. 3-1) on page 42. Imagine the changes you would make and draw them in detail. If necessary, move on to additional pages. As you inspire coworkers to join you in making environmental changes, have them try the activity. Brainstorm and collaborate. Then do it.

An effective learning environment serves every team member. If the environment serves the lone registered nurse working at night as well as the full staff scrambling during peak discharge and admission times, you have done your job well.

 If you want to know more:

De Muth, J.S. (1989). Patient teaching in the ambulatory setting. *Nursing Clinics of North America, 24*(3), 645–654.

Gilpin, L. (1993). Creating an educational environment in a hospital setting. In B.E. Giloth (Ed.), *Managing hospital-based patient education* (pp. 55–75). Chicago, IL: American Hospital Publishing.

Kaiser, L. (1997). *Creating healthy human habitats.* Unpublished presentation at the Eighth Annual Clinical Practice Model (CPM) International Conference. Minneapolis, MN: CPM Resource Center.

Mead, V.P., Rhyne, R.L., Wiese, W.H., Lambert, L., & Skipper, B. (1995). Impact of environmental patient education on preventive medicine practices. *Journal of Family Practice, 40*(4), 363–369.

Reid, A. (1998). Conquering time—the formidable teaching foe. *Patient Education Management, 5*(8), 101–103.

Venolia, C. (1988). *Healing environments: Your guide to indoor well-being.* Berkeley, CA: Celestial Arts.

Whitehouse, R. (1979). Forms that facilitate patient teaching. *American Journal of Nursing,* July, 1227–1229.

You're Not Alone

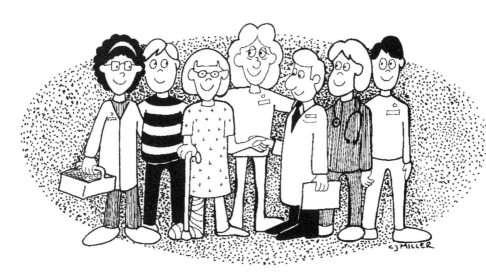

*W*ho is responsible for teaching families about equipment and procedures that they will be involved with after discharge?"

"What is the role of the RN versus nutrition and other departments in the process of teaching?"

"What is available to nurses as backup in educating patients and families?"

—questions from RNs

....

The loneliness associated with patient and family education is filled with conflicts and inconsistencies, pride and insecurities. It is our job! We often feel responsible for every aspect of patient and family education, but when will we find time to do it? There is so much to do, so little time. It's one thing to ask for overtime to stay with a patient until a bone marrow aspiration is done, but it's quite another to ask for overtime to finish evaluating a patient's understanding of how to care for an ostomy. What does management value? What will the organization pay for?

Feeling so alone can arouse an overwhelming sense of helplessness and hopelessness. Some nurses don't even begin teaching, believing that someone more capable will do it. Instead, they focus on things they can complete, like giving medications and treatments. Why set yourself up for failure when you can do things that make you feel successful?

Nurses are resourceful professionals. Rather than ask for help, we do our jobs as best we can with what we have. We have no time to waste quibbling over details. Patients are waiting for our care.

We realize that other members of the health care team are teaching, too. Some team members, in fact, may be better teachers in their areas of expertise than we would be. However, if they're teaching, what have they told our patients? Is there any evidence that they've taught the patients?

We're teaching all the time, but why take time to write down our assessments or evaluations? We have too much to do, and no one would read what we wrote anyway. No one else is doing teaching or cares about it.

Can you see the contradictions that contribute to our loneliness?

- I have no time to teach./I have to do it.
- Teaching is my job./Teaching is other people's jobs.
- No one is teaching./Teaching is done but not documented.
- Teaching is very important./No one cares about teaching.

This makes it hard even to start an interdisciplinary discussion on patient and family education. Priorities and responsibilities are hard to organize. This chapter opened with quotes from registered nurses from across the country. Nurses have a vague sense that others teach, but little clarity on who they are or how to work together.

> *"Too often we feel we [nurses] are the only ones on the battle lines, and we refuse to allow ourselves to ask for support when we need it."*
> —Rankin & Stallings, 1996, page 302

Can we break this cycle of loneliness? Yes. We can step out of our old behavioral patterns. If we initiate conversations with others on the health care team, we may find they feel alone in this too.

It may be difficult for us to admit vulnerability. We need to trust one another to feel safe. There is risk in taking the first step. Remember, our intention is to feel less alone, so we must use techniques that move us toward this goal.

Note the tone of the questioners at the beginning of this chapter: responsibility, RN versus nutrition and other departments, and available backup for nurses. They hint of blame, conflict, and hierarchy. If you express these viewpoints, you may push others away. These are not approaches that build partnerships.

Have you ever felt alone in a crowd? Being surrounded by people does not dispel loneliness but partnerships do. Partnerships remove the sense of loneliness. Build partnerships, and you don't have to feel alone any more.

Patient and Family Head the Team

If you need to teach and you feel alone, remember you practice patient-centered care. The patient and family head the team. They are the learners. It is not you *against* the learner. It is you *with* the learner. You cannot teach without the learner's involvement. How do you know what to teach if you don't assess the learner's knowledge and needs?

Partner With the Learner

> *"Nurses can only pretend to know what is right for clients if there is no mutuality."*
> —Henson, 1997, page 80

Mutuality means forming a partnership, building an alliance, and working together toward a shared goal. It takes time to get to know your learner, but it's the only way to individualize teaching. When you join with the learner, you will not waste time teaching information the learner will ignore. Teaching becomes conversation instead of lecture.

> *"Mutuality is shown to balance power and respect, and to promote productive provider-client communication. This interaction style for partnership relationships fosters positive and lasting health care outcomes."*
> —Henson, 1997, page 77

When you take time to partner with the learner, your teaching becomes relevant. When you involve the learner in the process, learning occurs faster.

Help Patients and Families Adapt

Unlike other team members, patients and families are often unprepared to join a team, let alone lead a team. A change in health forces them to become team leaders. The balance of their lives becomes upset. New choices are presented to them, and they may feel stressed.

> *"People involved in a crisis situation experience a period of disequilibrium."*
> —Tripp, 1987, page 168

This disequilibrium motivates learning. New circumstances create questions. The answers to those questions help people adapt to the new circumstances.

> *"Adaptive learning . . . [is] a dynamic, ongoing cycle of adult learning related to adjusting in a difficult circumstance. The designation of 'learning' as opposed to 'education' would denote an active as opposed to a passive form of obtaining new knowledge, attitudes or skills. The concept of adaptive learning would not require an adult learner to assume primary responsibility for planning, controlling, and supervising a learning project related to a situational transition. The concept would, however, assume learner activity toward understanding the new situation."*
> —Tripp, 1987, page 169

Patients and families who head the health care team are motivated to learn. At first, they may be too overwhelmed to plan, control, or supervise their own learning. They may not even know what questions to ask.

At this point, engage the learner in conversation and listen. Listen with the goals of patient and family education in mind. What information does the learner need to make an informed decision? Which self-care skills need to be assessed? Does the learner know how to recognize problems and know how to respond? What are the learner's resources for information?

It is unusual for a learner to have no questions. If none are written, explore why. The learner may be unable to write or may spell poorly and feel uncomfortable sharing this with you. Give this learner opportunities to ask questions. Stimulate conversations by presenting situations that may occur, and explore the learner's understanding. Ask open-ended questions, such as, "If your leg starts to itch under the cast, what would you do?" and teach from there.

Create a Learning Environment

Give the learner permission to ask questions by creating a learning environment. Instead of diversionary materials in waiting rooms, fill them with educational materials that invite learners to explore.

Offer the learner a paper and pencil to record his or her questions or concerns. Review the list with the learner periodically, and build your teaching from that base.

> *"When patients accept responsibility for their own health and share in decision-making, it takes a lot of the pressure off you. These patients relate to you in a way that makes practice more enjoyable. I've even found that difficult patients become less difficult with this approach."*
> —Grandinetti, 1996, page 84

Keep in mind that your workplace may be foreign to the patient and family. The rules are unwritten, so be sure to share them. Inform the learner that one of your responsibilities is to teach. Learners do not necessarily know this. A study of patients before and after elective spinal procedures determined, "the neurosurgeon was anticipated to be the sole source of information by an overwhelming majority of patients" (Holmes & Lenztyle, 1997, page 85).

Some organizations make patient and family education visible by formally contracting with the learner into the process:

> *"Each (Eaton Hospital) patient is asked to sign the protocol, agreeing to the learning process, becoming an active participant in his or her well-being. This commitment also serves to elevate the patient education process, making it an integral part of the hospitalization, and an important step on the path to a successful outcome."*
> —Integrating patient education . . ., 1998, page 2

However, this level of commitment may not always be necessary. Under most circumstances it is adequate simply to inform the learner that health care team members will provide information to support self-care as part of the treatment plan.

Focus on the Patient's Needs

Occasionally, you may have a patient who does not want treatment and does not want any information. Very few people prefer to know nothing and take no responsibility. Most often, refusal occurs when the partnership does not develop, despite your efforts to form an alliance.

> *"'How much responsibility to learn does the patient have?'*
> *When all factors are considered, it is the patient who must ultimately decide whether he is going to accept our attempts to teach him, whether he accepts selectively, or whether he completely ignores us."*
> —Rankin & Stallings, 1996, page 301

Center your care on the patient and family. Remember, the goals of patient education arise from the needs of the patient, present and anticipated. Consequently, they are the heads of the health care team. They determine the course of action.

> *"Patients . . . are not just recipients of the care we give, but rather, they and their families are at the head of the health care team. We develop this shift in focus by recognizing their right to choose their own futures and by willingly sharing our knowledge with them. This is known as* patient education, *a practice based on influence, not control."*
> —Rankin & Stallings, 1996, page 4

We're All in This Together

The patient and family head the health care team. Their decisions determine the direction of movement, and they control the breaks. The interventions of all the health care providers involved depend on the choices of the patient and family. From the emergency department to the intensive care unit (ICU) to the floor to home care to the doctor's office, specific team members may transition in and out, but teaching continues. The process of patient education is much bigger than preparation for procedures and discharge teaching. It extends beyond a hospital admission or an office visit. It is continual, over time and space.

You Can't Do it Alone

"Patient education is a process . . . it considers the patient holistically, with all his needs and concerns, and sets goals with the patient for desired outcomes. The process of patient education also includes an evaluation of the patient's learning, its usefulness to him, and the ease with which he has integrated it into his self-care practices."
—Rankin & Stallings, 1996, page 300

No matter how great a nurse you are, you cannot do it alone. You should not do it alone. By definition, one nurse in a limited amount of time cannot complete patient education. It's too big.

On the other hand, patient teaching can be done quickly, in short bursts.

"Patient teaching refers only to one component of the patient education process—the actual imparting of information to the patient . . . the total process of patient education is much more important than the teaching itself. The transfer of knowledge that occurs with patient teaching does not ensure behavioral change."
—Rankin & Stallings, 1996, page 300

Even if you find or make time to do all the teaching, it is only one part of patient education. To ensure behavioral change, your patient's knowledge needs to be evaluated and reinforced. Health care providers must facilitate integration of this knowledge into self-care practices over time. No one person can do this alone. The team must be involved. Relationships between interdependent health care team members are necessary to achieve effective patient and family education.

Work Together

Every individual on the health care team may know that if we work together the job gets done faster and better; however, that knowledge alone is not enough to make teamwork happen.

"Psychiatrists, for instance, know intellectually the benefits of a 'therapeutic community.' Yet almost never do psychiatric treatment units fulfill their potential in this regard. Neither physicians nor nurses desire to make themselves vulnerable to each other, much less to the patients. So the necessary authority system is also a specialized caste system in which the patients—supposedly the ones being served and most in need of self-esteem—are a kind of untouchables at the bottom of the heap . . . Nonetheless, . . . we are moving."
—Peck, 1987, page 260

Awareness of the problem brings hope. We each know we have a role in patient and family education. We probably also know that we will be most effective if we work together, sharing a goal and building on one another's experiences and evaluations; however, we're not there yet. One study found,

"Patients met many different health care providers during their hospital stay. All these different faces with different functions and responsibilities eventually confused patients, making it difficult for them to obtain the desired information from the most appropriate person. It is concluded that the large variety of health care providers patients met hindered them in their attempts to obtain appropriate patient education."
—Breemhaar, van den Borne, & Mullen, 1996, page 40

Collaboration between team members to provide patient and family education is not as common as it should be. Not only are teaching tools not standardized, but teaching content is not discussed. More often, we see isolated teaching by team members or multidisciplinary teaching, in which each discipline does its own thing. Health care professionals in a multidisciplinary practice are like 2-year-olds engaged in parallel play, side by side, not interacting. Each child has his or her own agenda and is playing alone. Collaboration on an interdisciplinary team is more like older children playing together, agreeing on the rules and roles of the game. They interact and adapt to one another. They collaborate.

Get to Know the Team

How do you know who is on the health care team, supporting this process of patient and family education? Not every team has every member. Not every member plays an equal part. Box 4-1 on page 53 lists individuals who may be included on your team.

It's a long list. How can you tell if you are communicating with everyone who needs to be involved? How do you know if your team has integrity? Has someone important been forgotten?

"If you wish to discern either the presence or absence of integrity, you need to ask only one question. What is missing? Has anything been left out?"
—Peck, 1987, page 256

Has any health care team member along the continuum been left out of communications? How can you include that member in the future? Put competitions and rivalries aside. What is best for the patient and family?

BOX 4-1   Who Is on the Team?

- [ ] Patient
- [ ] Patient's family and significant others
- [ ] Attending physician
- [ ] Specialists and consultant physicians
- [ ] Primary care physician
- [ ] Staff at primary care physician's office
- [ ] Bedside nurses
- [ ] Patient care assistants
- [ ] Certified nursing assistants
- [ ] Unit secretaries
- [ ] Housekeeping personnel
- [ ] Clinical nurse specialists
- [ ] Psychiatric liaison nurses and physicians
- [ ] Pharmacists
- [ ] Language interpreters
- [ ] Child life specialists
- [ ] Nurse practitioners
- [ ] Dietary and nutritional services
- [ ] Rehabilitation services, including physical therapy, occupational therapy, speech therapy
- [ ] Case managers
- [ ] Chaplains, clergy, spiritual counselors
- [ ] Social workers
- [ ] Community agencies and supports
- [ ] Telephone follow-up programs
- [ ] Home health care providers
- [ ] Quality assurance/improvement program staff
- [ ] Hospital administrators
- [ ] Nursing administration
- [ ] Nurse managers
- [ ] Public relations department
- [ ] In-house education department
- [ ] Third-party payers, including health maintenance organizations
- [ ] JCAHO
- [ ] And others!

"When the hospital gives discharge instructions to the patient or family, it also provides these instructions to the organization or individual responsible for the patient's continuing care."
—Joint Commission on Accreditation of Healthcare Organizations (JCAHO), 1998, page 10

This standard for practice reinforces teaching and promotes follow-up and a seamless continuum of care. Tell the primary physician where your teaching left off, where the learner had trouble, what instructions you gave. This helps develop that team approach, that community of providers of health care.

"A community is a group of all leaders."
—Peck, 1987, page 259

Coordinate With Other Team Members

Communication between disciplines across the continuum of care is essential to avoid wasting time. It is useless to teach details of a low-sodium diet with a learner who does not believe he has dangerous chronic hypertension. Coordination of teaching efforts gives us the freedom to individualize teaching, not just to the person, but also to the time.

"Patient readiness is another area of concern. It is unrealistic for the patient educator to wait for the educable moment or to expect that he or she will be able to keep the patient in the hospital until the patient is deemed 'educationally' ready for discharge. Shorter lengths of stay and the greater use of outpatient services mean that more patients are discharged to continue their recovery at home."
—Menke, 1993, page 162

The best way to help learners integrate new information into self-care practices and to support behavioral changes is to coordinate patient and family education across the care continuum. Team members need to build on the teaching of others. We must share understanding about the patient's story to individualize teaching. We need to present information to the learner in an organized manner. We should clarify and reinforce teaching that has come before. This will help us avoid several common problems, such as those found in one study:

"Information giving by different health care providers to one and the same patient was not well coordinated . . . . Patients received too much information on the day of admission, while they received little information at discharge."
—Breemhaar, van den Borne, & Mullen, 1996, page 42

By sharing the responsibilities of patient and family education, teaching is spread out to be more meaningful to the learner. If the admission is planned, why do we have to wait until the day of admission before orienting the patient to the unit? When discharge is set, why can't home care nurses meet the patient and begin their teaching? Some organizations have initiated these loosening of boundaries with great success.

Focus on the Goals

However, there are challenges along the way to collaboration. Often, historical relationships between disciplines make it difficult to initiate the collaborative effort.

"Too frequently and humanly we work out our own personal problems on the clients. Far worse, clients can become a human battleground for interdepartmental squabbles in which all sight of anyone's human needs is obscured."

—Brandon, 1976, page 44

Disciplines or individuals may fight for power and control, turning the workplace into a political arena. We focus on how things are done or who does them, instead of what is done or why we are doing it. The solution? Put the focus back on the mission, back on the goals. Put the focus back on the well-being of the patient and family.

"Things that matter most must never be at the mercy of things that matter least."

—Goethe

Creating mission statements and goals for our organizations may seem like a waste of energy when there's barely enough time to do patient care. However, when mission statements and goals are created collaboratively, they are wonderful tools for getting players back on track. Once everyone agrees on what matters most, it is easier to direct energies toward working together.

Have you ever been in a multidisciplinary meeting where professionals disagree on treatment plan and discharge path? Such chaos can be pulled together by a staff nurse (you) who reminds the team of what matters most: the best decision for this specific patient and family, as defined by this patient and family. You can refocus everyone on the shared goals.

As we focus on the shared goals, we may need to redefine who belongs on the health care team. Sometimes, work done in the hospital can be undone after discharge. Home health care may have different supplies and teach different techniques. Primary care providers may do things their own way. Insurance companies may not pay for what is ordered. Family members may undermine lifestyle changes.

> *"Patient education should no longer begin and end at the hospital door."*
> —Menke, 1993, page 163

What Can You Do?

What can you, one lone member of the team, do to help teams develop? Build relationships with the other team members yourself. Get to know the other members of the team. This includes nurses and people in other disciplines. Focus on the values you share. Listen. Acknowledge the skills of others. Ask them questions. Learn from them. Thank them for their help. Tell them your insights into the patient or family. Include them in your care.

This will take effort, and in the beginning, it may not be very rewarding. Keep it up, and the effects will be amazing. You will be recognized and remembered. Trust will build. Communication will increase. Cooperation and collaboration will flow. Others will be caught up in the transition, and your role modeling will be imitated. You can make a difference.

The long-term goal of building partnerships is to create a true health care community. Details on how to build a community are beyond the scope of this chapter. However, specific steps and stages are described in M. Scott Peck's book, *The Different Drum.* If partnership building inspires you, read it.

Interdisciplinary Partnerships

> *"When you have a diabetic not following her prescribed regimen and find she's encouraging the same behavior in her child, how do you get through?"*
> *"How can we decrease patient demands for frequent pain medication?"*
> —questions from RNs

Think of a difficult patient care situation in which you have been involved: a demanding patient or family member, a lack of cooperation with the plan of care, poor coordination between disciplines. If it was resolved, one person's actions probably were not solely responsible.

Generally, it takes interdisciplinary efforts to change a difficult situation.

The team approach is especially useful with holistic interventions, which deal with physiological, biobehavioral, spiritual, and interpersonal aspects of care. Insights from team members can be compiled to create a clear picture of the issues and resources and can assist problem solving. This helps the team unify and move toward a shared goal.

A sign in a neonatal ICU nursing station says, "What's best for the patient? What's best for the family?" When the shared mission is clear, partnerships develop. Focus on giving each patient and family consistent, supportive care.

Does interdisciplinary cooperation impact patient care? Yes. It promotes educational and treatment continuity. It sends a consistent message, which has a positive impact.

"A multidisciplinary treatment strategy significantly increased compliance rates."
—Rich, Gray, Beckham, Wittenberg, & Luther, 1996, page 274

In addition, there is evidence that collaborating on issues of patient and family education is cost-effective.

"On the average, for every dollar invested in patient education, $3 to $4 were saved . . . None of the studies reported that education cost more than it saved."
—Bartlett, 1995, pages 89 and 90

The patient and family head the team and direct the efforts. Health care providers work within that framework to use resources efficiently to obtain the best outcomes. Everyone on the team plays a role. Everyone has responsibilities.

"Accountability by both providers and clients is necessary to manage health care costs and outcomes."
—Henson, 1997, page 77

Building partnerships takes time and practice. It's a process, not an end. It can all begin with you, a staff nurse, or even a part-time staff nurse. Here are some examples of the sorts of challenges you may encounter, and actions you can take to build a better team.

Bringing Nurses Together

At Phoenix Children's Hospital, I was talking to another nurse about the frequency of phone calls from families of discharged patients requesting information that should have been covered during hospitalization. We thought about why this might be happening and realized the few teaching materials we had on the floor were disorganized. We went to the senior nursing administrator and explained why the current teaching system was not meeting our patients' needs. She asked us to get additional feedback from our colleagues.

We took a survey, developed a wish list, created a task force, formulated a plan, requested money, and spent it wisely (Kennis, 1996). We assembled and organized resources that supported the teaching we do most frequently. Our accomplishments were so impressive, nurses from other units came to us to borrow supplies. When the NG, trach, and CVC teaching dolls never came back, it became clear the need was not just on our unit, but hospital-wide.

Our task force became the Patient/Family Education Committee, open to any health care provider who wanted to improve patient education in the hospital, both inpatient and outpatient. Even a parent representing the Parent's Advisory Council is an active member. We assessed barriers to teaching and staff needs, furnished report rooms to store teaching materials, advocated for computers, and revised the education documentation record. The scope has expanded too. Our committee is now initiating a process improvement initiative, looking to improve the continuity of patient and family education between the hospital and home care providers.

And it all started with just us—two nurses having a conversation. You are not alone.

"Greater team efforts and support within nursing would improve patient education efforts and act as a motivator to inexperienced nurses looking for guidance."

—Rankin & Stallings, 1996, page 302

Even if you don't start an internal minirevolution in patient and family education, as these two nurses did, you can be incredibly effective. Be a role model and motivate others. Inexperienced nurses need this most obviously, but each of us needs mentoring from time to time. See Box 4-2 on page 59 for tips on how to mentor your colleagues better.

Partner with the nurses around you in some way every day. This will help each one of us feel less alone, and even small efforts add up.

BOX 4-2   Mentoring

Our jobs are so complex, intense, and stressful that support, kindness, and mentoring between nurses are vital. Each of us can be mentors or the recipients of mentoring at different times in our careers. The real benefit of mentoring is not an end result, but rather the ongoing process of professional intimacy, respect, cooperation, and interdependence that the mentoring relationship distills.

Mentor is defined as a wise, loyal advisor or a teacher or coach. Here are some things you can do to be a better mentor:

M—Mindful attention. Give thoughtful and sympathetic professional attention to the nurses around you.

E—Encouragement. Give positive encouragement to those with whom you work, especially those who are struggling professionally.

N—Nurture professional growth. Attend professional inservices and continuing education offerings together. Focus on the positive aspects of the experience.

T—Teach with joy. Share your experiences, and give your knowledge.

O—Observe and orient as needed. Compassionately observe other nurses, especially those new to the profession, and guide them through their struggles.

R—Recognize and respect the accomplishments of your colleagues, from novice to expert.

Through mentoring, we can connect with the ideals that drew us to nursing. Through mentoring, we gain a sense that one nurse can have a positive, lasting, and meaningful effect on our workplace and our profession.

(Adapted from Sitzman, K. [1998], Mentoring. *Home Healthcare Nurse, 16*[1], 20.)

Physicians and the Team

> As a Family Health Information Specialist in a consumer health library, it is my job to provide families with information about the health care needs of their children. Once they have the information, I make myself available to help them understand what it is they may be learning about.
>
> In talking with a physician one day, he voiced concern that a family would still have questions after he and his nurse provided the family with education. He felt that sending the family to obtain written, video, or audio information along with explanations from him and his nurse should be sufficient education.

The physician described in this situation seems unaware that often learning that leads to deeper understanding may generate more questions. Patient and family education is not a significant aspect of medical education. Consequently, physicians may have minimal expertise in teaching skills, especially assessment of knowledge and evaluation of understanding.

Sometimes health care providers use medical terminology when teaching and forget to define the terms for their patients and families. Learners may feel too intimidated to ask physicians for clarification or may not want to waste their time with unimportant questions. If the physician does not evaluate understanding, he or she is unaware that the teaching was not clear.

Other physicians worry that patients and families will make unwise decisions if they have access to information. These physicians are most comfortable when patients are just recipients of care, rather than active partners. These physicians may not trust their own teaching skills and may be unsure whether they can clarify issues so that the learner will make the best decisions. However, their feelings do not change the fact that patients and families have final accountability for care. They live with the outcomes.

Sometimes, physicians are concerned that other team members offer the patient and family conflicting information. Different team members may anticipate different discharge needs or may teach techniques differently. Their response may be autocratic.

In all of these situations, it is important to keep each team member focused on the goals of patient and family education and away from interpersonal issues. It would be difficult for any physician to argue against the appropriateness of informed consent, self-care skills, recognizing and responding to problems, and accessing resources to get questions answered.

Ask what is best for the patient and family. Resolve concerns about consistency of information through team collaboration, enhanced team communications, and clear documentation. Talk it out. Explore alternatives.

There is no one information gatekeeper, for there are far too many gates. However, you can develop a unified team plan that addresses issues consistently. This will be especially important as more people access the internet and health care consumers advocate for themselves. Learners will bring you information and ask you to help them make sense of it. As recently as 1996, however, this quote appeared in the literature:

> *"We most likely still will be confronted by physicians who absolutely refuse to allow any of their patients access to patient education . . . It may be necessary to have the patient himself request patient teaching and put pressure on the doctor to provide it."*
> —Rankin & Stallings, 1996, page 308

What is missing? Has anything been left out? The rest of the health care team is missing! Who decides what is best for the patient and family? The patient and family, of course. Most health care is self-care, not performed by a licensed professional. Most people's knowledge of health and illness is learned through life experience, family, friends, and lay media, not from a physician's teaching. Any health care provider who does not acknowledge this is disillusioned. A physician cannot refuse patients access to information any more than they can refuse them access to music. It is all around us.

A physician does not need to write an order for education to occur, and an order that "no education may occur" is meaningless. Patients and families learn during each interaction with a health care team member. Besides, it is inappropriate for anyone to limit the scope of practice of other licensed professionals on the team. Here, the multidisciplinary approach needs to become interdisciplinary. This whole team needs to come together and build partnerships, with the shared goal of improved patient outcomes.

Fortunately, most physicians recognize the importance of patient and family education in obtaining positive outcomes and collaborate with team members to optimize teaching. They appreciate the contributions of other team members and understand that collaboration enhances the quality of patient care.

Nonprofessional Members in Patient and Family Education

In these times of financial constraints, many tasks are being taken over by nonprofessional members of the health care team. While the roles of licensed health care professionals in education may be clear, how do patient care assistants, certified nursing assistants, care technicians, unit secretaries, and other personnel contribute to patient and family education?

These nonprofessional team members maintain the environment. They support the systems of communication, and they contribute to the emotional tone of the space. When these factors are out of control, teaching is difficult.

In addition, nonprofessional team members are in prime positions to identify teachable moments. They are often with the patient and family when licensed health care professionals are not. They may hear the questions or observe the distress.

Educate nonprofessional team members in identifying teachable moments. Explain that their role is to inform an appropriate licensed health care professional of the patient's or family member's need before the moment passes. If the patient fell out of bed, the assistant or technician would tell the nurse. In the same vein, if the patient has a concern or question, it, too, needs to be communicated in a timely manner.

Telephone Follow-up Programs

"It is recommended that routine, posthospitalization nursing care include follow-up, such as the follow-up telephone call."
—Holmes & Lenztyle, 1997, page 85

Learners take time to process information. Information that seemed clear at the time of teaching may not make sense at home. Problems come up that were not anticipated. Telephone follow-up programs not only improve patient satisfaction but are an effective tool for continuity in patient and family education. Communicate your concerns about the learner to the team member making the call. Evaluation can then hone in on potential problem areas.

The Home Health Care Advantage

"The different data that discerning health care professionals can gather on home visits far surpass in quality and quantity what they can assess in the hospital."
                                                    —Rankin & Stallings, 1996, page 309

Home health care providers have the assessment and evaluation edge on other team members. They are also in a unique position to individualize teaching. Relationships form easily in the nonthreatening environment. Patients and families are more likely to let down their guard when at home. In addition, simple observation of the environment can reveal a great deal of information. A bag of cookies on a diabetic's kitchen counter tells more than reviewing weeks of food diaries. Home health care providers can be a great resource to the rest of the health care team.

Consequently, they also provide a special link in continuity of patient and family education. The more detailed and accurate the information they receive from the rest of the health care team, the more effective their work can be.

Providers of Orientation and Continuing Education

"We also discovered that many of the nurses had never received formal training in patient education, including the proper way to document the teaching they were doing."
                                                    —Smalley, 1997, page 19

The patient teaching project we did in nursing school barely resembles real-life patient and family education. We were given time to research and prepare, teach, evaluate understanding, and document.

Providers of in-house orientation and continuing education are essential members of the health care team. They are in a position to address system-wide problems at their roots. They can teach staff how to teach, how to build interdisciplinary relationships, and how to communicate effectively. There are so many skills involved in effective patient and family education that most subjects they cover can probably include a patient education component. There are teaching implications for equipment, policies and procedures, treatments, and customer service topics. They can reinforce patient and family education skills for new employees and preceptors, in annual reviews, and in special programs.

BOX 4-3   Patient and Family Education

DISCUSSION QUESTIONS
- When do you do patient and family education?
- What's the best way to understand whether a learner understands your teaching?
- How can you help patients and families make informed decisions?
- How can you help patients and families learn basic self-care skills to survive?
- How can you help patients and families learn how to recognize problems and know what to do in response?
- How do you teach patients and families how to get questions answered and find resources for answers?
- Where can you find teaching materials to give patients and families to reinforce your teaching?
- What are your personal challenges in teaching patients and families?

"One or 2-day workshops offered to all health professionals are an effective means of imparting teaching and learning principles and securing interest in patient education."

—Rankin & Stallings, 1996, page 302

How can an educator engage staff in a discussion about patient and family education? A list of questions is listed in Box 4-3 on this page.

Health education week, nurse's week, hospital week, heart month, nutrition month, acquired immunodeficiency syndrome (AIDS) day, and other observances can each be opportunities to promote teaching. Efforts of in-house educators can greatly enhance patient and family education throughout the organization.

Reach Out to Community Resources

"People want to understand what is happening to them and how it will affect their future, so that they can make informed choices about their lives. They need time and space to discuss any anxieties and fears they have and to raise questions. They want honest and appropriate information. They want to talk to other people who are facing a similar future. They want the services to be available for their individual needs and to take account of what they are as a person. They want to promote research into their illness

and improve understanding and treatment and to make their own
contribution to this research. In all these areas the lay associations are a
major source of help and support to anyone embarking on this journey."
—Heijman, 1995, page 279

Not every patient sees a social worker. Community resources, if considered at all by hospital health care providers, are often considered as an afterthought. However, they are significant contributors to patient and family education.

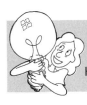

Many communities issue a directory of local resources. The federal government provides directories of national resources. Have them in your patient care area, ready to access easily.

Community resources obviously include lay associations and advocacy and support groups. They also include public libraries, consumer health libraries, the world wide web, school nurses, occupational health nurses, community agencies, government agencies, medical and nursing schools, senior centers, hospitals, and providers of integrative, complementary, and alternative medicine.

It's not just nice to do, it's the standard for practice:

"Patients are informed about access to additional resources in the
community."
—JCAHO, 1998, page 106

Learn the community resources most appropriate for your patient population. Build relationships with them, and promote continuity of patient and family education through them.

Organization Managers and Administrators

"The hospital plans, supports, and coordinates activities and resources for
patient and family education."
—JCAHO, 1998, page 10

It's a patient care standard. Hospitals have resources for patient and family education. Hospitals plan, support, and coordinate education. Obviously, this is done, not by buildings, but by health care team members working together.

A commitment to patient and family education from the top of the organization can contribute greatly to the efforts of the health care team.

Partner with your administrators to help them understand that patient and family education promotes health, saves money, and increases patient satisfaction.

Once they understand that teaching is a good investment, they should be motivated to provide the supporting structure. They may consider teaching needs when calculating staffing, providing continuing education, or assigning support services. Remember the example described previously in which two nurses who went to their nursing administrator were able to accomplish much more than they could have done without her. Her sanctioning of a needs assessment started significant organizational changes.

> *"One of the potentially most valuable mechanisms . . . is the establishment of a multidisciplinary institutionwide policymaking committee. This committee should bring together representatives of administration, the medical staff, and all departments directly concerned with patient teaching. The presence of a top-level administrative person on such a committee should make a statement about the institution's commitment to patient education that will be heard throughout the organization."*
> —Ruzicki, 1984, page 6

Patient and family education could be incorporated into daily rounds, nursing rounds, and grand rounds. This would contribute to interdisciplinary communications and increase visibility of teaching assessments and evaluations.

Administrators can also support patient and family education through policies and procedures that define who teaches, when, and the documentation required. Patient and family education reward and incentive programs would demonstrate organizational support. Compliance with policy can be considered during performance evaluations. Patient and family education skills can be evaluated through a performance-based development system clinical assessment. Clinical career ladder programs, which evaluate expertise, should include evaluation of teaching skills. These all show that patient and family education is important, expected, and supported.

What's JCAHO Got to Do With Patient Education?

The standards set by JCAHO evolve over time. Recently, JCAHO has been encouraging an interdisciplinary approach to patient and family education.

Two standards that specifically encourage professional teamwork follow:

- "The patient and family educational process is collaborative and interdisciplinary, as appropriate to the plan of care."
- "When the hospital gives discharge instructions to the patient or family, it also provides these instructions to the organization or individual responsible for the patient's continuing care" (JCAHO, 1998, pages 10–11).

It's easy to view JCAHO visits as an annoyance, telling us how to do things, making busy work, taking us away from our tasks of patient care. However, we can reframe the standards set by JCAHO and use them to our advantage. We can consider JCAHO as part of the health care team promoting our patient and family education efforts.

For example, hospitals often share their site visit experiences, warning the next organization where the surveyors focused. One such informal communication from an anonymous source suggested staff should be prepared to answer questions such as:

- How are physicians involved in patient teaching?
- Where would you find documentation of patient education?
- Where do you chart patient readiness to learn? What do you look for as cues of readiness?

The sheet also listed questions surveyors may ask patients:

- What have you learned?
- Will you be able to care for yourself at home? How?
- I see you have an IV hanging there. Do you have medicine in your IV? What is it for?

Can you see how impending JCAHO visits can be used to motivate improvement in patient and family education in your organization?

"In-house, mini-mock surveys will reveal any gaps in your patient-education procedure. Actively involve all interdisciplinary staff."
—Miller & Capps, 1997, page 58

If your preparations for the site visit reveal that changes are needed to meet patient and family education standards, this can motivate administrators and caregivers to collaborate to improve the system. Financial support, improved communications, and enhanced teamwork may, amazingly, appear. JCAHO is, indeed, on the health care team.

How You Can Promote Teamwork

The criteria for successful teamwork in patient and family education are:

- *"Communication (verbal and written), facilitated by planning meetings, care conferences, telephone consultation, good documentation and the 'willingness to go out of our way to communicate with one another.'*
- *Mutual respect among disciplines, recognizing respective areas of expertise, knowing one's limits, and teaching each other.*
- *Desire to work as a team in recognition of a common goal."*
  —Rankin & Stallings, 1996, page 18

No matter where you work or what sort of nursing you do, you are in a position to promote interdisciplinary teamwork. First, frequently review the potential health care team members listed early in this chapter. As you identify additional members, add them to the list. This will help you remember you are not alone. Here are some actions you can take to partner with those other team members:

☐ Think of yourself as a coordinator of patient and family education. Look at the big picture.
    ☐ What does this learner know?
    ☐ What does this learner need to know?
    ☐ How does the learner learn best?
    ☐ How are you communicating this to other team members?

Role model good patient and family education skills. Set a tone for cooperation.

☐ Partner with the learner. Make teaching visible, and engage the learner in the process. Support learning that promotes adaptation to new circumstances.
☐ Partner with other health care team members. Acknowledge and appreciate their areas of expertise. Compliment them on jobs well done.
☐ Solve problems together. Identify the constraints of institutions, and work within the environment to optimize patient care.
☐ Think big. Who else can you involve in the patient and family education process? Go beyond traditional organizations and boundaries. Who can you invite to join this health care team?
☐ Enhance interdisciplinary communications with creativity and flexibility. "Look for alternatives such as conference calls, voice mail, or e-mail to exchange information and to initiate changes in care" (Sherry, 1996, page 479).

☐ Whenever discussing a patient's physical, emotional, and spiritual status with other health care team members, include status of education. These conversations may occur formally or informally, in anywhere from a shift-change conversation to an interdisciplinary patient care conference.

☐ Read the chart and save teaching time by building on the efforts of other team members.

☐ Encourage other health care team members to view documentation of patient and family education as a way to communicate their patient and family education. When a health care team member tells you of an effective teaching method to use with a specific learner, ask him or her to document it for the rest of the team to read.

☐ Often, assessments and responses to treatment need to be evaluated before a long-term plan is in place. Until you know future needs, teach about the present. If the learner understands tests, medication, and treatments, he or she will be able to make informed decisions.

☐ When health care team members document patient education, let them know you read their notes and built on their efforts.

☐ If health care team members are not communicating with you about the teaching they are doing, either verbally or in writing, ask them.

☐ If you perceive the team's behavior as more multidisciplinary than interdisciplinary, call a patient care conference, and invite all the appropriate health care team members. Specifics on how to do such a meeting are described in Box 4-4 below.

BOX 4-4   Tips on Organizing a Patient Care Conference

"A general planning meeting can be useful in saving time for everyone and avoiding replication of efforts. If this meeting is set up around the physician's scheduled time on the unit or in the agency, the process will be facilitated. Mutually derived goals should be written at the planning meeting. Notifying the patient's family of a time to be present for planning is also helpful, and because the focus of the team is the patient, he should also be present."
—Rankin & Stallings, 1996, page 309

One way to pull a health care team together is to meet to collaborate on patient care. Here are some tips to help you organize a patient care conference.

• When communications and actions need to be coordinated, any member of the health care team can organize a patient care conference.

Box 4-4 *(Continued)*

- Focus on outcomes. Instead of rehashing problems that cannot be resolved, direct energy toward achievable goals.
- Set the ground rules. Don't assume everyone knows how to participate. Be clear on the purpose of the meeting, the expectation that everyone will participate, the time allotted, and the agenda. Often, the patient is introduced or identified, each member reports progress toward goals, new problems are brought up for discussion, and the goals, plan, and responsibilities are revised.
- Put patient and family education on the agenda. Share assessments and evaluations of understanding and insights into individualizing teaching.
- Pick a facilitator. A person in charge of running the meeting can schedule the meeting time, reserve the space, and keep discussion on the agenda and on time.
- Pick a recorder, or use a form on which each team member summarizes his or her assessments and plans. The summary of the meeting should fit on one page.
- Involve patients and family. Whenever possible, invite them to the meeting. Occasionally, a patient care conference is used to resolve conflicts between health care providers. In these cases, the patient and family members may not be invited but should be informed of the meeting and of any changes in the plan of care.
- If it is impossible for all the team members to meet in one room at one time, be creative.
  —Those who cannot be there may participate through a speaker phone on the table. More than one team member can be connected this way to listen and contribute to the discussion.
  —A member who cannot participate can submit a written summary for the facilitator to read at the meeting. Record the meeting on tape so the member who misses the meeting can hear the discussion and understand any changes in plan.

(Adapted from Sherry, D. [1996]. Patient care conferences with pizazz. *Home Healthcare Nurse, 14*[6], 478–480.)

☐ Anticipate learning needs. Find and conveniently place appropriate teaching materials so that you or other team members can use them as teachable moments occur.

☐ If a long-term plan is falling into place and details are not communicated to you, ask the team members determining the plan. The sooner you know the details of medications, equipment, nutrition, modifications to activities of daily living, rehabilitation, follow-up care, and community resources to be used, the sooner you can address them in patient and family education.

☐ When orienting or precepting new members to the health care team, include expectations about communication of patient and family education.

☐ Organize with other health care team members who are striving to enhance patient and family education. Actively participate in appropriate committees. If no appropriate group exists but is needed, start it. Focus on actions you can take that will enhance a learning environment.

☐ Be a continuous learner yourself. Learn from those around you. Share your insights into the process of patient and family education with your colleagues.

"There are many proven methods to keep patient education workload within reasonable limits, and still more need to be developed in order to efficiently use team-approach and referrals, to work with groups of patients, and to integrate community and clinic-based programs."
—Grueninger, 1995, page 52

You will have more time to teach if you partner with those around you and share the load. Work together toward the same goals, build on one another's teaching, and reinforce one another's messages.

Be creative and flexible. Be patient. Be persistent. Transitions from separate health care providers to multidisciplinary teams to interdisciplinary teams to health care communities take time. Remember that each step of the way, you are promoting quality patient and family education and quality patient care.

As we work together toward shared goals,

"the fact of our unity becomes more real and powerful to us than the belief in our separateness."
—Dass & Gorman, 1985, page 228

You are not alone.

If you want to learn more:

(1998). Integrating patient education into the continuum of care. *The Exchange: A Forum for Patient and Family Educators, 1*(2), 1–2.

Bartlett, E.E. (1995). Cost-benefit analysis of patient education. *Patient Education and Counseling, 26,* 87–91.

Brandon, D. (1976). *Zen in the art of helping*. New York: Arkana of Viking Penguin.

Breemhaar, B., van den Borne, H.W., & Mullen, P.D. (1996). Inadequacies of surgical patient education. *Patient Education and Counseling, 28*(1), 31–44.

Dass, R., & Gorman, P. (1985). *How can I help? Stories and reflections on service*. New York: Alfred A. Knopf.

Goethe, J.W. http://ur.utenn.edu/context/Sept97Context/quote.html

Grandinetti, D. (1996). Teaching patients to take care of themselves. *Medical Economics, 73*(22), 83–91.

Grueninger, U.J. (1995). Arterial hypertension: Lessons from patient education. *Patient Education and Counseling, 26*(1–3), 37–55.

Heijman, A. (1995). The role of lay associations: Difficulties encountered. *Patient Education and Counseling, 26*, 277–280.

Henson, R.H. (1997). Analysis of the concept of mutuality. *Image: Journal of Nursing Scholarship, 29*(1), 77–81.

Holmes, K.L., & Lenztyle, E.R. (1997). Perceived self-care information needs and information-seeking behaviors before and after elective spinal procedures. *Journal of Neuroscience Nursing, 29*(2), 79–86.

Joint Commission on Accreditation of Healthcare Organizations (JCAHO) (1998). *1998 Hospital Accreditation Standards*.

Kennedy, M. (1995). Making patients part of their healthcare team. *The Quality Letter for Healthcare Leaders, 7*(2), 2–12.

Kennis, N. (1996). Maximize your patient teaching potential. *RN, 59*(2), 21–23.

Menke, K.L. (1993). Linking patient education with discharge planning. In B.E. Giloth (Ed.), *Managing hospital-based patient education* (pp. 153–164). Chicago, IL: American Hospital Publishing.

Miller, B., & Capps, E. (1997). Meeting JCAHO patient-education standards. *Nursing Management, 28*(5), 55–58.

Peck, M.S. (1987). *The different drum: Community-making and peace*. New York: Touchstone.

Rankin, S.H., & Stallings, K.D. (1996). *Patient education: issues, principles, practices* (3rd ed.). Philadelphia: Lippincott-Raven.

Rich, M.W., Gray, D.B., Beckham, V., Wittenberg, C., & Luther, P. (1996). Effect of a multidisciplinary intervention on medication compliance in elderly patients with congestive heart failure. *American Journal of Medicine, 101*(3), 270–276.

Ruzicki, D.A. (1984). Motivating patient care staff to teach: A plan for action. *Promoting Health, 5*(4), 6–8.

Sherry, D. (1996). Patient care conferences with pizazz. *Home Healthcare Nurse, 14*(6), 478–480.

Sitzman, K. (1998). Mentoring. *Home Healthcare Nurse, 16*(1), 20.

Smalley, R. (1997). Patient education. We have a better system now. *RN, 60*(6), 19–21.

Tripp, K.R. (1987). *Perspectives on adult learning: Maternal coping with a monitored child in the home*. Unpublished doctoral dissertation, Arizona State University.

Wesorick, B., Shiparski, L., Troseth, M., & Wyngarden, K. (1998). *Partnership council field book: Strategies and tools for co-creating a healthy work place*. Michigan: Practice Field Publishing.

Wills, E.M. (1996). Nurse-client alliance. *Home Healthcare Nurse, 14*(6), 455–459.

The Teachable Moment

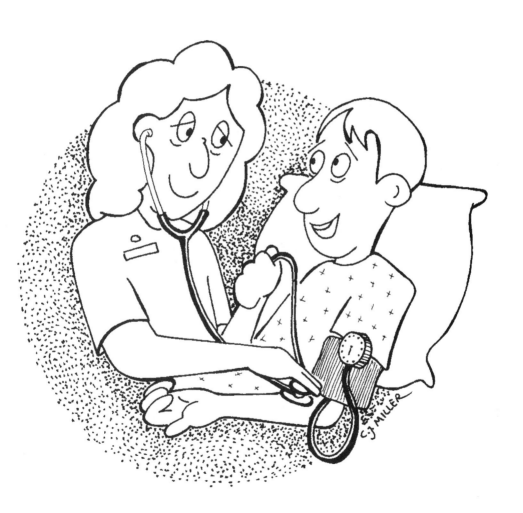

If we have a new piece of equipment, there is always a little information about the patient education that goes with it. . . . Instead of making patient education a stand-alone issue, we're trying to incorporate it into all practice."

—O'Conner Finch, 1998, page 9

Just think about the barriers we encounter to teaching.

First, we are trained as nurses, not teachers, yet we have to teach information that can impact life or death choices.

In addition, our learners are not students, but patients and family members. They don't come to health care providers to learn; they come for treatment.

However, our most important service is our teaching. Our learners provide most of their own health care. Up to 80% of all illnesses are managed by patients themselves (1997). Our job is to promote quality self-care.

As if that were not enough, our opportunities for teaching are limited. Box 5-1 lists qualities commonly found in learners. Check the qualities you have seen in your learners.

Some of these conditions are temporary and some permanent. Some make teaching difficult, but some can motivate the learner. How do we work within these limits? When can we teach?

BOX 5-1

What Qualities Have You Seen in Your Learners?

☐ Sick
☐ Worried
☐ Scared
☐ Anxious
☐ In pain
☐ Upset
☐ Angry
☐ Lonely
☐ Dependent
☐ Hopeless
☐ Helpless
☐ Depressed
☐ Apathetic
☐ Nauseous
☐ Medicated with narcotics
☐ Medicated with sedatives
☐ Medicated with antipsychotics
☐ Experiencing side effects of medications
☐ Sleeping
☐ Distracted by the foreign environment
☐ Distracted by interpersonal issues
☐ Distracted by financial issues
☐ Distracted by ethical issues
☐ Distracted by mortality issues
☐ Developmentally delayed
☐ Confused
☐ Disoriented
☐ Psychotic
☐ Experientially limited
☐ Educationally limited
☐ Illiterate
☐ Vision impaired
☐ Hearing impaired
☐ Mobility impaired
☐ Memory impaired
☐ Not fluent in English
☐ In denial
☐ Not interested in learning

Go With the Flow

- Do you find patient and family education an unpleasant chore?
- Are your learners sometimes disinterested, resistant, or rebellious?
- Do your learners sometimes take an awfully long time to "get it?"

Check the sentences you often say:

☐ "Read this now."
☐ "My name is _____ and I'm here to teach you about _____."
☐ "I know you're tired, but you have to learn this before you can go home."
☐ "Stop watching that (game show/soap opera/talk show) and change your TV to channel 3. Watch the video on _____. I'll be back in to talk to you about it later."

The more checks you had, the more likely you need to learn to go with the flow. You can waste a lot of teaching time by trying to teach a learner who is not ready to learn.

Why Wouldn't a Person Be Ready to Learn?

Have you ever been to a mandatory inservice that felt like a waste of your time? If so, why did you feel that way? Did you know the information already? Did learning this information not change any of your behaviors or viewpoints? Did you have other, more important concerns no one was addressing?

This is what it feels like to be taught against the flow. When you don't perceive the need for information, educators inefficiently use their time and yours.

Think About Yourself as Teacher

The right perspective can save you teaching time. When you shift your attention from what you need to teach to what the learner needs and wants to know, teaching becomes quicker.

Sometimes a learner has a question or concern we do not address. The learner may continue thinking about that concern without hearing what we are saying. When this occurs, our teaching time is wasted.

"Mothers cited numerous examples . . . where their questions were evaded, 'blown off,' not answered, or answered superficially. Those situations generated feelings of insecurity, anxiety, and frustration; and became barriers to the learning process."

—Tripp, 1987, page 173

Children expect adults to tell them what to learn. Children are too young and inexperienced to understand always how new information will be useful later in their lives. That's why teachers decide what children need to learn.

Adults, unlike children, know enough to function independently. Unless they perceive that new information is relevant to their changing situation, they may not feel the need to learn. After all, adults get along just fine with what they know right now.

Adult learners want to know right away why new information is important. If the new information does not fit with what they know and believe, it will be even more difficult to convince them to learn. Adults need individualized teaching.

Because the framework of this book is built around adult learning principles, a summary of what they are and how to apply them appears on the inside covers of this book. Read it if you aren't familiar with adult learning principles or if you need a review.

How do you go with the flow? Teach in context. Establish shared goals with the learner, and then let your teaching respond to needs as they arise. Remember the general goals of patient and family education:

- Make informed decisions.
- Develop basic self-care skills to survive.
- Recognize problems and know what to do in response.
- Get questions answered; find resources for answers.

As you go with the flow of learner-driven need, incorporate need-to-know information into your responses. For example, if a learner asks about a specific side effect of a medication, answer the question, and then expand your answer to include which side effects should trigger a call to the physician.

All essential information will fall into the mutually defined goals. Because adult learners are competent to decide what they learn and apply and the goals are mutually determined, you share educational responsibility with them. You are not alone.

Optimizing use of teachable moments can save you teaching time. Teach when the learner is open to information. By doing this, you will also integrate learning into your care. This generates an expectation for learning and facilitates additional learning.

What is a Teachable Moment?

"Teaching is most effective when it serves as a quick response to the need of a patient or family member. . . . Satisfy his immediate need for information; you can supplement your teaching with more details later."
—Cunningham, 1993, page 24J

A teachable moment is when the learner's readiness is at a peak. When teaching synchronizes with readiness, the most effective education occurs.

In a teachable moment, the learner is ready to learn, willing to change, and able to act.

Teachable moments are more easily recognized and responded to in a conversation than in a classroom. When we pay attention to the learner, we can nurture teachable moments and take advantage of them.

"The purpose of education is to assist learners to become independent."
—Brookfield, 1986, page 71

Often in our process of helping learners become independent, we are teaching. This teaching comes out of who we are. We use ourselves as instruments of teaching. By being warm, caring, and accepting of our learners, we create a nonthreatening environment.

Have patients ever asked you questions they should have asked their physicians, but didn't, because you were less threatening? Learners see nurses as their equals. They feel able to have casual conversations with us.

Teachable moments can happen anywhere, anytime. Teachable moments are opportunities. They most often occur in informal, casual moments. We may be performing a task or simply passing by. Often, in these instances, we do not perceive ourselves as teachers, so we don't acknowledge or document teaching done this way.

Teaching Informally

Teachable moments are all around you. Whether you know it or not, you often take advantage of them. Most of your teaching is on the run, embedded in casual conversations:

- Describing the procedure you are doing
  ("I'm putting the antibiotic in the IV.")
- Explaining why you are doing it
  ("I'm wearing gloves so the germs from my hands don't get on the incision.")
- Addressing something you observed in the interaction between patient and visitor
  ("If you leave the side rail down, he could roll out.")
- Answering a question
  ("Antibiotics don't kill viruses, and you have a virus.")
- Telling the patient what to expect in the upcoming test or procedure
  ("Before the test, you will get some medicine to make you sleepy.")
- Reassuring with information
  ("Oh, the needle doesn't stay in your arm! See, the IV catheter is made of a flexible plastic.")
- Providing anticipatory guidance
  ("Your baby won't be able to sit up by himself for another month or so. His muscles have to develop.")

If you define teaching as planned, formal patient and family education, you probably feel you rarely have time to teach. If you only document formal teaching, you probably don't document much on patient and family education.

> "But when do people really learn? We learn at moments rather than continuously, and it's the acceptance of moments of learning that allows you to make full use of them."
>
> —Wurman, 1989, page 154

Most patient and family education is informal. Unfortunately, informal teaching is often invisible teaching. The learner sees it as conversation and does not perceive that education has occurred.

> "I've been in the hospital six times and nobody ever taught me anything!"
>
> —A former patient

The nurse does not acknowledge that informal teaching is official patient and family education and does not document it. Without documentation, there is no indication to the rest of the health care team that teaching was done. This is invisible teaching.

Nurses then come away from their workdays frustrated because they had no time to teach, yet they were teaching all day long! Informal teaching can be invisible even to the person doing it, if the person doing it is not aware.

"Patient education is creative work, requiring astute assessment and energetic involvement with the patient and family to make every moment count."
—Rankin & Stallings, 1996, page 36

Looking for time to teach? Time to teach is handed to you with each teachable moment. Here are some ways to take advantage of these informal teaching opportunities.

- Learn to recognize teachable moments, and take advantage of them.
- Learn to recognize informal teaching. Take the quiz called in Figure 5-1 on page 81.
- Evaluate your learner's understanding so you know he or she understands and can apply what was learned. This helps learners become aware that teaching has taken place and makes teaching visible to them.
- Document both your informal and formal assessments and evaluations of understanding. Share your progress with other members of the health care team so that teaching can progress through teamwork.

Which statements are examples of the patient/family teaching process in action?

1. True False   "Here's that handout on your medication."
2. True False   "Let me show you how to change your wife's dressing."
3. True False   "This video will tell you all about that."
4. True False   "What would you do if your mother had trouble breathing?"
5. True False   "Show me how you feed him."
6. True False   "Have you tried putting your father's medicine in a small amount of juice?"
7. True False   "After surgery, your husband will go to the recovery room."
8. True False   "Where do you keep your medicine at home?"
9. True False   "How would you know if you have an infection?"
10. True False   "Most people who quit smoking gain only five pounds."
11. True False   "In a few months your baby will begin to walk."
12. True False   "Do you have any smoke alarms in your house?"
13. True False   "Here's a paper and pencil. As you think of questions for your doctor, write them down. This way you won't forget them when you see her."
14. True False   "It sounds like you feel all alone with this. Have you considered joining a support group?"
15. True False   "Where could you go if you had a question about this?"

Is It Teaching?—Yes!

1. True   "Here's that handout on your medication."
   • Handouts give learners something to refer to at home.
   • Many people cannot read, or may misunderstand medical terms, so be sure to review the contents of every handout with the learner.

2. True   "Let me show you how to change your wife's dressing."
   • Demonstration of a skill is an important part of teaching.
   • Don't forget to watch the learner do it, too.

3. True   "This video will tell you all about that."
   • Many people are visual learners; videos can be great teaching tools.
   • After the learner watches the video, ask the learner questions to be sure the contents were understood.

4. True   "What would you do if your mother had trouble breathing?"
   • Problem-solving scenarios are a great way to be sure the learner knows what to do.

Figure 5-1. Is It Teaching?

5. True   "Show me how you feed him."
   • It can save time and energy if you assess what is before you teach what should be.

6. True   "Have you tried putting your father's medicine in a small amount of juice?"
   • Sometimes they tried the intervention already.

7. True   "After surgery, your husband will go to the recovery room."
   • Most patients and families don't know hospitals and hospital routines. This sort of teaching helps them understand what is going on and feel more comfortable.

8. True   "Where do you keep your medicine at home?"
   • It helps to understand how the family plans to carry out instructions.

9. True   "How would you know if you have an infection?"
   • Evaluate knowledge. Can the learner apply information in real life?

10. True   "Most people who quit smoking gain only five pounds."
   • Teaching may include correcting misperceptions.

11. True   "In a few months your baby will begin to walk."
   • Teaching may include anticipatory guidance about normal growth and development.

12. True   "Do you have any smoke alarms in your house?"
   • Teaching may include prevention and safety topics.

13. True   "Here's a paper and pencil. As you think of questions for your doctor, write them down. This way you won't forget them when you see her."
   • Help the learner take control of the situation. Give permission and encourage the asking of questions.

14. True   "It sounds like you feel all alone with this. Have you considered joining a support group?"
   • Promote social support. Share the resources that are available. For those with a computer and modem, support groups are available on-line.

15. True   "Where could you go if you had a question about this?"
   • How will they find the answers when you're not there? Do they use the public library? Do they have access to an on-line resource?

Figure 5-1. *(Continued)*

Taking Advantage When the Learner Is Motivated

Teachable moments and the informal teaching that occurs in response can actually teach more effectively than formal teaching. This is because the learner is especially motivated and engaged in learning at that moment.

Once I took care of a 19-year-old male patient with abdominal pain in the hospital to rule out appendicitis. His white count was fine, and they couldn't figure out why his pain was so bad. Then, when we were alone, he asked me if his pain could be from acquired immunodeficiency syndrome (AIDS). I asked him why he wanted to know. He said his abdominal pain started after he and a male friend were talking about homosexuality, and then they impulsively decided to give it a try. His pain was not in his body, it was in his mind and spirit. He was feeling scared, guilty, and ashamed.

If this nurse kept to the care plan, she might have responded that abdominal pain is not a symptom of AIDS and switched the subject back to the diagnosis and treatment of appendicitis. She would have missed an incredible opportunity not only to teach and be heard, but to be therapeutic in this moment of vulnerability. It's almost impossible to get an adolescent to listen to teaching about impulsivity, risks, sexuality, and health. However, this young man offered this nurse a window of opportunity, a precious teachable moment.

"If . . . you only remember that in which you are interested, interest becomes a key word in assimilating information and reducing anxiety."
—Wurman, 1989, page 148

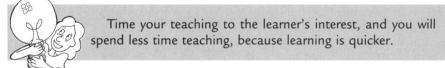

Time your teaching to the learner's interest, and you will spend less time teaching, because learning is quicker.

In the previous example, the doctor was ruling out appendicitis, but the patient was ruling out AIDS. If the learner is focusing on a topic you don't think is important, find out why it is so important to the learner.

To take advantage of teachable moments, we have to be with the learner in the present. Unfortunately, teachable moments may come when we're overwhelmed with tasks. At least initiate teaching during this window of opportunity to enhance engagement of the learner. This will be easiest to do if you have resources handy. Answer the question, and then take a second to grab a handout or video. An environment that supports learning can help you take advantage of teachable moments and save you teaching time.

> *"Delivering information to patients just when they need it is more effective than simply sending them a book when they first join your practice."*
> —Grandinetti, 1996, page 84

Learners are our biggest allies. The purpose of our teaching is to help them learn to take care of themselves. According to Maslow (1982, 1987) people are motivated by needs, which are felt states of deprivation. Maslow defines our needs to be as follows:

- Physiological
- Safety
- Belonging
- Esteem
- Self-actualization

Illness can create needs at each of these levels. People with asthma feel the need for oxygen (*physiological*). People with chronic, degenerative illnesses may feel the need for freedom from fear (*safety*). People with clinical depression may find their behaviors push people away, intensifying their needs for belongingness and love (*belonging*). People with visible deformities or those unable to live independently may feel a need for respect or competence (*esteem*). People who have come to grips with their illnesses on all levels may feel the need to express themselves, despite the obstacles (*self-actualization*).

A patient or family member with a need is motivated to act to satisfy it. Motivation begins with a cognitive and affective state. Feeling out of control creates a need. ("Why is this happening to me?") The first step in regaining control and fulfilling the need is to understand. ("What is happening to me?") This need to understand motivates the learner to learn.

Tripp (1987) explored how mothers of children with apnea learned to care for their infants at home. She says at one point in the mothers' experience, an event occurred that marked a transition from a generalized awareness of the potential infant death to a personalized awareness of the threat. At this point, they were motivated to learn. Learning helped them feel better, calmer, and more in control.

> *"If you master a situation you are in, wherever you stand, all becomes true; you can no longer be driven around by circumstance."*
> —Brandon, 1976, page 12

Always answer the learner's questions. The answer may be specific information or a resource for obtaining the information. If you do not know the answer, find out. Ask a colleague, or use a quick reference, like Mosby's Handbook of Patient Teaching (Canobbio, 1996). Listen to what the learner is really asking. Sometimes your answer may have to be, "Are you asking me to predict the future? I can't do that."

If the learner asks the same question several times, despite the fact that it has been answered, explore what is happening. Ask the learner to answer his or her own question, and offer to fill in the informational gaps. Find out if the learner does not understand the answer or if the learner has difficulty accepting the information.

Do not respond to a learner's question or concern with a verbal or nonverbal indication that it has been answered before or that it is minor, unimportant, or silly. If you do, you are not centering your care on the patient and family. In addition, you could harm the therapeutic relationship. Listen carefully. What is the learner asking?

Assessing, Colombo Style

Television's Lieutenant Colombo artfully used casual conversation to uncover information. His nonthreatening approach relaxed people who were protecting secrets. His informal questions ranged from superficial to probing. He sought to understand their motivations and capacities.

> "You must give permission to enable a patient to discuss unusual or deviant behaviors. Do this in a very specific manner: If you think a patient may be abusing some drug, say, 'Some people take only a tablespoon of milk of magnesia a day, some take 2 or 3 bottles a day. How much do you take?'"
> —Hammerschmidt & Meador, 1993, rule number 27

However, unlike us, Lieutenant Colombo's goal for uncovering details was to catch people in lies. He listened intently. Colombo's relaxed informality made murderers comfortable. They were not afraid of him and ultimately revealed their secrets. Nurses are naturals at making people comfortable.

> "Openness, intimacy and sensitivity . . . seeing deeply and directly into the other person and feeling his needs and wants."
> —Brandon, 1976, page 48

Health care providers could use the same artful conversation techniques to uncover self-care practices, attitudes, and understandings. Careful listening and paying attention to detail could help us understand our learners better so that we can best individualize our teaching, which improves teaching and saves time.

"The assessment considers cultural and religious practices, emotional barriers, desire and motivation to learn, physical and cognitive limitations, language barriers, and the financial implications of care choices."
—JCAHO, 1998, page 106

Constantly search for clues. Look for meaning in the ordinary. Recognize tips. Who is this learner? What does the learner care about? What does this learner want and need to know?

Assess and treat the human response.

Using Conversation

Conversation, the informal verbal interaction between two people, is an efficient and effective teaching tool. As described previously, it is a nonthreatening assessment method. In addition, it helps you engage with the learner and develop a rapport. Conversation is a wonderful way to demonstrate nursing compassion.

"Compassion means giving people room; opening doors rather than closing them; asking questions rather than giving answers. It means becoming sensitively aware of another person's situation and feelings. It means listening with your whole being and giving, if you can, what is relevant and appropriate to the relationship without self-consciously measuring what that is."
—Brandon, 1976, page 49

Our learners are adults and not students, so formal teaching styles are often inappropriate at the bedside, office, or living room. A superior sense of professional know-how can intimidate learners into passivity. It can arouse feelings of inadequacy that interfere with learning and make teaching and intended behavior changes take even longer.

"The aura of know-how in the helper can undermine our confidence as the helped in defining issues for ourselves. We're a little unsure of the ground, don't know the technical language, generally uncomfortable. It must be our fault. Best we lie back and take what's given agreeably . . . and end up feeling still more helpless."
—Dass & Gorman, 1985, page 130

Nurses know how to use conversation therapeutically. We treat human responses and intervene on the levels of body, mind, and spirit. We partner with patients and families in the present. We cherish those moments of connecting, of true conversation. In these conversations, we provide much more than emotional support. We assess readiness and need. We role model. We clarify. We teach.

> *"If 'people don't like to be should upon, they'd rather discover than being told,' then our invitation will probably be most effective when it communicates trust and respect. And honesty as well: We have to stay conscious of the ways in which our own lives still lack integrity and consistency. We're strongest when we act from what we have in common. We usually have to listen for that before we can really begin to act. Even the slightest bit of self-righteousness can get in the way."*
> —Dass & Gorman, 1985, pages 160–161

For example, let's say your patient is going home with a cast. One approach is to jump in and start a lecture on cast care. Another, the conversational method, means you discuss it.

Start with, *"Did you know you'll be going home with a cast?"*

Then find out what the learner knows: *"Have you or anyone in your family ever had a cast before?" "What kind of a cast was it?" "Tell me how you took care of that cast."*

Then clarify learning needs: *"Do you know what your leg will look like when the cast comes off?" "What bothers you about having a cast?" "What worries you about having a cast?"*

Each question helps you individualize your teaching to the needs of the learner. You can inject bits of information, as appropriate, and teach within the conversation.

In addition, listening helps you assess learning needs. You understand the influences of cultural and religious practices, emotional barriers, desire and motivation to learn, physical and cognitive limitations, language barriers, and the financial implications of care choices. Within this context, you take advantage of teachable moments.

Remember, adults already know quite a bit. The information you supply supplements their knowledge. Even if the patient has a rare diagnosis, some aspects of the symptoms or treatments are familiar.

 To facilitate learning, lead the conversation from the familiar to the new.

> *"New ideas are not so much discovered as uncovered by moving from what you already understand into the realm of what you would like to understand. Sometimes simply by reorganizing the information you possess, by using and comparing what you already know, you can uncover other information."*
> —Wurman, 1989, page 187

Do this through conversation. For example, a learner may express concerns about taking a pain medication because it is a narcotic. Explore what the learner knows about narcotics, feels about addiction, and experiences with the pain. Within this context, correct misperceptions and reframe the issue in quality-of-life terms. This reorganizes current knowledge and can help move the learner to a new understanding.

"You only understand information relative to what you already understand."
—Wurman, 1989, page 173

A two-way conversation is much more effective at changing health attitudes and behaviors than a lecture. Questions and conflicts arise when you hear new information out of the context of already known information. This makes it difficult to understand and accept the new information. This could result in wasted teaching time because even if the new information was heard, it may not be accepted and applied.

For example, notice how this book contains examples, not only from nursing practice, but also from popular culture. The references to movies, television programs, magazines, and a Broadway musical are intentional. They are meant to help you connect what you know to the contents of this book.

"Failing to make connections between the known and the unknown prevents us from grasping new ideas and new opportunities."
—Wurman, 1989, page 172

Because the goals of patient and family education are to promote healthful changes in attitudes and behaviors, simply relaying information is not enough. Quality teaching partners with the learner to enhance informed decision making. Conversation can also be used to present options, or questions, to help the learner explore possibilities.

"Part of the role of the helper is to bring people to an awareness that there are choices to be made at all."
—Brandon, 1976, page 108

Conversation is used in patient and family education to engage the learner and facilitate assessment and teaching through an informal, two-way relationship. This makes both teaching and learning pleasant activities. Baltasar Gracian gave this advice to learners:

"Make your friends your teachers and mingle the pleasures of conversation with the advantages of instruction."
—Wurman, 1989, page 155

Paying Attention

> When I was a new grad, I was amazed that one of my experienced colleagues could tell a patient who just had her appendix out the course of recovery: how to treat the incision site, how the diet and activity will advance, and how the pain diminishes, day by day. I never learned any of that in nursing school! Years later I realized she learned that on the job. I, too, could see patterns in certain admitting diagnoses.

The more experienced you are as a nurse, the more you will learn and the more answers you will have. Just by observing the course of many patients with the same treatments, you will learn about the interventions and the human response to them. Next time, you will have more answers.

"Living in the here and now . . . means concentrating more fully on tasks as they are being done rather than longing for them to be over. Normally we live our lives sandwiched in time between important events. The decision as to what is important and exciting is ours. Most of our living goes by almost without noticing."

—Brandon, 1976, page 98

Pay attention. Look for patterns. Look for the unusual. Increased awareness will help you identify teachable moments, learn how to individualize teaching, and help you evaluate understanding accurately. It will also help you teach better next time.

Listening

Do you listen in a hurry? Do you know your answer before the learner is done asking the question? Do you keep things moving, interrupt, or blurt out your response? Are there some topics you don't want to discuss? Are there some people you just don't want to listen to because they bother or annoy you?

"So we jump between listening and judging. But in our zeal to help, we may increase the distance between the person and our own consciousness. We find ourselves primarily in our own thoughts, but not with another person. Not only are we listening less, but the concepts our mind is coming up with start to act as a screen that preselects information. One thought rules out another. One of the results of all this mental activity is that there's less room to meet, less room for a new truth to emerge, less room to let things simply be revealed in 'their own good time.' The mind tries to do too many things at once. It's difficult to know which mental vectors are useful and which are distractions, static on the line, bad connections."

—Dass & Gorman, 1985, page 99

When you listen, who has the loudest voice, the speaker or the voice in your head? Do you listen in a hurry?

If you want to save teaching time, listen to your learners. They tell you what you need to know. They tell you about their abilities, skills, social and physical resources, lifestyle, beliefs, culture, and spiritual views.

They tell you what they feel is important: what bothers them, what worries them, and what they need to know. Listen, and they will tell you what and how to teach them most effectively. At the same time, you will strengthen therapeutic bonds and build partnering relationships.

"The more deeply we listen, the more we attune ourselves to the roots of suffering and the means to help alleviate it. It is through listening that wisdom, skill, and opportunity find form in an act that truly helps. But more than all these, the very act of listening can dissolve distance between us and others as well."

—Dass & Gorman, 1985, page 112

How do you learn to listen deeply? See Box 5-2 on page 91. What do you listen for? You want to assess learning needs and obtain information that will help you individualize teaching so it will be most effective. You want to listen for the learner's story. Information about who the learner is and how this medical event fits into the context of the learner's life will also help you individualize teaching. The more relevant your teaching, the more efficiently and effectively you can teach. This, again, saves teaching time. For specifics on what to listen for, see Box 5-3 on page 92.

How to Listen Well

"All we have to do is listen—really listen."
—Dass & Gorman, 1985, page 69

The less you know about your learner, the more likely you will teach inappropriate or already known information. You can avoid wasting teaching time by listening more. The better you understand your learner, the more individualized, targeted, and streamlined your teaching can be.

- Want to listen.
- Tune out distractions.
- Listen to the whole message. Don't interrupt the speaker.
- Listen actively. Listen to learn. Hear what is being said and think about it.
- Don't just show interest, be interested.
- Listen on many levels. Listen to what the speaker is telling you and what the speaker is communicating about himself or herself.
- Acknowledge your feelings, but tune them out. If what the speaker says arouses your emotions (such as making you upset or excited), don't focus on your reaction. You will not be able to listen.
- Listen for meaning. Listen to what isn't being said, too.
- Listen for feelings.
- If you refer to a feeling a speaker defined, such as "scared," use the same word the speaker used to describe it.
- Read nonverbal messages, such as body position, expression, tone, and breathing.
- Remember important points the speaker is making.
- Repeat important points to the speaker to confirm you understand the intended meaning.
- Nod your head. Lean forward a bit. Show you're attentive.
- When appropriate, cue for details. Say, "Go on," "Tell me more," or "And then what happened?"
- If you want specific information, ask a close-ended question, such as, "Which daughter are you talking about?" or "Did you have the x-ray?"
- Repeat the essential details to confirm that you understand. An example would be, "You felt the pain in your chest but thought it wasn't serious?"
- If you get confused or aren't sure of the intended meaning, paraphrase the learner's statements. Listen and repeat what you think was meant. Avoid the stereotypical format of, "What I hear you say is (repeat the exact words)." Instead, say, "Sounds like you're feeling . . ."

Box 5-2 *(Continued)*

- If appropriate, make physical contact, either in the context of a task or within the conversation. Touch an arm or shoulder. It communicates a sense of connection.

"A university study found that when students asked for information in a library, they were able to retain the information longer when the librarians made physical contact with them by lightly touching their arms while answering the student's questions."

—Wurman, 1989, page 321

- Silence is OK. It helps you or the learner collect thoughts or emotions, review what was said, or decide what to talk about next.
- Speakers repeat themselves when they feel they were not heard. If this happens, clarify that you heard and understand the message so the learner can move on.
- Don't give advice. Give information. Information helps learners make informed decisions. Advice is not helpful. If your advice works, you encourage dependency instead of independence. If your advice doesn't work, you lose trust.

BOX 5-3   Patient and Family Education Assessment Guide

I. Physiological data
   A. Chief complaint
   B. History of present illness or problem
   C. Review of systems
   D. Functional, cognitive, and sensory abilities (anxiety, ability to concentrate)
II. Family profile: a word picture of the family
   A. Household composition
   B. Gender and age of members
   C. Occupations of family members
   D. Health status of family members; physical limitations
   E. Genogram: a diagram showing family relationships
III. Resources available to the family
   A. Ability to provide for physical needs
      1. Home: space, comfort, safety
      2. Income: sufficient for basic needs and important extras?
      3. Overall ability to perform self-care
      4. Health insurance: available to the family?

Box 5-3 *(Continued)*

   B. Neighborhood/community resources: friends, neighbors, church, and community organizations helpful and involved?
      1. Kinds of support provided?
IV. Family education, lifestyle, and beliefs
   A. Educational backgrounds and attitudes toward education
      1. Do all adult family members have basic reading and writing abilities? Check ability to read aloud from patient education material.
      2. To what extent is education, formal or informal, valued? How much education does each family member have?
      3. Are there language barriers to verbal communication among the patient, family members, community, and medical personnel?
   B. Lifestyle and cultural background
      1. Does the family subscribe to folk medicine beliefs?
      2. Is there a conflict between cultural and lifestyle approach and the health professional's teaching?
      3. What are the normal diet patterns of the family?
      4. What are the family's sleep habits?
      5. What are the activities, exercises, occupations, and hobbies of family members?
   C. Learning abilities of family members
      1. Do they assimilate information easily?
      2. Are they able to apply what is taught?
   D. The family's self-concept
      1. Are family members lacking in self-esteem?
      2. Do they have feelings of powerlessness as a result of either life situation or patient's sick role?
V. Adequacy of family functioning
   A. Ability to be sensitive to the needs of the family members
      1. How is the identified patient perceived?
      2. What are the relationships of other family members to the identified patient and each other?
   B. Ability to communicate effectively with each other
   C. Ability to provide support, security, and encouragement, especially pertaining to the learning environment
   D. Ability for self-help and acceptance of help from others when needed
      1. How open is the family to the health professional's teaching?
      2. How likely are family members to request help in the future, if needed?
   E. Ability to perform roles flexibly
   F. Ability to make effective decisions

Box 5-3 *(Continued)*

   G. Ability of the family to readjust ideas about family status, goals, and relationships
   H. Ability of the family to handle crisis situations
      1. Has the family been confronted with chronic illness in the past?
      2. How has the family reacted to situations such as accidental injury or death? Who helped them through it?
 VI. Family understanding of the present event
   A. Current knowledge about the problem: eight questions
      1. What do you think has caused your problem?
      2. Why do you think it happened when it did?
      3. What do you think your illness does to you? How does it work?
      4. How severe is your illness? Will it have a short course?
      5. What kind of treatment do you think you should receive?
      6. What are the most important results you hope to receive from this treatment?
      7. What are the chief problems your illness has caused for you?
      8. What do you fear most about your illness?
   B. Point in the life cycle of the family at which the problem occurred
   C. Type of onset of the illness or problem: gradual or sudden
   D. Prognosis for survival or prognosis for restorative training
   E. Nature and degree of limitations imposed on the patient's functioning
   F. Level of the family's confidence in the health system with which they affiliate
VII. The identified patient, health problem, and educational needs
   A. The patient's educational and cultural background, especially if different from the family's
   B. The patient's self-concept and reaction to stress
   C. Physical limitations that are barriers to learning or self-care
   D. Information base of the patient
      1. Does he or she understand the health team management and the health team's advice?
      2. Does he or she know others with the same problem and have knowledge of their treatment?
      3. What is his or her position and his or her role in the family?
      4. Has he or she had past illnesses?
      5. What kind of physiological feedback is he or she using?
   E. Are the patient and family members willing to negotiate goals with the health care team?
   F. Are the patient's perceptions and expectations congruent with those of family members?

(From Rankin, S. H., & Stallings, K. D. [1996]. *Patient education: Issues, principles, practices* [3rd ed.]. Philadelphia: Lippincott-Raven.)

Noticing Teachable Moments and Using Them

Teachable moments offer the best teaching opportunities. Readiness to learn is optimized during teachable moments. If you use them, you will get more teaching done in less time.

The following are teachable moments:

- When the learner asks a question
- When the learner makes a provocative statement, such as, "This always happens to me."
- When you are giving a medication. Describe what it is and why it is given.
- When you are giving a treatment. Describe what it is and why it is given.
- When you are performing a procedure. Talk through what you do so the learner understands your thought processes.
- When the learner asks for specific foods. Discuss nutrition.
- When you and the learner see something on television that relates to the learner's situation. Use it to initiate a conversation.
- When others demonstrate appropriate behaviors. Point these out, such as a physician washing his or her hands before examining the patient.
- When the learner demonstrates knowledge that has been acquired informally. Affirm accuracy of information and appropriateness of application.
- When the learner expresses misinformation or lack of information. Teach the correct information.
- When the learner expresses a need for change. Offer information that can support that process.
- When the learner performs a self-care behavior. If the job was done well, say so. If safety is jeopardized, state your observation, and teach how to perform the behaviors correctly.
- When the learner discusses lack of supports. Mention available community resources.

Perhaps you have noticed that nearly every interaction with a learner can offer a teachable moment. Use the general goals of patient and family education and the goals you established in partnership with the learner to decide on which teachable moments to act. Prioritize your teaching.

Creating Teachable Moments

Sometimes you have to prime the learner for teaching. Sometimes patients and family members don't ask questions because the challenges are too new and too big to comprehend. They don't know what they don't know or need to know. The stress of diagnosis or illness can make it difficult to think ahead, to formulate questions. In these cases, you have to create teachable moments by giving enough information to help learners discover what they don't know.

"Teaching involves creating conditions where learning can occur."
—Redman, 1993, page 197

Sometimes you will not get an opening for a bit of information that is essential to convey. For example, your learner may not be internally motivated to find out if a certain medication has side effects, yet that learner may need to learn the potentially dangerous side effects of a medication and how to respond. Your job, as facilitator of education, is to set the stage for learning.

"The emergency department visit may provide a teachable moment in which to communicate the message of appropriate passenger restraint use. During the ED visit and at the time of discharge we can teach and instruct at a time when our patients and their caregivers may be particularly likely to pay attention. This heightened attention may result from the circumstances that prompted the ED visit (e.g., motor vehicle injury) or because the ED provides a dramatic milieu in which to deliver messages related to injury prevention."
—Todd, 1996, page 242

First, identify what information the learner needs to know to meet the goals of patient and family education. See Box 5-4 on page 97 for tips on identifying essential information to convey.

What skills or competencies will your learner need to reach the goals? Broadly define skills and competencies; they occur in the realms of body, mind, and spirit. What challenges will your learner face?

What resources will be necessary to achieve the goals? Resources include facilitators, time, information, and learner ability.

What are your learner's opportunities for learning? Does the learner believe he or she can meet the goals? Does the learner feel he or she needs permission to act? Can he or she practice and perform the skills?

You can also use the environment to create teachable moments. Tools in the setting can stimulate learner involvement. For example, they can be inexpensive and "low-tech":

BOX 5-4   What Do I Teach?

What do you teach? How do you know the difference between information that's nice to know versus information that the learner needs to know? Go back to the general goals of patient and family education, mutually agreed upon by the learner and health care team:

- Make informed decisions.
- Develop basic self-care skills to survive.
- Recognize problems and know what to do in response.
- Get questions answered; find resources for answers.

These goals will help you **identify the content** that the learner needs to know.

- What decisions will the learner have to make? Are there any tests, procedures, or surgeries scheduled? Will any consent forms need to be signed? Ask the learner what he or she knows about these procedures. Prepare the learner to make informed decisions.
- What self-care skills will the learner need to survive? What has changed? What is new? Will the learner need to perform any procedures or operate any equipment? Will the learner need to take or give any medications, modify diet, or modify activity? What could make it hard for the learner to implement the plan? For example, does the learner lack electricity or running water, money to buy medications or supplies, or ability to travel? What feelings might the learner expect to experience? Ask the learner to talk through each step of implementing the plan. Listen for misunderstandings and potential barriers to implementation. Teach as needed.
- Identify problems that could occur, such as side effects or complications. What psychosocial responses would be a concern and need follow-up? An example would be signs and symptoms of depression. Ask the learner if _____ would be a concern. If so, why? What should the learner do in response? Prepare the learner to recognize potential problems and know how to respond. When should the learner call the doctor or an ambulance? Provide a list of resources for the learner.
- Identify the learner's concerns. What does the learner want to know to feel safe and comfortable at discharge? Individualize the content of what you teach to the learner's needs.

Don't Unnecessarily Repeat Information
Check what others on the health care team have documented about the education they provided. Evaluate understanding of previously taught information, and pick up from there.

Box 5-4 (*Continued*)

Evaluate Knowledge

Pick one subject, and ask what the learner already knows about it. "Tell me what you know about . . ." or, "You need to be able to care for this incision at home. I don't want to bore you with things you already know. How would you know if it was infected?"

Teach and Document

Correct misperceptions and misunderstandings immediately. Fill in details for the learner, as necessary.

Remember, the most effective way to prepare a learner for a procedure is to describe the sensory experiences rather than the technical details. Then, as the learner goes through the experience, he or she will watch for the signs and be reassured that all is well, going according to plan. For example, tell the learner a blood pressure cuff, when pumped up, feels tight around the arm for a short time. The stethoscope may feel cool in the bend of the arm. There will be a slight hissing sound as the pressure is released, and the pulse may be felt in the arm. Use objective, nonevaluative terms to describe the sensations, like pressure and pinch instead of pain.

If you don't know how to use equipment the learner is going home with or don't know the answers to your learner's questions, who would know? Ask other members of the health care team. Use your resources. Document your assessment of the learner's readiness and ability to learn and your evaluation of the learner's understanding of essential information. Note areas that need reinforcement and further evaluation.

"While the patient sits in the waiting room, he (or she) notices on the wall the colorful, attractive . . . waiting room poster, which states 'We Put Prevention into Practice, Please Ask Us for Details.' This develops a prevention 'mind-set' and alerts the patient that he will hear about prevention during each visit. Probably he is being seen for an acute illness, but it is important to take advantage of every patient encounter and 'teachable moment' for prevention."

—"Put prevention," 1994, On-line

In the case of computer-assisted learning, you can stimulate learner involvement in ways that are more expensive and more technical:

"Technology assists learning by providing additional motivation and rewards at the 'teachable moment.' Technology helps shift the responsibility for learning, so that it is more evenly balanced between the teacher and student. It allows students to become more self-directed; it breaks down barriers between the teacher and learner."

—"A dialogue," 1996, On-line

Precaution About Using Teachable Moments

A neighbor called me Saturday afternoon. Her husband was discharged from the hospital late that morning. Some of his meds were changed. At discharge, no one explained why the changes were made or what meds he got that day and which were due when. And she just realized she didn't know what she needs to give him. I told her to call the floor and ask to speak to the nurse who discharged him.

This learner did not get all the information she needed to carry out the treatment plan at home.

Teachable moments are wonderful opportunities, but if you use them exclusively, you risk incomplete teaching.

How do you plan ahead when you don't know how the treatment plan will change and what the learner needs to know? See Box 5-5 on page 100 for details.

BOX 5-5   How Can I Start Discharge Teaching From Admission?

"How can I start discharge teaching from admission? My patient is acutely ill. With these short stays, I don't know what my patient has, let alone what meds or equipment he will go home with . . ."

—An RN

From the first day of nursing school you heard, "Discharge teaching starts at admission," but what does that mean? If you don't know what the patient has or what medications he or she will be on or what equipment he or she will need, what do you teach? What can you teach?

There's more to discharge teaching than meets the eye. Here are some tips on how to do discharge teaching throughout the admission. These work even if the patient is admitted to the intensive care unit!

1. Start the first step of teaching: assessment.
   - Find out what the learner knows about the symptoms, possible diagnoses, tests, and treatments.
   - Complete the history form to get the story of the patient's living conditions, lifestyle, environment, and potential challenges at discharge.
   - Identify the learner's concerns. What bothers or worries the learner? What does the learner want to know?

2. You don't know the future, so focus on the present.
   - What you do in the hospital will relate to what the learner will do at home. Teach about the assessments you are making and for what you are looking. Teach about the tests and procedures, medications you give, and equipment used. This will prepare the learner. It will not only keep the learner informed, but help the learner understand what the problem is, which will provide a context for home care he or she will give.
   - As the condition changes and physician's orders change, teach. Why was that medication changed? Why are they doing this test now? Why is that procedure performed?
   - Refer the learner to relevant resources, both in the hospital and within the community.
   - Most teaching you do will be in casual discussions, but don't let the informality fool you. The information you share is still important enough to document.
   - Make sure your teaching is a two-way conversation. Find out what the learner knows and wants to know. Things you are saying may not make sense because the learner is making certain assumptions. Something obvious to you may not be so clear to a learner.

Box 5-5 *(Continued)*

3. As you learn more about the diagnosis and prognosis, anticipate learning needs. As discharge comes closer, think about how learners might need to be prepared. What has changed for the learner?
    - Teach as you do care. Teach the learner how to do assessments, like taking a temperature or identifying respiratory distress. Explain the medications you are giving. Explain the steps in the dressing change.
    - Evaluate learning. Ask the learner to tell you the purpose for that medication or what comes next in the dressing change. Document learning that has occurred so other members of the health care team can build on your teaching.
        —The more patients you work with, the more you see patterns in discharge plans. The more experienced you become, the easier it is to anticipate discharge teaching needs. In time, you may even learn to anticipate the discharge orders of certain physicians.
        —If you don't know the specific discharge orders yet, teach from general to specific.
    - You may expect dressings will be changed at home but not know which dressings will be ordered. Therefore, teach about the purpose of dressing changes and clean or sterile technique.
    - Not every person with asthma goes home on the same medications, but you can teach about the roles of different types of asthma medications.
    - As discharge comes closer, anticipate how nursing care might relate to home care.
        —Reinforce the importance of follow-up care and involvement in the care plan for home. Teach which signs and symptoms need to be reported to the doctor. For example, how to tell if there could be an infection.

4. Communicate with other health care team members.
    - Ask the physician who will write the discharge orders what he or she anticipates will be ordered so you can teach more specifically. Tell the physician you want to know so you can teach early, reinforce it, and evaluate learning.
    - Document what the learner knows and wants to know. Read documentation about the teaching done by your colleagues, and build on it. Evaluate learning before teaching more. Continue this throughout hospitalization.

Box 5-5 *(Continued)*

Discharge teaching is more than a list of medications, equipment, and follow-up appointments! The discharge teaching you begin at admission involves getting to know the abilities and needs of the patient and family so your teaching can be relevant and individualized. It involves familiarizing the learner with symptoms, assessments, tests, procedures, and treatments throughout the hospitalization so informed decisions can be made. It involves listening to the learner's concerns and helping the learner understand what is happening.

This may not seem like preparing for discharge, especially when you work with acutely ill patients, but it provides a context and prepares the learner for home care. It gives the learner an understanding of the connection between illness and treatment, symptom, and response. This background also helps with problem solving. If an odd situation comes up at home, the learner may understand enough of why things are done to be able to think through a solution.

Begin discharge teaching at admission, and the teaching done at the hour of discharge will merely be a review, supplemented by some details provided in the discharge orders.

If you collaborate with your colleagues on the health care team to do discharge teaching throughout each admission, you'll find more discharges will be a breeze instead of a hurricane.

Check for completeness by evaluating learning. For example, if this nurse asked, after teaching, "When will you give him meds next, and what will they be?" he or she would have discovered the omission.

When you teach in the teachable moment, you are cutting out the planning stage, which includes your research. If you teach what you know spontaneously, make sure what you know is complete and accurate. If you don't know the answer or if you have any doubt about your facts, say you're not sure, and find a book or a team member who does know. Learn the answer and follow up.

When Not to Teach

If you get any resistance to teaching, stop and reassess the situation. Again, by taking advantage of teachable moments and not planning teaching, you may inadvertently skip an essential assessment step.

Sometimes you encounter what looks like an unwillingness to learn. This is frustrating because your job is to teach! Fortunately, returning to conversation and listening skills can help resolve this challenge. For details, see Box 5-6 on page 103.

BOX 5-6

How Do You Teach Someone Who's Unwilling to Learn?

If you try to teach someone, and find he or she is unwilling to learn, stop what you are doing. Resistance is a red flag. Resistance says you have skipped a step in the teaching process. Have you assessed the following?

- The learner's need for information
- The learner's readiness to learn
- The learner's ability to learn
- Barriers, such as the learner's beliefs

Have you partnered with the learner to set short-term goals for teaching, including information to help him or her in the following ways?

- Make informed decisions
- Develop basic self-care skills to survive
- Recognize problems and know what to do in response
- Get questions answered, and find resources for answers

Have you checked your assumptions?

- Will someone else provide care? Perhaps you are trying to teach the wrong person. Even if the patient is a competent, functional adult, the spouse may provide the care. If the patient is a child, mom and dad may visit in the hospital, but grandma, who is home with the other children, may be the primary caregiver.
- What does the learner know and do already? Does the learner need to know what you are trying to teach? Are you offering new information? Perhaps you are teaching information that conflicts with the learner's current understanding and practices.

What does the learner know? What are the learner's concerns? Seek to understand, then to be understood. Teach in conversation, not a formal lecture.

Discuss situations the learner may experience at home, and ask how he or she would problem solve. For example, ask how the learner would recognize an infection. Teach from the answer. Confirm correct signs listed, and add signs the learner missed. When discussing fever, ask if the learner has a thermometer and have the learner show you how he or she reads it. Ask when the learner would call the doctor.

Why would a patient or family be unwilling to learn?

- They may feel intimidated, insulted, belittled, or afraid you will find out they are uneducated, illiterate, or have no electricity. These barriers can be overcome by forming an alliance with them before you start to teach.

Box 5-6 *(Continued)*

- They may feel the information you are offering is irrelevant, impractical, incorrect (not in agreement with their beliefs), or impossible (they do not have the resources to follow through with your expectations). They may feel powerless or incapable. These barriers can be avoided if, in your assessment, you determine how best to individualize teaching.

Obviously, assessments and alliances take time. These are done not at the moment of teaching, but during every encounter with the patient and family.

Document your findings to share them with other members of the health care team. If necessary, call a patient care conference to collaborate. If team members partner with the patient and family, unwillingness to learn may never be an issue.

If you sense resistance, step back and return to focus, not on your own frustrations, but on the needs of the learner, the needs of the patient.

"So we are called upon to take what is valuable from our training, but not let it constrict the helping relationship itself. We need to enlist the service of the intellect, but not let it block the intuitive compassion of the heart. Not easy, this task. For the temptation to identify ourselves as What We Know is especially formidable when it comes to helping."
—Dass & Gorman, 1985, page 130

Adapt Your Teaching to the Individual Learner

Patient and family education is not just teaching. Sometimes giving information is not the most direct way to increase a learner's awareness to lead to a change in behaviors and a good outcome.

Listen to your learners. How do they make decisions? How do they decide what to do?

Not everyone buys major appliances or cars based on the hard data of Consumer Reports magazine. Even though this magazine identifies the best buy, some people will spend money on the more expensive, less effective model just because it feels good.

Sometimes people make choices by their feelings, not by objective information. When we see this, our teaching strategy needs to accommodate it.

If we don't adapt our strategy, we will waste teaching time. We will spend time giving information that will not be appreciated. Our information will not be applied because we did not listen and did not present information in a way that makes it relevant to the learner.

"A patient's resistance to receiving therapy needs to be respected, listened to, and dealt with."
—Hammerschmidt & Meador, 1993, rule number 44

Don't teach until you understand who you are teaching. Listen to the learner to identify the most efficient and effective way to teach. Steamrolling in with facts against feelings of resistance does not change health behaviors. It hurts the partnership and impairs long-term therapeutic potential. It prevents us from meeting the goals of patient and family education.

This listening takes time, but preserving the relationship and individualizing the teaching will save you time. It is efficient teaching. It takes more time if you steamroll in, damage relationships, repair relationships, than it takes to individualize the teaching. Besides, it will not only take more time, it may not work or may not work as well. The quality of care is best when you listen first and adapt your teaching from the beginning.

How do you know if you're steamrolling? Listen to yourself. Are you feeling the learner is wrong and you are right? Are you arguing with the learner? If so, stop speaking. Ask the learner questions about his or her point of view and understanding of the situation. Do you and the learner share teaching goals? If so, will the learner's choices work toward meeting those goals? If you don't share goals, why are you not accepting the learner's goals? Is your teaching coming out of your feelings and not objective information?

Explore, observe, and understand. You will then have time to teach and teach well.

"But perhaps there will be nothing we can do. Then we can only be, and be with the person in his or her pain, attending to the quality of our own consciousness. . . Hearts that have known pain meet in mutual recognition and trust. Such a meeting helps immeasurably."
—Dass & Gorman, 1985, page 88

Sometimes it is not the right time to teach. Respect your learner's right to refuse teaching, whether temporary (to get much needed sleep) or not (emotionally unable to perform certain tasks). Maintain an atmosphere of respect, open communication, and access to information, and promote self-care at the highest level possible at that time.

Sometimes, a damaged relationship between you and the learner may mean you need to step aside and let someone else on the health care team teach. Learn to recognize these times and respond appropriately.

"Manipulation hinders the authentic growth of both. My experience as helper, but more poignantly as one who has been helped, gives me a great confidence in the community's own ability for caring. Love is all around. Helpers are in a real sense, people who sell water by the river. Compassion flows all around them although we find it difficult to channel and irrigate it."

—Brandon, 1976, pages 108–109

Example of a Teachable Moment

This book intends to catch you in a teachable moment.

As I speak to nurses around the country about patient and family education, the issue that consistently comes up is that nurses have no time to teach. If you bought this book, you are ready to learn, willing to change, and able to act.

"Without prior knowledge, without training, you can find your way through information by making it personal, by deciding what you want to gain from it, by getting comfortable with your ignorance."

—Wurman, 1989, page 165

You don't have to read the whole book straight through. You could if you want, but you don't have to. You're busy and may not have time to read a book straight through. So instead, jump around. Check the index. Look for the information you need right now. Keep the book handy, and come back when you're ready for more.

This book is not meant to be passively read. It's meant to get you actively involved in the process of improving your teaching skills. When you read this book and find information you need, apply it right away. Think about how it worked and how you can make it work better. If you own this book, take notes in it, in ink, not pencil.

This way it won't just provide short-term cognitive stimulation, which is only forgotten tomorrow. This book becomes a tool for thinking, for changing behaviors, for improving the quality of the care you give.

If you want to learn more:

(1994). Put prevention into practice (PPIP). *Journal of the Academy of Nurse Practitioners.* (On-line). http://www.hhs.gov/PPIP/man9.html

(1996). A dialogue on the impact of technology on learning. *Maricopa Center for Learning and Instruction* (On-line). http://hakatai.mcli.dist.maricopa.edu/ocotillo/itl/impact.html.

(1997). Collaborative care requires new approaches, says internist. *Mental Health Weekly, 7*(44), 4.

(1998). Patient education only as good as staff teaching. *Patient Education Management, 5*(1), 8–10.

Brandon, D. (1976). *Zen in the art of helping.* New York: Arkana of Viking Penguin.

Brookfield, S.D. (1986). *Understanding and facilitating adult learning: A comprehensive analysis of principles and effective practices.* San Francisco: Jossey-Bass.

Canobbio, M.M. (1996). *Mosby's handbook of patient teaching.* St. Louis: Mosby-Year Book.

Cunningham, D. (1993). Improving your teaching skills. *Nursing93, December,* 24J.

Grandinetti, D. (1996). Teaching patients to take care of themselves. *Medical Economics, 73*(22), 83–91.

Hammerschmidt, R., & Meador, C.K. (1993). *A little book of nurses' rules.* Philadelphia: Hanley & Belfus.

Joint Commission on Accreditation of Health Care Organizations (JCAHO) (1998). 1998 Hospital Accreditation Standards.

Maslow, A.H. (1982). *Toward a psychology of being* (2nd ed.). New York: Van Nostrand Reinhold.

Maslow, A.H. (1987). *Motivation and personality* (3rd ed.). New York: Harper and Row.

O'Conner, F.M. (1988). Patient education only as good as staff teaching. *Patient Education Management, 5*(1), 8–10.

Scobey, S. (1994). *Focused listening skills: How to sharpen your concentration and hear more of what people are saying.* (Cassette recording). Boulder, CO: CareerTrack Publications.

Stamler, L.L. (1996). Toward a framework for patient education: An analysis of enablement. *Journal of Holistic Nursing, 14*(4), 332.

Todd, K.H. (1996). Air bags and the teachable moment. *Annals of Emergency Medicine, 28,* 241–242.

Tripp, K.R. (1987). *Perspectives on adult learning: Maternal coping with a monitored child in the home.* Unpublished doctoral dissertation, Arizona State University.

Wurman, R.S. (1989). *Information anxiety: What to do when information doesn't tell you what you need to know.* New York: Bantam Books.

Never a Dull Moment

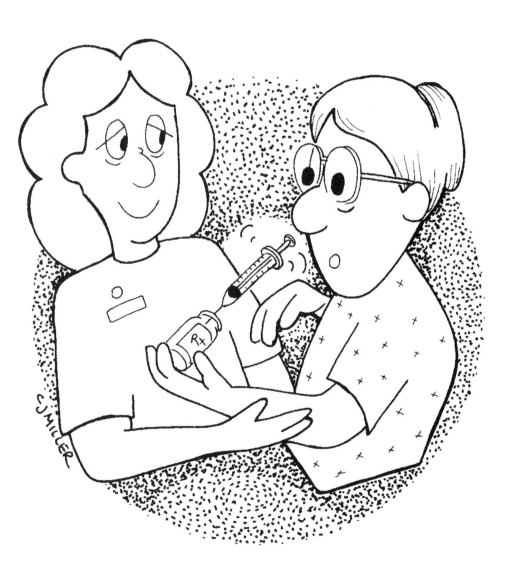

L earning can be seen as the acquisition of information, but before it can take place, there must be interest; interest permeates all endeavors and precedes learning. In order to acquire and remember new knowledge, it must stimulate your curiosity in some way."

—Wurman, 1989, page 14

Did you ever nod off to sleep in a lecture hall? Would you agree that dullness does not promote learning?

Think about your favorite learning experience. Was it dull? It probably wasn't. Most people's favorites were classes like nursing clinicals, biology lab, art, or physical education. They enjoyed stimulating classes that actively involved them, either with cognitive challenges or physical activity.

The Secret: Active Involvement

Lectures may seem like a direct and efficient way to teach. However, patients and family members are not in a student state of mind. They are sick, at risk for getting sick, or giving care to the sick. They are often worried, frightened, or in pain. They are dwelling on their feelings or problems, not attending to your lecture. How do you get and keep their attention?

Get Them Involved

"Make instructions interactive—i.e., the patient must do, write, say, or show something in response to the instruction. This greatly increases interest in and recall of information, and should be a standard feature in the design of nearly all instructions. Medical science has shown that interaction causes a protein change in the brain that stimulates information retention for long-term memory."

—Doak, Doak, & Root, 1996, page 24

Learning, obviously, involves the brain. The biochemistry of the brain proteins change during learning. When people actively interact with information during the learning process, the chemical change that takes place enhances learning and memory. Therefore, actively involving your learners shortens teaching time.

Even the Joint Commission on the Accreditation of Healthcare Organizations (JCAHO) thinks you shouldn't give patients dull lectures:

"Interactive patient education is an integral part of patient care."
—JCAHO, 1998, page 110

The JCAHO goes even further, saying *you* also need to be part of the process:

"An 'interactive' education process is one in which hospital staff, while imparting information to patients and families, continuously elicits feedback to ensure that the information is understood, and that it is appropriate, useful and usable in practical terms."
—JCAHO, 1998, page 110

Lecture may seem straightforward, but it wastes teaching time. Lecturers keep talking, even if the content is inappropriate, misunderstood, rejected, or ignored by listeners.

When you teach interactively, you continuously observe and evaluate the learner's responses. This helps you constantly individualize teaching to the learner's needs. In the long run, this saves teaching time.

For example, one patient was repeatedly admitted for a problem related to impaired self-care.

The adolescent with spina bifida kept getting readmitted with serious infections from skin breakdown on her legs. Each time she was discharged, we taught her and her mother about the need to change position and how to watch for skin breakdowns and respond. But we'd send her home, and she'd come back with new sores. Finally, we asked her what caused the skin breakdown.

She told us. The pathways in her home were too narrow for her wheelchair, so she got around by dragging herself across the floor!

Interaction shortened teaching time by directing the nurse to the right subject. The adolescent knew how to take care of her skin. She didn't know how to get around the house without hurting her skin. A home visit and a new wheelchair solved the problem. There were no more readmissions.

Keep it Brief

Another way to prevent dullness is to avoid long teaching sessions. (This, of course, is not hard, because it's difficult to find time to schedule long teaching sessions.) Teach in brief, informal interactions. Teach the smallest amount necessary to do the job. This is often referred to as "need to know" information instead of "nice to know."

Space out instruction and review. The rest periods help the learner think about and get used to the new information.

> "Two half-hour sessions are more desirable than one hour-long session. Shorter sessions also allow the patient an opportunity to integrate new information and formulate questions for the next teaching session."
> —Rankin & Stallings, 1996, page 317

Make Connections

> "In teaching or communicating anything, we have no choice but to make connections between a new idea and that which is already known."
> —Wurman, 1989, page 172

People learn faster when new information builds on old. When new information fits, it makes sense and connects. When it doesn't fit, it may be rejected.

We learn not just with our brains, but with our whole bodies. When we learn, not only do thoughts connect (cognitive), but muscles (kinesthetic) and feelings (affective) connect and learn new ways to respond.

The more pathways new information makes into the brain, the more connections and associations it makes. The more associations it makes, the more ways the information can be recalled.

For example, did you ever hear an old song and remember details of your life when that song was popular? These are associations. You used the music association pathway, your brain's cross-referencing system. You could have also brought back that same time of your life if you thought, "What was I doing in 1981?" This is a different path for recall.

Involve your learner by creating sensory connections. Think of ways you can present the material that involve vision, hearing, touch, smell, and if appropriate, taste. Then, when those sights, sounds, feels, odors, and flavors are reintroduced, the information has other pathways for recall. For example, when teaching about dressing changes, comment on the smell of the alcohol or antiseptic solution, and be sure the learner is consciously aware of it.

Involve your learner by creating connections through physical activity. You can create kinesthetic memory pathways by practicing skills.

Involve your learner by creating connections with feelings. Teach with a sense of fun, and the information will be associated with positive emotions.

Also, break up information in simple, doable steps that build on one another. This will help the learner understand and succeed at each step. Success is comfortable and enhances learning. Fear, embarrassment, and failure interfere with learning.

Even cognitive connections help people learn. Guide the learner through problem solving. For example, we often tell patients to take antibiotics until they are all gone, and this message is reinforced on the medication container. One survey of more than 2000 patients found that 33.7% misunderstood written instructions to take all the pills in a bottle (Williams et al., 1995).

A conversation is a better approach. It involves the learner, enhances understanding, creates connections, and improves the chances for behavior change:

Nurse: *This antibiotic will kill the germs that are making you sick. Have you ever heard that you're supposed to take all the pills of an antibiotic until they're gone?*

Learner: *Yes.*

Nurse: *Do you know why?*

Learner: *No.*

Nurse: *Well, when you're sick, you have lots of germs. Some germs are strong and some are weak. Does that make sense?*

Learner: *Yes.*

Nurse: *So you start to take the antibiotic that kills the germs. Which germs do you think get killed off first, the weak ones or the strong ones?*

Learner: *The weak ones.*

Nurse: *Right. And when you kill off enough germs, you start to feel better. But you still have some pills left and you haven't killed off all the germs. Which germs are left, the weak ones or the strong ones?*

Learner: *The strong ones.*

Nurse: *That's right. You feel better, but there are strong germs left. So if you stop taking the pills before the strong germs are all killed, what do you think they will do?*

Learner: *Make me sick again.*

Nurse: *Right. And you'll be sicker this time, because stronger germs will be making you sick. That's why you're supposed to take all the pills, even if you feel better.*
Learner: *I never thought of it that way.*
Nurse: *So why should you take all the pills in this prescription?*
Have the learner explain it in his or her own words.

It seems like it takes longer to have learners interact with the material, but it actually saves time. Learners pay attention, process the data, and are more likely to understand the information so they can use it to change behaviors.

Encourage Application of Knowledge

Next, you need to encourage application of this new knowledge. Have the learner apply the new information right away so the connections are strengthened. In this case, you might ask the learner the following questions:

- If you take the first pill now, when will you take the last pill? (Answer: In 7 days.)
- What should you do with leftover pills? (Answer: There will be no leftover pills.)
- When you feel better, is it time to stop taking the pills? (Answer: No.)

"Allow immediate application of knowledge. Encouraging the patient or family member to apply his new knowledge reinforces learning and builds confidence."
—Cunningham, 1993, page 24J

Encourage Active Participation

Learners may participate passively or actively. Passive participation is internal and personal. Active participation is external and often interpersonal.

Passive participation includes listening to an audiotape, watching a video or slide show, or thinking of an answer to a question. Passive participation is thinking. It is internal. This book uses passive participation every time it asks you, the reader, a question. When you read, "did you ever hear an old song and remember details of your life when that song was popular?" and answer the question in your mind, you are participating passively.

Active participation includes activities that can be observed. They may be writing, physical activities, or interpersonal activities. Active participation includes filling in a blank, circling the right answer to a multiple choice question, putting photos of steps of a skill in order, or having a discussion.

People learn better and faster using active rather than passive participation techniques. Whenever you teach using passive participation, follow it up with an active method for reinforcement and evaluation of learning.

Here's an example. For every videotape you use to teach, create a handout that reinforces the key information. Every time you use the videotape to teach, give the learner the handout that summarizes the main points and uses a puzzle, game, or quiz to test recall and understanding.

> *"Use booklets that are brief, interactive, and designed to involve the patient as a partner in treatment planning."*
> —Robinson et al., 1997, page 570

How can you make your teaching active? Conversation is easiest and most convenient and is always appropriate. Actually, you can't avoid conversation, because every activity uses discussion for clarification and evaluation.

> *"All real change comes out of conversations. For both sides the conversation should be somewhat of a surprise."*
> —Whyte, 1992

Here are a few other possible activities you can consider using. Choose activities appropriate to the content, learner, and situation. Prepared materials are worth creating only for information you teach repeatedly, such as:

- Patient rights and responsibilities
- Advance directives
- How to take medicines
- Self-injections
- Catheter care

Prepared activities are especially useful as follow-up to reading booklets, watching videos, or attending group presentations.

Make sure your learner can read and write before initiating an activity that involves reading or writing.

Arrange the Pictures Game

The learner must arrange pictures of steps in a skill in order of implementation.

How to Use it
1. Identify key steps in skill.
2. Illustrate each step in a line drawing or photo.
3. Ask the learner to arrange steps in order.
4. Discuss results with the learner.

Example
After demonstrating a dressing change, give the learner shuffled photos of closed supplies, open supplies, removing the old dressing, cleaning the wound, putting on the new dressing, and disposing of waste.

Tips
- Keep skill photo collections of commonly taught skills for use in your work area. For example, a heme-onc unit may have picture sets of photos on central line flushing, cap changes, dressing changes, and blood draws.
- Use an instant-picture camera to create photos of the learner doing the skills (correctly). Individualized photos can then be mounted and given to the learner as a guide for doing the skill at home. This could be especially useful for learners with low literacy skills.

Cartoon Sharing

The learner reads a caption on a cartoon.

How to Use it
1. Find cartoons that illustrate how a learner may feel about the diagnosis, treatment, or prognosis.
2. Show the cartoon to the learner.
3. Encourage the learner to discuss his or her feelings about the cartoon and the medical situation.

Example
Show your patient a cartoon showing one man's perception of impending quadruple bypass surgery (Fig. 6-1). If you're not sure the patient can read, read the cartoon aloud. Laugh together, and ask the patient what the relationship is between fat intake and quadruple bypass. Teach from there.

Tips
- Carefully consider appropriateness of cartoons. How to judge appropriateness appears later in this chapter.
- As you find cartoons relevant to your patient population, cut them out and glue them in a looseleaf scrapbook. Then, when

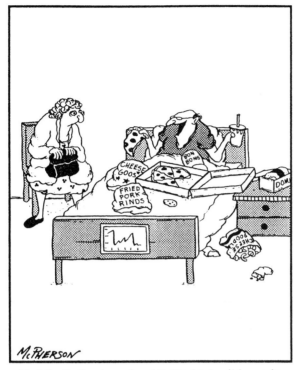

"But that's the beauty of it, Rita! I don't have to worry about my fat intake today. I'm having a quadruple bypass tomorrow!"

Figure 6-1. Show your patient a cartoon like this to initiate conversation.

a situation arises, pull out the relevant cartoon to initiate a discussion, or draw your own!

Sort True and False Statements

The learner sorts a group of written statements into true and false.

How to Use it
1. Identify key statements and misconceptions on a subject.
2. Print the statements on heavy paper.
3. Cut statements into individual strips.
4. Label one full piece of paper "true" and another piece of paper "false." The statements will be sorted onto these.
5. Ask the learner to sort the statements.
6. Discuss results with learner.

Example
Statements about acquired immunodeficiency syndrome (AIDS) to be sorted may include, "I can get AIDS by donating blood" and "I can get AIDS by shooting heroin."

Tips
- This activity works best with subjects that are often misunderstood.
- If you include many statements that are easy to identify as true or false, this activity can build a learner's confidence in an area.

Sort Problems With Follow-up Resources

The learner associates problems that may occur after discharge with appropriate responses.

How to Use it
1. Identify key situations that may need follow-up (excessive bleeding, uncontrolled pain, missed doses of medications, signs and symptoms of infection, anxiety, grief, and fear) and the appropriate follow-up responses and resources for each.
2. Print situations and responses on different colors of heavy paper.
3. Cut into individual strips.
4. On the back of the situation strips, assign a number to each. Put that number on the response that should be assigned to it. If several situations have the same response, put the numbers of all the situations on each of those response strips. If the response for four situations is "call your doctor," four "call your doctor" strips have situation numbers "3, 4, 8, and 12" written on the back.
5. Lay out the situation cards. Ask the learner to put the appropriate follow-up resource under it.
6. Discuss the results with the learner.

Example
"Yellow pus oozing out from the incision" should match up with "call your doctor," and "constipation" should match up with "eat more fruits, vegetables, and whole grains and drink more water."

Tips
- This activity can build a learner's confidence in an area if you include many situations that are easy to assign to responses.

Crossword Puzzle

The learner completes a crossword puzzle.

How to Use it
1. Decide content to be reviewed by the learner.
2. Identify key terms in content.
3. Use definitions of these terms as the clues.
4. Construct a crossword puzzle, either by computer or by hand.
5. Ask the learner to complete the crossword puzzle.
6. When the learner completes as much of the puzzle as possible, review the remaining terms with the learner.

Example
You may provide the following clue: "This kind of participation includes filling in a blank or having a discussion." The answer to be filled in the puzzle would be "active."

Tips
- Create puzzles only for topics you teach frequently. A puzzle may be used to review contents of a handout or video or for health-promotion topics.
- Do not offer a puzzle unless you are absolutely sure the learner can read and write.
- There are many inexpensive computer programs that create puzzles from your clues and answers. With a good program, you can create a puzzle quickly if you have the content. One such program, Puzzle Power, is referenced at the end of this chapter.
- Variations include fill-in puzzles, word-search puzzles, and anagrams. Instead of individual clues, present a paragraph with missing key words that appear in the puzzle. For example, "When you teach (7 across), you continuously observe and evaluate the learner's responses. This helps you constantly (4 down) teaching to the learner's needs." The answer for 7 across is "interactively"; for 4 down, the answer is "individualize."

Flash Cards

Show the learner one side of a flash card. The learner responds with the answer on the other side.

How to Use it

1. Decide content to be reviewed by the learner.
2. Opposite sides of the card can show:
   Medical term/definition
   Picture of equipment or supply/picture of item in use
   Question/response
   Problem/solution
3. Show the learner the card. Ask the learner to read the term.
4. You say the term again.
5. Ask the learner to repeat the term.
6. Explain the meaning of the term and how the learner may hear it used. For example, "white blood cell count is one of the lab results the doctor looks at to measure response to treatment."
7. If another term can be used interchangeably with this one, introduce it. For example, "WBC" means "white blood cell count."
8. After going through each card, go through again, and ask the learner to tell you the meaning of each word. If necessary, add information or explanation. If the learner knew the answer, respond positively and put that card aside. Success is reinforced as the active pack gets smaller. If the learner did not know the answer, discuss the topic more fully, and put that card on the bottom of the pile.
9. When the learner understands the terms, review them in the context of the illness or treatment.
10. Give the learner the cards to review on his or her own.
11. At the beginning of the next session, review these flash cards first.

Example

A flash card that addresses a problem and solution might say, "What would you do if your cast started to feel tight?" The other side would say, "Keep my limb on pillows, raised above my heart. If that doesn't help the cast feel more comfortable within an hour, call my doctor."

Tips

- Create flash cards only for topics you teach frequently. A puzzle may be used to review contents of a handout, video, or for health-promotion topics.
- If you are using flash cards to teach new words, teach no more than seven words in a session.
- Flash cards can be created by writing on index cards or by printing them on a computer.

- If appropriate, have the learner create his or her own flash cards. Writing the information on the cards adds another sensory pathway to the learning process.
- The learner can use the flash cards alone to practice and learn the material.

Cloze Activity

The learner fills in blanks in sentences from a group of key words.

How to Use it
1. Write seven sentences that describe key points in your teaching.
2. Replace one key word or phrase in each sentence with a blank (underline) to be filled in.
3. Under the sentences, put an out-of-order list of the terms you removed.
4. Ask the learner to fill in the blanks, using the terms in the list.
5. Discuss results with the learner.

Example
"_____ is a food with very little fat." The list of out-of-order terms includes "peanut butter" and "apple."

Tips
- There should be only one right answer for each blank. Review the terms and blanks for interchangeability, and adjust sentences and words accordingly.
- Following is a shortcut: Your word processor (for example, Word) may have a feature under Tools called autosummarize. Use this to obtain a quick summary of the key points in your written material, as perceived by your computer. Choose your seven sentences from the summary that include concepts the learner needs to know.

Practice a Procedure on a Doll or Model

Have the learner practice a skill on a doll or model before doing it on a human.

How to Use it
1. Tell the learner you will demonstrate the procedure on the doll or model and then you will talk the learner through doing it.

2. Do the procedure on a doll or model slowly, explaining what you are doing as you are doing it. Encourage the learner to ask for clarification as needed while you are demonstrating.
3. Have the learner do the same procedure on the doll or model while you talk him or her through the steps.
4. When the learner is done, discuss the procedure. Help the learner express feelings about performing the skill and specifics of technique.
5. Ask the learner to perform the skill again, this time explaining what he or she is doing. If the learner demonstrates techniques that could cause harm, problem solve with the learner through that part of the skill.
6. When the learner is done, identify what was done correctly, and if necessary, discuss the procedure in more detail.

Example
The learner may use a mannequin to learn cardiopulmonary resuscitation.

Tips
• Learners who succeed will gain confidence. Let the learner practice under your support before asking for an independent return demonstration that you evaluate. For details on how to use return demonstration, see Chapter 13, Measuring Outcomes.
• Provide a written list of the steps in the skill, each step illustrated with line drawings, if possible.

Directions for Performing a Skill

Create an audiotape that talks the learner through a self-care skill.

How to Use it
1. When a learner practices a skill, record yourself talking the learner through the process, or record the learner talking himself or herself through the process.
2. This tape may include discussions of potential problems and solutions.
3. Give the learner the tape to use when repeating the skill at home.

Example
This method is useful for dressing changes, injections, tube feedings, intravenous medications, self-catheterization, and other skills.

Tips

- Before creating the tape, make sure the learner knows how to use a tape player and has access to a working tape player in the situation where the skill will need to be performed.
- This is a good support tool for learners with low literacy skills or when your teaching involves a language interpreter.
- Next time the learner performs the skill, have the learner use the audiotape, and observe to evaluate and teach further, if necessary.
- If the learner is hearing impaired, substitute a videotape, if you have the ability to record and the learner has the ability to play the tape at home.

Written Quiz

The learner answers written questions.

How to Use it

1. Keep the quiz brief (7–10 questions) and nonthreatening. The quiz may include usual test question formats: multiple choice, matching, or fill in the blank.
2. Write the questions based on contents of a teaching handout, booklet, or video. Make the questions clear, and be sure there is only one correct answer for each question.
3. Tell the learner before he or she views or reads the material that a self-scored, written quiz will follow.
4. Have the learner answer the questions.
5. Give the learner the answer sheet to score the quiz himself or herself.
6. Discuss the results with the learner.

Example

After watching a video on self-care after a hip replacement, the learner is given a written quiz that evaluates learning of key points.

Tips

- Because this method is similar to tests given to children in school, other methods of encouraging active participation are preferred. However, some adults thrive on demonstrating they can do well on tests. This is a fine teaching method when used appropriately.
- Do not offer a written quiz unless you are absolutely sure the learner can read and write.
- Do not treat adults like school children. If the learner does not want to take a written quiz, discuss the key points instead.

- A variation is to present questions on a computer, with mouse or touch screen, which provides immediate feedback and scoring when the choice is entered. This can make the quiz feel more like a game than a test. However, if the learner is fearful of computers, discuss the key points instead.

Use checklists of signs and symptoms to help a learner understand and accept a problem or diagnosis, and provide motivation for treatment or behavior change. For example, symptoms checklists for diabetes, clinical depression, attention deficit disorder, alcohol addiction, and grief could help learners see that they meet criteria and get help.

Keep pads of note paper and pencils for use by patients and family members in examination and treatment rooms. They can write questions or take notes.

There are variations on the techniques listed previously and other ways to involve the learner. Individualize the methods you use to the content, readiness, and abilities of the learner. Once you start looking for ways to help learners actively participate in the learning process, you will discover which ways work best in your professional practice. Indeed, your learners may lead you down new paths.

Use Your Creativity!

"Help has become collaboration. In this collaboration we see just how much we ourselves have to offer: our own perseverance, honesty, openness, gratitude, humor. And we may be amazed to find out how hungry people are for these qualities."

—Dass & Gorman, 1985, page 147

Nursing is an art and a science. Few nursing activities have the opportunities for applying creativity that patient and family education offers.

How do you get in touch with your creativity? You can start by answering these questions: What do you do for fun? If you couldn't be a nurse, what would you do? Incorporate these impulses into patient and family teaching.

- For example, if you would be an elementary school teacher, consider creating educational bulletin boards for your waiting rooms.
- If you would be a writer, consider writing teaching materials.
- If you would be a cruise ship activities director, consider creating a BINGO game to reward health-promoting behaviors.

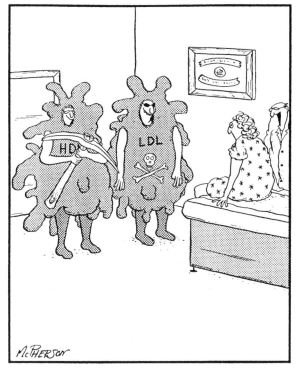

"To help you better understand this good
cholesterol/bad cholesterol thing, Nurse Bowman
and Nurse Strickling are going to
do a little skit for you."

Figure 6-2. Learn to recognize when you've taken things
too far.

NYLCare Health Plans (1996) used a DiaBINGO game to track
preventive screenings for diabetics, such as retinal and food
exams, hemoglobin AIC monitoring, and urine testing. When
each screening test is done, the card is signed by a physician. A
full card entitles the participant to a gift bag of food and
seasonings recommended by the American Diabetes
Association. In 4 months, screenings increased by 14% to 20%.

Assuming your teaching is accurate and appropriate, the only limits
to using your creativity are practicality and good taste. For example,
the nurses in Figure 6-2 have probably gone too far.

My biggest challenge was a patient who was on several medications and could not read. No one in his family could read at all. They couldn't even measure out doses of liquid medicines! They also didn't speak English. But they could tell colors. So I used different colored stick-on dots to color code the medicine bottles, the dose on measuring spoons, and a chart with pictures which told what time to take each med. It worked!

Do you need to stimulate your creativity a bit? Look at the list of items that can help lighten the mood (Box 6-1) and create an environment that invites participation. Have fun with it.

BOX 6-1   Stuff to Lighten the Mood

Here are some items that may help inspire your learners to participate. Think about the sorts of things you most often teach. Look at the list and mark those that fit your frequently taught topics. If the choice feels right to you, you will be able to introduce the item without awkwardness. Choose one or two of your favorite items and bring them to work. Keep them handy for the right moments. When the moments come, test them, and see if they work for you. If not, try to figure out how you can make them work. You can always go back to the list and try something else.

If you feel the urge to stock your workplace with all of these items to use in teaching, step back. Are you doing it for your learners, or do you need to schedule more play time in your life?

If none of these items feels right to you, skip this section completely. Not every nurse needs props. If you feel most comfortable with conversation, then stick with that!

☐ Art supplies
  —Cardboard
  —Crayons
  —Colored chalk
  —Colored pencils
  —Markers
  —Paints
  —Paper

Box 6-1 *(Continued)*

☐ Cassette player and headphones
☐ Audiotapes of
  —Animal sounds
    Does your patient feign sleep to avoid physical therapy? A rooster crowing might provide enough surprise to rouse a laugh.
  —Applause
  —Laughter
    These can be used to celebrate success.
Sound effects tapes are readily available. Check your local music store or public library. Or make your own!
☐ Balls
  —Rubber
  —Sponge
☐ Bean bags
  Balls and bean bags can be used to vent frustration safely.
☐ Bells
  Wake them up with a gentle tinkle!
☐ Boxes
  —Applause box
  —Suggestion box
  —Surprise box
  —Wish box
  —Unusual medical word box
    These can be shoe boxes with reinforcers inside. Pediatric nurses might put stickers in a surprise box. An applause box could contain an audiotape player that plays applause in response to success. An unusual medical word box would contain a word for the learner to define, such as "mastication." Creative nurses could festively decorate such boxes.
☐ Bulletin boards
☐ Photographs
  —Great quotes board
  —Happy outcomes
    One bone marrow transplant unit posts photos and letters from previous patients.
☐ Instant camera
  Catch those happy moments! Use with discretion and good taste.
☐ Cartoons
☐ Certificates
  Celebrate your learner's success with an award! Ragland (1997) suggests
    "The 'Keeps on Ticking' Award" and "The 'Think I Can' Award."
☐ Costume pieces

Box 6-1 *(Continued)*

☐ Hats
  —Decision-making hat
  —Reminder hat
    Is your patient having difficulty deciding whether or not to have surgery? Offer a silly hat to help. Offer your patient a straw hat to wear while drinking GoLitely, so he or she can pretend it's some exotic tropical beverage.
      (Word of caution: One nurse wore a costume to work for Halloween, then found herself needing to tell a parent her son's surgery was not going well. If you use a costume, make sure it can be removed easily.)
☐ Games
☐ Masks
  —Animal noses
  —Clown nose
  —Groucho nose and glasses
    Put one on, and then go about your business as normal.
☐ Mobiles
  Hang an illustrated version of the care pathway over the bed to inspire progress.
☐ New Year's noisemakers
  This is another way to celebrate.
☐ Oversized props
  —Pill the size of a pillow
  —Syringe, 50 mL
  —Stethoscope, clown-sized
    Cut the tension by getting outrageous.
☐ Posters
  —Affirmations
  —Inspiring
  —Nature scenes, especially with water
    Consider putting them on walls, ceilings, and floors.
☐ Symbols
  —Traffic signs
  —International symbols
  —Unique hospital symbols
    Play with it! Draw a mouth, put a red circle and a slash through it, and call it "NPO."
☐ Flags and banners
  Put your symbols on fabric. Creatively name your workspace. Use a flag or banner to announce attractively "no blood draws in left arm."

"Choose to have fun. Fun creates enjoyment. Enjoyment invites participation. Participation focuses attention. Attention expands awareness. Awareness promotes insight. Insight generates knowledge. Knowledge facilitates action. Action yields results."

—Oswald B. Shallow
from Wooten, 1994, page 31

Have Fun With it

As mentioned previously, you can also involve your learner by creating connections with feelings. Teach with a sense of fun, and the information will be associated with positive emotions.

"Two [nursing] instructors demonstrated how humor can be used to reduce a patient's anxiety during preoperative care. The 'nurse' said, 'You look as though you'd like to get out of bed and run. You remind me of a cartoon I saw. There is an operating room with six gowned and masked figures standing around an empty operating room table. The surgeon is looking around and saying, "Come, come, now, one of you must be the patient.'"' The role-playing 'patient' giggled and said, 'Yeah, that's what I'd like to do, hide.' A discussion of her fears ensued."

—Robinson, 1991, pages 207–208

In this case, humor released the tension of fears, created the interpersonal connection, and invited participation in learning about what to expect before and after surgery. Humor was the grease, the lubricant for learning.

There are many ways humor works to facilitate learning:

1. Cognitive
   Captures and maintains attention
   Stimulates the right and left sides of the brain
   Coordinates function between the right and left sides of the brain
   Promotes insights through new associations
   Promotes interaction with the material
   Enhances short- and long-term memory
2. Affective
   Releases anxiety and fear
   Releases anger, aggression, and hostility in a socially acceptable way
   Avoids or denies painful feelings
   Decreases perceived intimidation (environment, subject, people)

Reduces tension
Lowers defenses
Promotes a sense of control and mastery
Promotes a sense of safety
Facilitates acceptance
Promotes rapport and trust
Facilitates relationship building
Makes learning pleasurable
Promotes positive emotions and increases a feeling of hope
Promotes healthy coping
Facilitates communications and enhances readiness to learn
3. Psychomotor
Improves coordination
Improves dexterity

"Humor in education sets the tone for a caring environment that promotes openness and facilitates communication . . . [The learner is more willing to] shift patterns of thinking, generate creative solutions to problems, perceive double meanings, understand analogies, and examine paradoxes. Flexible and creative ways of thinking emerge; the corollary benefits are critical thinking and independent problem-solving."
—Cannella, Missroon, & Optiz, 1995, page 61

Do you ask patients to cough, turn, and deep breathe? Instead, try laughter, which accomplishes similar ends with added emotional benefits. Laughter is a wonderful therapeutic tool for the busy nurse. It treats the body, mind, and spirit simultaneously!

Humor is Not Necessarily Laughter

"By injecting fun and some levity into the learning situation, we can make the pleasure of learning become a positive force."
—Rankin & Stallings, 1996, page 300

Generally, when we think of fun and humor, we think of laughter, but laughter is not easy to elicit! Comedians have talent, but they have to work hard to get laughs regularly. Do nurses really have to develop this skill, too?
Fortunately, they don't.

Clifford Kuhn, a psychiatrist, defined in detail the 15 stages of laughter (1994):

1. Smirk
2. Smile
3. Grin
4. Snicker
5. Giggle
6. Chuckle
7. Chortle
8. Laugh
9. Cackle
10. Guffaw
11. Howl
12. Shriek
13. Roar
14. Convulse
15. Die (as in "die laughing")

Note that an actual laugh is in the middle the list. Most humor actually stimulates us below the laughter stage. Even on a day when we're in the best of moods, we bounce around between stages 1 and 8, only occasionally, if ever, bursting into higher stages. Can you even remember the last time you guffawed, let alone convulsed, in laughter? It's hard to maintain shrieking for very long, but we can comfortably smile for much of the day.

We do not need to set our humor goals very high to reap the benefits.

"A mere smile results in an observable stimulation of the immune system, as well as the release of those naturally occurring 'feel good' substances, endorphins. Thus, very early in this progression the body receives a physiological benefit."

—Kuhn, 1994, page 34

There's one more reason we don't have to work very hard to use humor in our professional practices. Laughter depends on tension. Comedians have to build up their audiences' tension so they can introduce the surprise that releases the pent up energy in laughter. Our audiences are already tense. They are primed to release that tension through laughter.

Physiological Effects of Laughter

Another physician, William Fry, has written extensively on the physiological effects of laughter (1992). He opened the doors for scientists to look seriously at humor and laughter, and research is increasing in this area. Here's a summary of what has been found so far.

The first phase of laughter stimulates the following:

- An increase in pulse rate
- An increase in respiratory rate
- An increase in catecholamine and endorphin production
- Some contraction in skeletal muscles, but muscles not participating in the laughter remaining generally flaccid (This is associated with the side effect of laughter, incontinence.)
- Both hemispheres of the brain producing a unique level of consciousness and the brain processing in a higher mode

The second phase of laughter accomplishes the following:

- Relaxes muscles, eases tension
- Reduces blood pressure
- Helps respiration, heart rate, and muscle tension return to below normal levels
- Enables greater coordination between right and left hemispheres of the brain

Laughter in general promotes the following:

- Aids ventilation
- Clears mucous plugs
- Accelerates exchange of residual air, enhancing blood oxygen levels
- Exercises the myocardium
- Increases arterial and venous circulation
- Promotes movement of immune elements and phagocytes through the system; helps fight infections
- Enhances venous return, reducing vascular stasis and the risk of thrombus formation
- Controls pain by (1) distracting attention, (2) reducing tension, (3) changing expectations, and (4) increasing production of catecholamines and endorphins

Contraindications to Laughter

- A few people have neurological symptoms when they laugh: seizures, cataplectic, and narcoleptic attacks.

- Laughter creates a brief, sudden increase in blood pressure. This could lead to cerebrovascular accidents or myocardial infarction in susceptible people.
- In some situations, the large increases in abdominal and thoracic pressure associated with laughter are contraindicated. For example, patients who have just had abdominal or pelvic surgery, those with acute rib or shoulder girdle fractures, or those with acute respiratory disease, such as asthma, should refrain from laughing.

Accidental Humor

Let's get back to patient and family education. How do you teach with humor?

"We're living in the land of Catch 22. The challenge is to turn it into M*A*S*H*."

—Dass & Gorman, 1985, page 198

The easiest way is to take advantage of accidental humor. Keep a humorous mind-set and situations will offer you opportunities to respond spontaneously. In your interactions with patients and families, frustrating Catch 22 situations come up all the time. Use them. In the movie and television program M*A*S*H*, the humor emerged from the experiences. (Not counting the practical jokes, but those were never aimed at innocent patients.)

Observe the learner's sense of humor for cues. You may not hear laughter, but you can note the smirks and smiles. The best examples of spontaneous humor are in your personal experiences with patients. They do not translate well into anecdotes, because the words spoken were not necessarily funny. The mood and attitudes are funny.

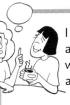 I can remember one admission interview where the patient and I laughed straight through. I have no memory of what we were laughing about. He was coming in for surgery, was anxious and coped with humor. I only remember his surgery was successful and his hospitalization went as planned.

"Life does not cease to be funny when people die any more than it ceases to be serious when people laugh."

—George Bernard Shaw
from Wooten, 1994, p. 4

Take notice when you laugh with patients. Note when humor happens. Then, think about the elements that created the moment. The more aware you are of the details of successful spontaneous humor, the better prepared you will be to take advantage of future opportunities.

Intentionally Use Humor to Teach

"Always remember that we all have distinctive humor styles and preferences. What works for one person does not necessarily help another."
—Bittman, McGhee, Berk, & Wooten, 1997, page 11

The easiest way to use humor intentionally is to take advantage of the work of a professional humorist in a therapeutically appropriate way. Cartoons are the most available of these resources. Cut out cartoons from your newspaper, or buy the books of artists who often address medical issues. There are many examples, including Jim Unger (Herman), John McPherson (Close to Home), and if you're tastefully selective, John Callahan (Callahan).

You can hire a cartoonist to create teaching materials custom-made for your program. One hospital gives pregnant teenagers a cartoon booklet drawn by the makers of the comic strip Baby Blues. The section on telling your parents begins: "For some girls, this seems like the scariest part of being pregnant. But it doesn't have to be. Here are a few things you can do to make it easier." The first item on that list is "Do it now!" It says, "Tell your parents that you're pregnant early so you can get medical care early. In other words, don't wait until you can't see your shoes to break the news" (Scott & Kirkman, 1995, page 8).

If you're more comfortable with a lower key of humor, cartoon-like illustrations add an element of fun and interest with minimal risk. For example, nurses Zerwekh and Claborn (1994), have created Memory Notebook of Nursing, illustrated by C. J. Miller, RN. Although intended for teaching nursing students, in the right context, some could be used for teaching patients (Figs. 6-3, 6-4, and 6-5). Translate the medical terminology into lay language, and use the images to reinforce the messages through visual pathways.

"The use of humor in patient/client education is a positive tool. A little story, cartoon or joking sets the stage for decreasing the anxiety and increasing the receptivity to learning, to listening and to hearing the facts about a serious subject."
—Robinson, 1991, page 20

BLOOD SUGAR MNEMONIC

Hot & Dry = Sugar High

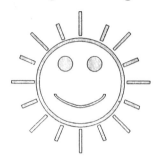

Cold & Clammy = Need Some Candy

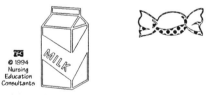

Figure 6-3. Zerwekh, J., Claborn, J.C. (1994). *Memory notebook of nursing.* Dallas, TX: Nursing Education Consultants, page 50.

Another way to introduce humor and fun into teaching is by using props. In the right situation, pulling out a 20-cc syringe for an intramuscular injection or offering a pill the size of a pillow could break the tension.

Of course, the ultimate humor prop is the rubber chicken. How can you use it to help you evaluate the learner's understanding of teaching?

RIGHT SIDED FAILURE

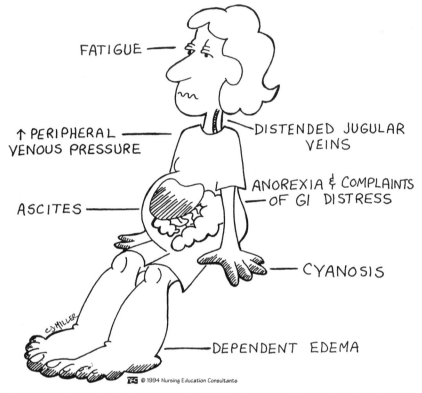

FATIGUE

↑ PERIPHERAL
VENOUS PRESSURE

ASCITES

DISTENDED JUGULAR
VEINS

ANOREXIA & COMPLAINTS
OF GI DISTRESS

CYANOSIS

DEPENDENT EDEMA

© 1994 Nursing Education Consultants

Figure 6-4. Zerwekh, J., Claborn, J.C. (1994). *Memory notebook of nursing.* Dallas, TX: Nursing Education Consultants, page 77.

"Have the patient draw his or her afflicted internal organs on the rubber chicken with water-based markers, and describe the pathophysiology and treatment."

—London, 1996, page 5

Maybe you don't have to teach about pathophysiology, but you get the point.

Would you prefer to be less outrageous? Use natural humor sources in the room as props for humor, such as the room temperature, the amount of light, the toilet, the emesis basin, or the get well cards. A simple observation can lighten the mood. Ultimately, a lighter mood facilitates teaching faster and more effectively because it helps engage the learner.

ATROPINE OVERDOSE

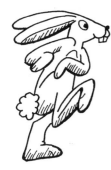

Hot as a Hare
($\uparrow$ temperature)

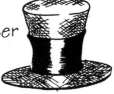

Mad as a Hatter
(confusion, delirium)

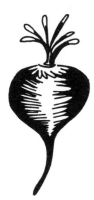

Red as a Beet
(flushed face)

Dry as a Bone
(decreased secretions, thirsty)

Nursing
Education
Consultants
From: Robert W. Malone, RN

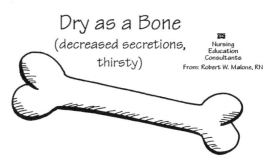

Figure 6-5. Zerwekh, J., Claborn, J.C. (1994). *Memory Notebook of Nursing.* Dallas, TX: Nursing Education Consultants, page 19.

The following is an imprint on a toothbrush provided by Gary Stanton, a dentist:

"Brush for 3 minutes. Use fuzzy end."

This probably originated one day when a dentist looked into a mouth and thought, "The patient says he brushes regularly. It doesn't look like he does. What end of the brush is he using?"

Be Sensitive and Use Humor in Moderation

"How do you use humor effectively with family members who are upset/ distressed and might not appreciate the attempts at levity?"

—an RN

It's easy. When in doubt, don't use humor.

In some ways, using humor is very simple and natural. In other ways, it can be quite a sophisticated tool in the hands of an expert. Know where your skills are in the continuum, and apply the sense of fun at the level of your ability. Move slowly and surely. If you jump in beyond your skill level, you may meet with an embarrassing situation that will make you hesitant to use humor again. Don't let this happen to you. Humor is too valuable a tool to eliminate from your repertoire.

These three rules can help guide you:

1. Unless you are taking a photo, never, never tell anyone to smile. Inspire smiles from within.
2. Don't force humor.
3. Don't make anyone participate in humor.

Be especially careful with using humor with people who may not get it or who are likely to misinterpret it. Use caution in using humor when the learner's primary language or culture is not the same as yours, has low literacy skills, is mentally ill, or is developmentally delayed, demented, delirious, or confused.

Use humor as a condiment, in moderation. Do you have trouble telling when humor is appropriate? See Box 6-2 on this page for details.

BOX 6-2   Appropriate Humor Versus Inappropriate Humor

Appropriateness of humor refers to its therapeutic usefulness. This is not an issue of political correctness. Whenever you use humor professionally, it must always be used appropriately.

Appropriate Humor
- Laughs with people
- Is constructive
- Is timed appropriately
- Is aware of the recipient's ability to receive it
- Is aimed at yourself, your foibles, or things in the environment
- Decreases stress
- Decreases anxiety

Box 6-2 *(Continued)*

- Promotes hope
- Shares frustrations
- Puts a problem into perspective
- Enhances good feelings
- Establishes emotional bonds between people
- Brings people closer together
- Is therapeutic and healing

Inappropriate Humor
- Laughs at people
- Is destructive
- Is delivered at the wrong time
- Is delivered to the wrong people (Certain jokes between health care providers can be therapeutic, but if they are shared with patients, they could be misunderstood and hurtful.)
- Is aimed at other people
- Increases stress
- Increases anxiety
- Decreases hope
- Creates problems
- Hurts others
- Creates communication barriers
- Distances people from one another
- Is not therapeutic and interferes with healing

"In many cultures humor is not used when dealing with serious health problems. The perception of non-English speakers may be that the information is not serious or 'you don't care about me.' Test any material of this type with the intended audience before using it."

—Doak, Doak & Root, 1996, page 69

Choosing appropriate humor is a learned skill. Where did you learn your humor skills? Did those sources use appropriate or inappropriate humor?

If you are told you have used humor inappropriately or the response to your humor tells you it was perceived as inappropriate:

1. Immediately apologize, briefly and sincerely.
2. Identify for yourself why the humor was inappropriate.
3. Maintain awareness when using humor in the future to keep your humor appropriate.

"How do you know when a patient is ready to accept humor?"

—an RN

"What type of assessment would you use to determine the appropriate kind of humor for each patient?"

—an RN

Obviously, the best way to assess readiness and type of humor to use is to listen to the learner. When the learner uses humor, the time could be right. The type of humor used gives you insight into the learner's humor style. If the learner uses humor inappropriately (see Display 6-2 for details), do not lower yourself to the same level. However, if the learner uses humor appropriately, that may suggest the sort of humor you could try.

Conversation is the most efficient assessment tool. If you prefer, and have time for, a more formal way to assess humor style and readiness, Herth (1984) provides questions to ask when doing a Funny Bone History. If you have access to a computer with Windows, try the Subjective Multidimensional Interactive Laughter Evaluation (SMILE) (Bittman et al., 1997). After the learner answers 40 questions about humor preferences, the program prints out a summary of the learner's responses and resources for a personalized humor program. This survey is not specific for patient and family education, but you may be able to apply some of the report's information when you teach.

"Always remember to carefully and sensitively gauge your humor intervention and adapt it to the specific needs of the subject. Be prepared to advance slowly and cautiously. Develop an awareness for the need to slow down or step back and reassess your approach if the subject becomes uncomfortable at any time."

—Bittman et al., 1997, page 10

Timing is essential in humor. The funniest joke will crash if told at the wrong time. Assessment is as necessary before application of therapeutic humor interventions as it is before medical treatments or teaching. You need to know where and why you are intervening before you act so you can ensure appropriateness and assess effectiveness of the intervention.

"Humor is tragedy plus time."

—Mark Twain
from Klein, 1991, page 92

If you act too soon, you're dealing with tragedy, not humor. As patients and families process the little and big tragedies, their humor emerges. Travel with them. When used properly, a sense of humor can be an exceptionally professional therapeutic tool.

"Most of us know how supportive it is merely to be in the presence of a mind that is open, quiet, playful, receptive, or reflective. These attributes are themselves helpful. Moreover, there is something we frequently experience—perhaps we can call it intuitive awareness—that links us most intimately to the universe and, in allegiance with the heart, binds us together in generosity and compassion."
                                          —Dass & Gorman, 1985, page 94

Share Your Successes

If you use humor in teaching, document its effectiveness. Does the learner respond best to puns? Let other members of the health care team know. This will help everyone individualize teaching.

Close With a Cloze

How well did you understand the key points of this chapter? Test yourself. Fill in the blanks, using the words in the list. All words will be used.

The answers are at the end of the section called, "If you want to learn more."

_____ shortens teaching time. When you teach interactively, you continuously _____ and evaluate the learner's responses. This helps you constantly _____ teaching to the learner's needs. When people actively interact with information during the learning process, the _____ change takes place that enhances learning and memory. Involve your learner by creating _____ connections. Have the learner apply the new information right away so the _____ are strengthened. Choosing appropriate humor is a _____ skill.

Fill in the blanks with these words:

chemical
connections
individualize
interaction
learned
observe
sensory

If you want to learn more:

(1996). NYLCare diabetic screening rates jump with senior bingo game initiative. *News and Strategies for Managed Medicare & Medicaid, 2*(31), 1, 4.

(1997). *Puzzle power: The all-in-one puzzle maker.* Centron Software Technologies. E-mail: centron@ac.net

Berk, R.A. (1998). *Professors are from Mars, students are from Snickers: How to write and deliver humor in the classroom and in presentations.* Madison, WI: Mendota Press.

Bittman, B., McGhee, P., Berk, L., & Wooten, P. (1997). *SMILE (Subjective Multidimensional Interactive Laughter Evaluation): The computer-based guide for creating personalized humor programs.* Meadville, PA: TouchStar Productions.

Callahan, J. (1989). *Don't worry, he won't get far on foot: The autobiography of a dangerous man.* New York: William Morrow and Company.

Cannella, K.S., Missroon, S., & Optiz, M. P. (1995). Humor—An educational strategy. In K. Buxman & A. LeMoine (Eds.), *Nursing perspectives on humor* (pp. 51–86). Staten Island: Power Publications.

Cunningham, D. (1993). Improve your teaching skills. *Nursing 93, 24J.*

Dass, R., & Gorman, P. (1985). *How can I help? Stories and reflections on service.* New York: Alfred A. Knopf.

Doak, C.C., Doak, L.G., & Root, J.H. (1996). *Teaching patients with low literacy skills* (2nd ed.). Philadelphia: Lippincott-Raven.

Fry, W.F. (1992). The physiologic effects of humor, mirth and laughter. *Journal of the American Medical Association, 267*(13), 1857–1858.

Herth, K.A. (1984). Laughter: A nursing Rx. *AJN: American Journal of Nursing,* August, 991–992.

Joint Commission on Accreditation of Healthcare Organizations (1998). *1998 Hospital Accreditation Standards.* Oakbrook Terrace, IL: Author.

Klein, A. (1991). *Quotations to cheer you up when the world is getting you down.* New York: Wings Books.

Kuhn, C. (1994). The stages of laughter. *Journal of Nursing Jocularity, 4*(2), 34–35.

Leidy, K. (1992). Enjoyable learning experiences—An aid to retention? *The Journal of Continuing Education in Nursing, 23*(5), 206–208.

London, F. (1996). *A nurse's guide to therapeutic uses of a rubber chicken.* Mesa, AZ: JNJ Publishing.

Loomans, D., & Kolberg, K.J. (1993). *The laughing classroom: Everyone's guide to teaching with humor and play.* Tiburon, CA: H.J. Kramer.

Lorig, K. (1992). *Patient education: A practical approach.* St. Louis, MO: Mosby–Year Book, Inc.

McGhee, P. (1998). Rx: Laughter. *RN, 61*(7), 50–53.

McPherson, J. (1998). *The get well book: A little book to make you feel a whole lot better.* Kansas City, MO: Andrews McMeel Publishing.

Ragland, G. (1997). *Instant teaching treasures for patient education.* St. Louis, MO: Mosby–Year Book, Inc.

Rankin, S.H., & Stallings, K.D. (1996). *Patient education: Issues, principles, practices* (3rd ed.). Philadelphia: Lippincott-Raven.

Robinson, V.M. (1991). *Humor and the health professions: The therapeutic use of humor in health care* (2nd ed.). Thorofare, NJ: Slack.

Robinson, P., Katon, W., Von Korff, M., Bush, T., Simon, G., Lin, E., & Walker, E. (1997). The education of depressed primary care patients: what do patients think of interactive booklets and a video. *Journal of Family Practice*, 44(6), 562–571.

Sherman, J.R. (1994). *Creative caregiving*. Golden Valley, MN: Pathway Books.

Scott, J., & Kirkman, R. (1995). *Now what? How to survive being a pregnant teenager*. Phoenix: Good Samaritan Regional Medical Center.

Thaler, M. (1995). *The school nurse from the black lagoon*. New York: Scholastic.

Unger, J. (1992). *Herman VIII: A Herman treasury*. Kansas City, MO: Andrews and McMeel.

Whyte, D. (1992). *Images of fire: Creativity and personal passion*. Boulder, CO: Sounds True Recordings.

Williams, M.V., Parker, R.M., Baker, D.W., Parikh, N.S., Pitkin, K., Coates, W.C., & Nurss, J.R. (1995). Inadequate functional health literacy among patients at two public hospitals. *Journal of the American Medical Association*, 274(21), 1677–1682.

Wooten, P. (1994). *Heart, humor & healing*. Mount Shasta, CA: Commune-A-Key.

Wooten, P. (1996). *Compassionate laughter: Jest for your health*. Salt Lake City, UT: Commune-A-Key Publishing.

Wurman, R.S. (1989). *Information anxiety: What to do when information doesn't tell you what you need to know*. New York: Bantam Books.

Zerwekh, J., & Claborn, J.C. (1994). *Memory notebook of nursing*. Dallas: Nursing Education Consultants.

Answers to the Closing Cloze

Interaction shortens teaching time. When you teach interactively, you continuously *observe* and evaluate the learner's responses. This helps you constantly *individualize* teaching to the learner's needs. When people actively interact with information during the learning process, the *chemical* change takes place that enhances learning and memory. Involve your learner by creating *sensory* connections. Have the learner apply the new information right away so the *connections* are strengthened. Choosing appropriate humor is a *learned* skill.

The Teaching Toolbox

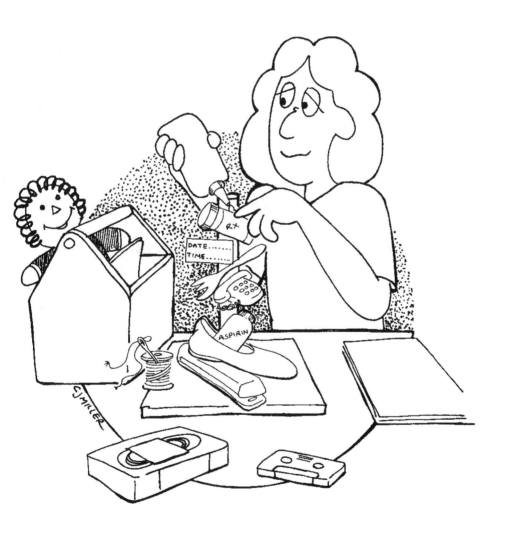

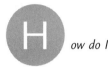 ow do I teach tube feedings quickly in the home care patient?"

—an RN

"If the only tool you have is a hammer, you tend to see every problem as a nail."

—Abraham Maslow
(Brass Tacks Quotations, [On-line])

"A good facilitator or teacher, says Carl Rogers, tries to 'organize and make easily available the widest possible range of resources for learning.'"

—Wurman, 1989, page 145

A tool is an instrument or device used to accomplish a task. An environment that promotes quality patient and family education contains a variety of teaching tools. To what sort of tools do you have access? Do they meet your needs?

If you work in a hospital and you don't have what you need, don't fret. You've got the support of the Joint Commission on Accreditation of Healthcare Organizations (JCAHO)! They tell us we must have the necessary tools:

"The hospital identifies and provides the educational resources required to achieve its educational objectives."

—JCAHO, 1998, page 10

You, as direct patient care provider and patient educator, are the part of the hospital qualified to identify educational objectives and resource needs. Point this out to the person or group controlling the budget. Make sure they understand that JCAHO expects you to have the educational resources you need.

Teaching Tools

Having the right tools available helps you teach more effectively and efficiently. You know what information you teach regularly. What tools do you need to support that teaching best?

"Only one what, but many hows."

—Wurman, 1989, page 81

This chapter lists some of the different types of tools available and how to use them. Note that tools do not replace you; they facilitate your work. Teaching tools don't teach. Teaching is an interactive process that involves a learner and a health care professional.

"Media should be carefully selected and should be consistent with instructional objectives."
                                              —Rankin & Stallings, 1996, page 184

Not everyone needs every tool. Look at your patient population, your environment, your resources, what you have to teach, and what resources are available. Take all the variables into account, and decide what you need to achieve your educational objectives.

"Media help deliver a message. A variety of media can be creatively used to help patients learn more, to help them retain better what they have learned, and to encourage the development of skills."
                                              —Rankin & Stallings, 1996, page 185

Medical Equipment and Supplies

"It's difficult to get patient education going, especially in a busy clinic. How do other people make time?"
                                              —an RN

Every time you are with a patient or family member is an opportunity to teach. If you can't make more time to teach, use the time you have well. Is your teaching environment disorganized? Use the teaching tools at hand. Thermometers, stethoscopes, dressings, medications, monitors, and pumps can all be the starting points for teaching. As you provide care, evaluate the learner's understanding of what you are doing and how it relates to the illness and treatment. Take your teaching conversations from there.

Handouts

Handouts are classic teaching tools. They could be fact sheets, discharge instructions, or detailed booklets. They could be written descriptions of anticipatory guidance, signs and symptoms, side effects of medications, descriptions of medical tests, self-care instructions, or information on when to call the doctor.

Handouts can be used during workup, when diagnosis is first established, during treatment, at discharge, and during maintenance. They can be in a binder in the waiting room, offered on racks, or posted on bulletin boards. They can be available in the examining room or given to the learner by a health care professional to reinforce or introduce teaching. They can be mailed to learners. They can be used creatively:

> *"The nurse attaches the daily key teaching points to the [patient's] mirror . . . it gives the patient an opportunity to review the information, thus reinforcing the lesson."*
> —"Streamline CHF education," 1998, page 6

Following are some advantages of handouts:

- Standardized, so everyone on the health care team teaches the same content
- Have spaces for individualization
- Reinforce interactive teaching
- Reference for learner; can look up answers to questions
- Learner can pick up handouts on topics of interest
- Can be purchased or created
- Relatively inexpensive
- Easily updated if you create them

Following are some disadvantages of handouts:

- Ability to read and understand written materials is necessary
- Need to be appropriate for the learner (content, culture, language, reading level)
- Need a handout on the specific topic you are teaching
- Need to be readily available at the right time
- Need a system for storage and personnel for maintenance

> *"I walk around the hospital and find piles of handouts under supplies and equipment.*
> *I know they're not being used."*
> —an RN

Handouts are important tools that may not be used as well as they could. Doak and Doak (1998) say that tailoring printed materials to the learner makes them more effective. They offer three suggestions for accomplishing this:

1. Highlight or underline key information as you discuss it. You or the learner may do this.
2. Write the learner's name on the front, except for materials on human immunodeficiency virus/acquired immunodeficiency syndrome or sexually transmitted diseases. This helps the learner perceive the information as personally important.
3. Ask the learner questions to verify that he or she has learned the key points.

Chapter 8, Say it in Writing, defines qualities of a good handout and specifics on how to create your own.

Multimedia

Multimedia means using a combination of media, such as film, tape recordings, slides, written words, and special lighting effects, to educate or entertain.

The term generally refers to their use simultaneously in a high-tech environment. However, different media can be also used one at a time. People learn best when several senses are stimulated and information is repeated in several different ways. Using several different media helps create more memory pathways.

> *"Audiotapes, flip charts, and videotapes are also useful supplementary materials for providing patient education. Some hospitals lend or provide educational audiotapes and videotapes to patients for use at home. This is an ideal way to supplement the patient education received in the hospital because the patients and/or families have control over the learning process. They can stop the tape when they need a break, and they can replay it as needed."*
>
> —Menke, 1993, page 159

Notice this quote repeated the word "supplement." Media enhance teaching. They emphasize important points. Use them to begin and add to discussions.

Binders and Photo Albums

A binder or photo album is useful to create when many of your learners will be going through the same experiences. A binder can include photos, illustrations, descriptive captions, and small objects, such as name bands or samples of dressings. It is portable and delivers a lot of information in a small amount of space. Photos attract and maintain learners' interest, especially if they are in color. Don't have too many nonessential details in the background. The more closely the images reflect your learners, the more your learners will identify with the messages. Show familiar places, age, gender, and sociocultural and racial backgrounds.

Binders' contents can be brief, such as a description of an electroencephalogram or a mole removal, or they can be longer, showing the stages of transplant, from waiting for the organ to recovery. A binder can be used by the learner alone, at his or her own pace, and then discussed, or the learner and health care provider can go through the binder together. Ask the learner to describe what he or she sees, and take the teaching conversation from there.

One hospital uses such a photo album to prepare parents for their baby's craniofacial surgery. Many parents reacted with shock when seeing how swollen their children's faces became after surgery. The photo album helped prepare parents, showing swelling right after surgery, 3 days later, 1 week later, 3 weeks later, and 6 months later. This reassured parents that their child's swelling was within normal limits and would eventually be gone.

One oral surgeon has a binder in his waiting room showing illustrations of impacted molars and the results of removal. Text describes the problems that can occur if these teeth are not removed and what to expect during and after surgery.

If you create such a binder, ask those who have been through the process what they feel should be described to prepare others. What do they wish they had known to expect? For what were they glad they were prepared? Be sure to get written permission to use the pictures of all who are photographed for the binder.

Some learners need more structure than others. Binders can also be developed for a single learner or family. Here's one nurse's story:

The baby was a 3-month-old near-SIDS patient, the son of a teenage single mom. His mother lived with her father (the baby's grandpa), who was also a single parent. The mother was very attentive to the infant in the hospital, staying night and day, and only left him for one afternoon to attend her high school graduation. This baby was neurologically devastated, requiring tube feeding, apnea monitoring, respiratory treatments with nasopharyngeal suctioning, specific handling, positioning and stimulation techniques, and seizure management. In effect, almost everything she learned about normal infant care was not applicable to her son.

We taught her how to care for her son throughout the hospitalization, with successful return demonstrations. The young woman was intelligent, and I had no concerns about her ability to perform any of the skills. My concern was with her ability to organize and prioritize her child's care and maintain some semblance of normal growth and development herself. I noticed that handouts, business cards, appointment cards, and equipment handbooks were everywhere, crumpled and food stained. When talking with the grandpa, he voiced concern about her ability to maintain the somewhat rigid schedule needed by the infant because, "I have to work long hours and can't be there. She might be a mother, but she is still a teenager. The baby was all right with her before, because he would sleep with her and she could feed him when he cried and then go back to sleeping or talking on the phone. She doesn't have a good sense of time."

The team (social worker, doctor, and nurse) felt placement in a facility, at least for a while, might be the best thing for this family. However, the mom didn't. What could we do? I sat down and talked with her for a long time. Earlier in the admission, we assessed that she learned best by doing, but how could we teach her the problem solving and time management skills she would need at home?

The solution was rooming in. She would be here around the clock, providing all the care for her child, using her home equipment, and independently contacting resources as needed. The nursing staff would get involved only if necessary. I wanted to provide her with a tool to help guide her in this endeavor. I knew her ability to read and comprehend was higher than a fifth grade level, so a book of some sort seemed the way to provide all of the information she would need at her fingertips.

I got a binder and placed a cute, colorful cover on the front. I used tabbed dividers to separate each topic. The topics included:

1. Daily schedule (devised in collaboration with mom)
2. Medication information
3. Respiratory information
4. Feeding information
5. Seizure information
6. Therapy information

Each section had all pertinent teaching handouts, equipment brochures, a page listing the most common potential problems, possible solutions, and resources in the form of the business card of each resource. I also included three other sections for business cards, appointments, and her notes.

The rooming in went well. The family was discharged with instructions to take this book to all appointments and add changes to it as necessary until she was comfortable with her unique parenting role. For a long while, I wondered how they were doing and if all my hard work made a difference for them.

About 3 years later, a young woman approached me in the hospital hall and told the young man with her, "This was our nurse when [my son] and I first came here." Trying to act like I knew who she was, I went to the room to see the boy. I saw a big, obviously developmentally delayed boy. He didn't ring a bell. Then I noticed the book on the over-bed table. It was a little smudged and dog-eared but well used by the looks of it. After catching up on her and the child, I asked if the book had been helpful. She opened it and showed me how she had added and deleted as things changed. "I take it everywhere I go. There are so many doctors and medical people in our lives that the information in the book helps to keep everyone from getting screwed up. I even helped one woman at school make one for her and her son."

Models and Illustrations of Anatomy

When you're describing a disease, test, or procedure, you sometimes talk about organs or body parts that are not readily apparent. Models and illustrations of anatomy can help make the abstract visible.

These are expensive, but if your teaching has regularly occurring themes (gastrointestinal or pulmonary system, orthopedics), models and illustrations are a good investment. Models may be realistic or symbolic, like the fabric dolls with removable organs often used in pediatrics. They attract and maintain interest. They show proportions and relationships. They clarify.

Use models to evaluate understanding as well. Ask the learner to use the model or illustration to describe, or pretend to describe, to a significant other what he or she has learned.

Posters

Posters can be used passively, in waiting rooms and hallways, offering information to those who are interested. Even those who are not interested will see that you encourage learning. Posters can also be used in interactive teaching sessions.

Posters can be purchased, or you can make your own. They are inexpensive and don't take long to make. Posters are great tools for summarizing and simplifying information. Consider posters that illustrate and describe topics often taught, like signs and symptoms of infection. Instead, you may consider signs that inspire thought. ("What do you need to know to take care of yourself at home? Ask your nurse." "Do you know what medicines you take, why, and when to take them?") Posters could also show a sequence of events, like how arteries get hard and how to intervene.

If you frequently walk patients up and down a specific hall after surgery, consider hanging posters along the way that announce distances ("You're halfway down the hall already!") or benefits of exercise ("Walking gets the gut moving!"). These can provide topics for discussion, reinforce teaching, and distract from discomfort.

Displays and Bulletin Boards

Displays and bulletin boards are similar to posters. Bulletin boards are most often used informally, in halls or waiting rooms. Both may present more information in smaller print than posters. Displays and bulletin boards are easy to update and can include small three-dimensional objects. Both may be used passively or actively.

Filmstrips and Slide-Tape Programs

Filmstrips are a length of film containing still photographs, illustrations, diagrams, or charts arranged in order, to be projected on a monitor, wall, or screen one at a time. They may be accompanied by an audiotape. Slide-tape programs coordinate sounds with the images. The projectors are relatively inexpensive, and they are easy to store.

You can buy both filmstrips and slide-tape programs. Slides and audiotapes can be inexpensive to create and easy to update. They may be used in groups or with individual learners. A learner can be taught how to use the projector and can study the contents at his or her own pace. They can be good teaching tools for some learners with low literacy skills.

Overhead Transparencies

Transparencies are best for teaching small or large groups. To use them, you will also need a projector and blank wall or screen. They come clear and in color, with or without frames.

Transparencies can be created on a photocopy machine from printed text or illustrations. They can also be hand written or drawn ahead of time or at the time of the presentation. They are very easy to update and rearrange, if necessary, even at the time of presentation.

Transparencies highlight key points well. Print should be large, with no more than four to six lines per sheet. Don't project the details, discuss them. Use transparencies with the lights on, so your audience will not fall asleep.

When using transparencies for a presentation, make sure you have a spare bulb, just in case the one in the projector goes out. Before the audience arrives, clean and focus the projector. Don't cover up parts of the transparency—it's distracting. Instead, use a separate transparency for each point, and if possible, illustrate each point with a reinforcing image. If you are going to speak for a while without changing transparencies, turn off the projector so the image does not distract the audience.

If you find you are using a lot of transparencies in a single presentation, check to see if you are presenting too much information.

Flip Charts

Use flip charts to present simple concepts in order and to summarize teaching. Flip charts use color and illustrations well. If you create them yourself, flip charts are easy to individualize and update.

Flip charts can be large for teaching groups or small enough to stand on a table top for individual teaching. Flip charts can be prepared ahead of time or written on at the time of teaching.

Do you want to look cool by writing and drawing the flip chart pages in front of the group? On the chart pages, write yourself reminders of what you want to discuss in very small, pale print at your eye level. You'll appear brilliant (unless you have trouble reading your own handwriting).

Small flip charts can be 8½ × 11-inch paper pads or stand-up binders of prepared materials. Each sheet can be placed in a plastic page protector so the flip chart can be used many times and still look fresh.

Chalkboards or White Boards

Boards are for teaching groups. They are best used if you need to show development or flow of connected information and everything you need to present can fit clearly on the board at the same time.

Even if on wheels, boards are not easily portable. You also need to be able to talk to the audience and write at the same time.

Audiotapes

Have you ever used an audiotape for teaching? They have the following advantages:

- Reliable
- Small and easy to transport
- Easy to use
- Easy and inexpensive to make and duplicate
- Adaptable to many environments (battery or AC power)

Many people have access to tape players. They can be used with or without headphones. Audiotapes can be individualized to reinforce facts, give directions, or provide support. They can be played over and over.

Audiotapes are good for the following learners:

- Those who are vision impaired
- Those with low literacy skills, especially when combined with a handout or booklet with pictures
- Those who speak in a foreign language or dialect, if you can make a tape in that language or dialect
- Those who prefer to listen
- Those who need standardized or introductory instructions

Audiotapes can be played in the following ways:

- On a tape player
- As a recorded phone message
- Over a public address system
- Over the radio

To be effective, the learner needs to know the language in which the audiotape is recorded and must be able to understand the message and follow spoken directions.

Doak, Doak, and Root (1996) give detailed directions on how to create an audiotape for effective patient and family education. These same criteria can be use for evaluating audiotapes you purchase from other sources.

Research indicates that audiotapes work best when the objectives are limited, focus on behaviors, and are interactive. You can make audiotapes interactive using a dialogue of questions and answers with a booklet or picture sheet the learner can mark in response to questions or cues on the tape. Listeners tend to lose interest after 5 minutes, so tapes should be 5 minutes long or less.

The following summarizes the steps for creating a tape:

1. Decide your topic, such as "nutrition for diabetics" or "how to stop smoking."
2. Decide your purpose. What behavior do you want to change?
3. Consult with learners. What information do they want the audiotape to address?
4. Address the essential points so the learner thinks through the change in this order:
   - I perceive that I am personally at risk, and the risk is serious.
   - I see a way to reduce my risk, and I believe I will benefit if I do it.
   - The barriers (such as pain or cost) are not too high for me to do it.

   Any information that does not support one of these three points is superfluous.
5. Write a statement defining the key message. State this at the beginning and the end of the tape. Write a rough outline of the topics to be covered and who speaks on them.
6. Choose two people to record the message as a dialogue. Get signed written releases from every person heard on the tape. Read the opening statement, and then have a conversation, following the outlined topics. Have an ordinary, natural conversation with short chunks, incomplete sentences, interruptions, repeating part of what the previous speaker said, and expressing either understanding or problems understanding.

7. End with the key message.
8. Play back the audiotape and revise it, if necessary.
9. Test the audiotape with a few learners. What are their reactions? Revise the audiotape, if necessary.

If you want to turn a handout or booklet into an audiotape, use the same process. Do not read the contents of the written material, but use it as your source for facts. Leave out any information that does not fit in with step 4.

Teach the smallest amount necessary to do the job.

For more details on how to create quality audiotapes and use them effectively with learners, see pages 129 to 143 of Doak et al. (1996).

Another way to use this tool is to audiotape teaching discussions and give the tape to the patient and family (Foltz & Sullivan, 1996). Minimal time is spent preparing the audiotape, and the learner has an individualized teaching tool.

Videotapes

Most of your learners are familiar with watching television. This will make it both easier and more difficult to teach with videotapes. On one hand, your learners are used to watching the monitor. On the other hand, they are used to entertaining productions made with high technical quality. These features include good acting, directing, sound, light, camera work, animation, text, and editing. Learners' expectations for videotapes may be quite high. Keep this in mind if you plan to make your own teaching videos.

Videotapes are a familiar teaching medium. Mail order companies sell them, and drug reps give them away. Hospitals use them in house (Rankin & Stallings, 1996) and for outreach programs (Clabots & Dolphin, 1992). Health maintenance organizations offer them to their enrollees as a perk (Borzo, 1994). Producers have even marketed teaching videos directly to learners in drug stores (Symons, 1996). Teaching videos cover the full range of topics, including diagnoses, treatments, home care, and health promotion. More titles come out every day.

Doak and Doak (1998) say that the way you present a videotape to a learner can make it more effective. Before you show a videotape, tell the learner the following:

1. Identify the purpose of the video and how the learner will benefit from it.
2. Point out what to look for in the video, with cues to help the learner know when this information appears. (For example, "After the baby cries, watch how the mom sets up the breastfeeding pump.")
3. After the video, come back in the room to answer any questions.

Following are qualities of a good teaching videotape:

- Is between 5 and 20 minutes long or 30 minutes if very engaging
- Role models desired behaviors
- Uses clear, direct, and accurate language
- Is entertaining; flows or tells a story
- Uses vocabulary below an eighth grade level with little medical jargon
- Keeps text on screen long enough to be read
- Addresses real-life situations, including emotional and social issues
- Shows how to solve problems; answers learner's questions
- Teaches only basic facts
- Uses dialogue instead of monologue
- Comes with prepared interactive activities, or can be easily created and inserted about every 5 minutes
- Uses culturally appropriate concepts and images; shows people like your learners
- Emphasizes what to do, instead of what not to do; is functionally appropriate
- Is paced appropriately for your learners (slower for older audiences, faster for adolescents)

Upon the birth of my first child, I decided I wanted to breastfeed instead of bottle-feed. I had a C-section and was sent home with my gorgeous, yet jaundiced, newborn son. Breastfeeding did not go well in the hospital, yet no one seemed concerned and thought I would just supplement feed him formula. I was sent home with videotapes on parenting and breastfeeding full of perfect mothers with breasts engorged and overflowing with milk, with infants who had no trouble at all with the task of feeding. My son, of course, had no patience with such activity since bottles poured out the formula with little effort, and no patience for the gas the formula gave him in the late evening. Nothing on these tapes was beneficial to me for they taught things I already knew from my nursing school education or were pure fiction. I am sure many women have watched these tapes and cried while thinking their experience should be so easy.

—a learner and RN

This points out many issues. No teaching tools, including videotapes, can replace the educator. Always follow up videotapes with conversation. If teaching tools are sent home with the learner, provide the telephone number of a health care professional who can answer questions. Better yet, follow up with a phone call. This learner was postpartum with her first child, recovering from surgery and childbirth, and was probably exhausted. Don't make assumptions, even when your learner is a health care professional. She was a learner, like any other new mom. In this case, the role modeling demonstrated in the video did not match the learner's experience, and she became discouraged and frustrated.

A videotape that looks great may not be appropriate for your learners. Doak et al. (1996) suggest you field test each video with a small sample of your patient population to see how it is understood and accepted. Find out if the video successfully presents what you want to communicate. You may also objectively evaluate a videotape using the Suitability Assessment of Materials instrument, designed for use with written materials. This tool is offered and discussed in detail in Chapter 8.

In general, videotapes that instruct can hold attention for 8 minutes. Videotapes with drama, scene changes, or humor can hold attention up for to 30 minutes, but these are rare. Viewers with low literacy skills lose interest in 4 to 6 minutes. Active involvement should occur about every 5 minutes. If a videotape lasts longer than 8 minutes, stop the tape at a good spot within 4 to 8 minutes, and involve the learner in an interactive activity. Discuss the key points or behaviors addressed in the video. Have the learner answer a few questions, presented in word or picture format, on a worksheet. You may use any of the activities listed in Chapter 6.

If you want to create your own videotape, keep in mind that they are expensive to produce, take a great deal of effort and time, and can be outdated quickly. (If the procedures and supplies don't change, fashion will.) If at all possible, use a professional production company. Learners' expectations for quality are high, and amateur productions may be easily criticized. Obtain a grant, if you can. Consider asking for a donation of production time or supplies, but keep in mind that volunteer producers may put paying jobs first.

All the nurses in our department worked on the script. They consulted with nurses around the country to make sure the content was universal, so they could sell the tape. Someone with a video studio offered to make the tape for us for free. We interviewed patients and families of various cultural backgrounds and got some very good footage. Taping of the procedures went wonderfully, but editing took forever, because the producer ignored our mutually agreed upon deadlines. Then he stopped returning our calls. His secretary made up excuses. Five years later, we have a partially edited video with outdated procedures and supplies, and families asking to see the video they were in. The time and efforts of a lot of nurses were wasted.

This personal experience is not meant to discourage you but to alert you to potential problems. With good planning, enough resources, and a cohesive team, you can create quality teaching videotapes. Maller, Twitty, and Sauve (1997) had great success with the video they created and showed to patients before surgery. They made this videotape available for viewing at home, in hospital clinics, in patient rooms, and in rural outreach clinics. They found that this delivery of available, accessible, and consistent information improved patient outcomes.

The steps for creating a videotape are similar to creating an audiotape. This is a general outline. It may differ slightly from your production company's procedure:

1. Decide your topic, such as "how to change a CVC dressing" or "cardiac catheterization."
2. Decide your purpose. What behavior do you want to change?
3. Consult with learners. What information do they want to see addressed in the video?
4. Address the essential points so the learner thinks through the change in this order:
   - I perceive that I am personally at risk, and the risk is serious.
   - I see a way to reduce my risk, and I believe I will benefit if I do it.
   - The barriers (such as pain or cost) are not too high for me to do it.

   Any information that does not support one of these three points is superfluous.
5. Write a statement defining the key message. State this at the beginning and the end of the tape. Write a rough outline of the topics to be covered and who speaks on them.

6. Write script (dialogue, not lecture), with text, visual components, format, timing, and transitions, like fade-ins and fade-outs. End with the key message. Computer software is available to facilitate script writing. Some are interactive programs, and some less expensive options are merely templates for use with your word processor. Remember to keep the script short. Show; don't tell. Add interest by changing the camera's view to flow with the content. Use the visual part of the medium. Maller et al. (1997) outline their video script in detail.

7. Have clinical experts review the contents for accuracy and clarity.

8. Plan props: what they'll be, where they'll be, how they'll be used, and how they should be filmed.

9. If you are planning to translate and dub the video in Spanish, remember that Spanish takes one-and-a-half times longer than English to say the same message. Leave enough time in the video portion to fit the Spanish dubbing, and speak the English slowly.

10. Plan graphics of summary terms or labels, using few simple words and large print that contrasts clearly with background color.

11. Choose at least two people to have a dialogue. Get signed written releases from every person seen or heard on the tape. Have them practice the script, with activities.

12. Videotape the speakers, the use of props, the activities, and the images several times, if possible. Have clinical experts available during the taping to ensure accuracy.

13. Edit the video to flow smoothly and clearly. Add the graphics.

14. Prepare the interactive activities to use with learners viewing the tape.

15. Test the videotape and activities with a few learners. What are their reactions? Revise the videotape, if necessary.

Closed Circuit Television

One way to show teaching videos is over closed circuit television (CCTV). Many systems exist. Videos may be shown on a schedule or on demand. To show purchased videos on these systems, make sure you buy the rights for broadcasting when you purchase the tapes.

Topics appropriate for CCTV should be those with many potential viewers, such as magnetic resonance imaging, how to stop smoking, and nutrition for a healthy heart. A bored patient may turn on the education channel for distraction. An inquisitive patient with little tolerance for talk shows and soap operas may seek them out.

"I always catch the teenage boys watching those breastfeeding films meant for new moms!"

—an RN

Closed circuit television may seem easier than using a video cassette recorder (VCR), but it still takes some effort to link your learner with the right video. If you want a learner to see a specific video, you need to read the schedule and plan for it or schedule the on-demand system.

Closed circuit television teaches passively, more like television than teaching videos. CCTV cannot be stopped and started to individualize time for interactive activities, nor can it be rewound and replayed as needed. If you ask your learner to watch a video on CCTV, be sure to follow it up with a discussion.

Satellite Systems

Satellite systems expand and elaborate the concept of CCTV. They offer teaching videos on demand; live video and audio interaction between learner and health care provider at different sites; and on-line evaluation of knowledge through multiple-choice tests, using a computer. The technology is currently available but expensive.

Telephone

Since the first time a patient called a doctor for advice, telephones have been used as tools for patient and family education. Many people own telephones or have access to them and know how to operate them. (We often assume all people have and use phones, but this is not true.) This tool can be used in one of two ways: The learner can initiate the telephone contact, or the health care professional can call the learner.

Telephone calls are initiated by the learner for various reasons:

• To get the answer to a question
• For reassurance
• For clarification
• For assistance

Examples include calling the following:

- A health advice service staffed by nurses
- A poison control or suicide hotline
- A pharmacist to find out what to do if an extra dose was taken by mistake
- A recorded message with information on a specific medical problem

You can purchase equipment that makes audiotapes available to learners with touch-tone telephones. Grandinetti (1996) describes a Parent Advice Line that provides recorded messages on 300 health care topics for parents. Each message starts warning parents to call 911 or their physician if the child is seriously ill and states the information is not a substitute for medical care.

Telephone calls are initiated by a health care professional for the following reasons:

- To gather information before a test or procedure
- To follow up after test, procedure, or discharge
- To evaluate understanding and application of knowledge
- With a reminder

Examples include the following:

- To find out how a newly diagnosed diabetic is doing with medications and diet
- To obtain a brief health history before a test
- To inform that it is time for a mammogram or flu shot

Telephones can be inexpensively used to involve, inform, and support learners with a brief interaction. The visual privacy of telephones may help some learners feel more comfortable asking questions. Telephones can reach learners in distant rural locations, those who are homebound, and those with low literacy skills.

On the other hand, much communication is nonverbal, and that dimension is absent in telephone conversations. Phone calls may seem impersonal, and some may view a call as an invasion of privacy. Those who cannot use telephones for whatever reason cannot be reached at all with this tool.

Dolls and Models

Are you thinking it would insult an adult to teach with a doll? When was the last time you renewed your cardiopulmonary resuscitation (CPR) certification? Did you practice and demonstrate your skill on a doll?

Some skills, like blood glucose monitoring, don't need the added step of using a doll or model. However, if anxiety or risk of potentially injurious errors is high, a doll or model can be quite useful for learning the basics and building confidence.

Learners feel safe learning and practicing skills on dolls and models. In addition to CPR, dolls can be used to practice maintenance of nasogastric tubes, gastrointestinal tubes, central lines, and buttons. Models can be used to teach skills like breast and testicular self-exams.

Anatomically correct dolls and models can be expensive but worthwhile if they are used often enough. Kennis (1996) describes how to create your own teaching dolls. Rankin and Stallings (1996) explain how one nurse made a breast model from a nylon stocking stuffed with cotton socks and Styrofoam particles as lumps.

Sculptures With Discussion Cues

"How or what can you say or do to discharge someone humorously?"
—an RN

Imagine, at discharge, sitting down with the learner and placing an odd sculpture on the table between you. Its base is a square of wood, and it has a stick up the middle. Glued on this stick are a variety of objects: a medicine bottle, a fork and knife, an appointment slip, a telephone, an old shoe, a threaded needle, a row of staples, and a bottle of aspirin.

Then you ask the learner what each item has to do with going home. Use the items as cues to discuss medications, diet, follow-up appointments, when to call the doctor, activity, care of stitches or staples, and pain management. Evaluate understanding, and fill in information as needed. Give the learner a written copy of the instructions.

The same sculpture technique can be used to cue conversations on admissions and preoperative preparation. You could paint the wood red, and glue on a match, a balloon, a thermometer, and a rubber finger with a nail through it. The topic is the signs and symptoms of infection: redness, heat, swelling, fever, and pain. Be creative. The opportunities for sculptures of conversation cues are unlimited.

Interactive Activities

The activities listed in Chapter 6, such as flash cards, puzzles, and games, are also tools for teaching. Return demonstrations are discussed in detail in Chapter 13, which looks at ways to evaluate learning. Other interactive activities include role playing and contests.

Hussey (1994) found that color-coded picture medication schedules were effective with learners with low literacy skills. After each dose was taken, the patient crossed off the picture. When the last set was taken, the patient erased the marks from the plastic protector and started over.

Nurses also use themselves as teaching tools in interpersonal activities. Sometimes our colleagues can be teaching tools too.

> We were teaching a mom about SQ shots for her infant. We did all the basic techniques: opening the syringe, cleaning the vial, drawing up the med, choosing a site. Then I ordered an orange from dietary so she could practice on something with texture. By that afternoon mom was good at SQ shots on oranges, but fearful of giving them to her baby. She couldn't do it. She said it was too different on a real person. Painful. So I talked to two peers, and the three of us walked in, rolled up our sleeves, and told her to give each of us an SQ shot of NS right then. She was scared but did it. That night she gave her baby the injection. No problems.

Clearly, teaching tools available to you are limited only by your imagination, creativity, and willingness to take calculated risks.

Computers and Videodiscs

Computers have many applications as tools for patient and family education. Use them to create handouts and booklets. Use them to access information from other health care providers, information databases, CD-ROMs, and the world wide web. They can illustrate medical information in two dimensions, video and audio, or even virtual reality, with the feel of three dimensions. They can be used interactively for computer-assisted instruction, tutorials, simulations, and games. They can test knowledge through quizzes and provide immediate feedback. They can be used for group presentations to project images, words, or video clips. Computers can also be used to disseminate information through documentation, e-mails, or websites.

Chapter 9 details the many uses for computers in patient and family education.

Learning Contracts

The ultimate goal of patient and family education is to improve health outcomes. Learning contracts increase commitment to both the educational process and behavior changes that enhance health. When a learner applies new behaviors, like drinking less alcohol, his or her health will benefit.

Learning contracts can be informal or formal. One example of an informal learning contract is when the learner tells you what, when, and how often he or she will perform a new behavior. The act of telling you increases the learner's commitment to follow through.

Another example of an informal contract is illustrated in Figure 7-1. This Education Care Path for Congestive Heart Failure describes a plan for teaching and includes a place for the learner to document weight, an important indicator in this diagnosis. This form can be used to establish mutual goals if the plan is reviewed and adjusted before teaching begins.

Formal contracts are mutually agreed upon, written, and signed. They work best when the learner is motivated but having trouble maintaining a behavior change. The learner can contract with himself or herself, using the health care provider as an advisor and support. The formality enhances motivation for behavior change. Family members can also be involved in supporting the learner in behavior changes. If so, they should sign the contract too.

These contracts can be used for all sorts of purposes, such as to promote weight change or exercise; decrease self-destructive behaviors, such as cigarette, alcohol, or drug use; or improve self-care management in chronic illnesses, such as diabetes or hypertension. See Box 7-1 for a possible format for a written contract.

A good behavior change contract is mutually agreed upon and includes the following:

- A clear and specific measurable goal
- Clear and specific measurable behaviors to be performed (with complex behaviors broken down into small steps), defining who, what, when, and where
- What reinforcements will be used, defining who, what, when, and where
- A clear and specific description of who will do what if the agreed upon behaviors are not performed
- A clear and specific description of who will do what if the agreed upon behaviors are performed beyond expectations
- Specific dates for start, renewal, modification, and end of agreement
- A copy of the signed contract for everyone involved

EDUCATION CARE PATH
FOR CONGESTIVE HEART FAILURE

FIRST DAY

Receive your education packet.

Review Care Path with your Doctor and care givers.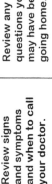

Your Weight Today

Write down any questions you or your family may have.

SECOND DAY

Watch CHF video.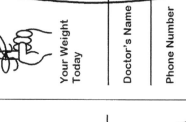

Discuss a low salt diet if ordered by your doctor.

Your Weight Today

Read Handouts in packet.

THIRD DAY

Learn about the signs and symptoms of CHF.

Learn about any medicines you will be taking at home.

Your Weight Today

Review any questions.

FOURTH DAY

Learn about activity and rest.

Review signs and symptoms and when to call your doctor.

Your Weight Today

Review any questions you may have.

FIFTH DAY

Review medicines.

Review any questions you may have before going home.

Your Weight Today

Doctor's Name

Phone Number

Figure 7-1 This care path is intended as a *possible* guide and time table. The information in this packet is not intended

BOX 7-1   **Possible Format for a Written Contract**

Goal: (*clear and specific measurable goal*)
Starting on (*date*),
I, (*learner's name*), agree to (*who, what, when, and where*) and if I do, to be rewarded with (*who, what, when, and where*) or if I do not, to pay the price of (*who, what, when, and where*).
If I succeed beyond the goal, I will be rewarded with (*who, what, when, and where*).
I will continue this contract until (*date*). At that time, I will review the goals, behaviors, rewards, and costs of this contract and adjust them, if necessary.
This contract will end on (*date*).
Signed: (*learner*)
Signed: (*health care provider or support person*)
Signed: (*family member, if applicable*)

Reinforcements should be meaningful to the learner. If successful, money or time could be spent on a treat (movie, book, meal out). If unsuccessful, money or time could be given to charity (either one the learner supports or one the learner does not support). The greatest reward, however, is self-management success and meeting the goal of improved health outcome.

Patient Education Programs

Often, when nurses talk about "patient education," they are referring to coordinated patient education programs. However, programs are specialized and comprise only a fraction of teaching actually done by nurses. A patient education program organizes and coordinates the teaching plan and tools for a specific population that shares a health experience, like arthritis, diabetes, cardiac rehabilitation, or childbirth.

Lorig (1996) describes in great detail how to develop such a program, with assessment, planning, implementation, and evaluation. Assessment includes defining the population that will be taught and determining the group's needs for information. Planning includes determining objectives, content, process, and materials and getting participants. Implementation is putting on the program and documenting it, and evaluation determines whether the goals have been met.

Programs may use group classes or progressive programmed instruction and often add an individualized one-on-one teaching component. Patient education programs have a wide variety of structures, because different populations have different needs.

Patient education group programs are only feasible if the population is large enough for new groups to begin as they're needed. For example, pregnancy occurs often enough to support teaching programs. On the other hand, the frequency of prenatally diagnosed multiple suture synostosis (Kleeblattschädel or cloverleaf skull) may not justify a group class. However, a clinical nurse specialist who works with a pediatric neurosurgeon may develop a collection of teaching materials on the diagnosis and treatment of multiple suture synostosis to use as the need arises.

Resources for Self-Motivated Learning

Many patients and families cope with stress by striving to understand what is happening and why and what they can do about it. Many are becoming health care consumers, taking an active role in looking for cutting-edge, complementary, and alternative treatments. These are super teachable moments! How are we, busy health care providers, taking advantage of these impulses to facilitate learning?

> *"Instead of 'telling' people everything they need to know, adults could be directed to alternative resources and given direction about how to find out what they may want or need to know. Formal instruction may be a part of the learning project along with other activities. Such an approach to patient education could facilitate relevant learning by providing structure to the learning process while simultaneously encouraging active learner participation."*
>
> —Tripp, 1987, page 174

So we need to provide the resources or direct learners to them; we need to provide structure for learning. These resources could include all the teaching tools described previously, plus the following:

- Self-learning modules
- Workbooks, with frequent review and self-tests
- Books, magazines, newsletters, and journals
- Bibliographies
- Lists of world wide web and internet resources
- Lists of local and national groups:
  - Support groups (like Alcoholics Anonymous)
  - Advocacy groups (like Planned Parenthood)
  - Community agencies (like Catholic Social Services)
  - Disease-specific groups (like the American Lung Association)

- Professional groups (like the local medical association)
- Health-promotion groups (like the American Red Cross)
- Government agencies (like the Department of Health and Human Services)
- Consumer health libraries
- Public libraries
- Academic libraries

"Health professionals could approach 'patient education' as a learning project and help adults choose, plan, and implement various learning activities relevant to and appropriate for particular learners in particular situations."

—Tripp, 1987, page 174

Assessment of the learner's readiness and motivation to learn is essential before suggesting self-directed learning. Learners have a range of knowledge, understanding, and problem-solving skills. To take advantage of self-directed learning, the learner needs to know enough to be able to articulate questions to search for answers. Learners need to be able to understand the information they find, evaluate its quality, and deal with conflicting information. They will need the help of health care providers to accomplish this.

"Self-directed learning takes time in order to plan and implement the learning project."

—Tripp, 1987, page 168

The degree of planning, preparation of resources, and assistance provided depends on how quickly the information is needed (is surgery scheduled for tomorrow?), how complicated the questions and answers are, and how much information is available on the subject.

When the medical problem is chronic, there is less urgency and less need for structure. One organization created a learning environment filled with a variety of teaching tools in which learners explore and discuss the medical problem of back pain.

"The patients are free to roam the education area and see firsthand what a pinched nerve is, or how an epidural steroid injection is performed. As we continue to grow and expand our office, additions to the Center will include interactive video models and computer-simulated programs."

—Weil, 1996, page 1

The site for self-directed learning can be far more complex and offer several levels of assistance. Kantz et al. (1998) describe a multidimensional learning center at Beth Israel Deaconess Medical Center in Boston. It consists of a consumer health library, services that support patients in learning needed care skills (Health Education for Living Program), and programming that addresses health education needs of the community (Partnerships for Health).

The health information library offers the public free access to books, videotapes, computer programs, and on-line services to promote independent inquiry into health issues. At the clinician's request, staff will also prepare customized information packets for patients. Staff members include nurses, a librarian, researchers, and specially trained volunteers.

The Health Education for Living Program helps patients and families better understand and participate in their care. It includes a learning lab, where nurses teach learners skills, group instruction programs, support and coordination of development, and translation of written materials.

Partnerships for Health helps meet the health education needs of the community by partnering with community agencies, like the local health department and public library.

The facilitation of self-directed learning in health care is a growing field. New sites are developing every day, and as evaluation studies are completed, we will hear more about them.

Documentation Tools

"Buckminster Fuller used to say that if you want to teach people a new way of thinking, don't bother trying to teach them. Instead, give them a tool, the use of which will lead to new ways of thinking."
—Senge et al., 1994, page 28

Because every health care professional is teaching patients and families all the time, the key to collaboration is communication. If your health care team members are not communicating as well as they could be, give them documentation tools that will lead to new ways of thinking. Is your current form multidisciplinary? Does it clearly define what has been taught and what needs to be taught?

"Who do I tell if I think of a way to improve the Education Record?"
—an RN

Speak to your representative on the committee that revises forms, or get on the committee and initiate the necessary changes yourself.

Care is coordinated when all team members know the diagnosis, treatment, and home care needs anticipated. Teaching is faster when the information you teach builds on former knowledge, learning is reinforced, and no mixed messages are sent. Then work is shared, not duplicated.

"Because patient teaching is universally regarded as an important nursing responsibility and will continue to grow in importance, more effort into structure and design for documentation is required. The form it takes can be creatively structured to the needs of the patient, the content to be taught, the learner outcomes that were achieved, and the time constraints of nurses."

—Casey, 1995, page 260

A good documentation form for patient and family education accomplishes the following:

- It organizes communication. It has a place for everything that needs to be communicated and enough space to communicate it.
- It is clear and easy to use. Rating scales and symbols are defined and not ambiguous. Everyone on the health care team can understand the language used on the form.
- It helps all team members focus on the same mutually determined goals.
- It reminds you what needs to be done.
- It helps you build on what others have taught and promotes continuity of teaching.
- It clearly evaluates progress toward goals. It's easy to identify the goals that are not achieved.
- It is accessible to everyone who needs the information.
- It avoids duplication and refers you to other documents, if necessary.
- It is used. A documentation tool doesn't serve its purpose unless it is written on and read, and professional behaviors are determined by the information.

Many organizations have created documentation tools that work for them. Figure 7-2 is the Congestive Heart Failure Checklist from Northwest Medical Center in Minnesota. It lists the video and handout and cues the interactive review of contents. It then lists the specific information the learner needs to know to ensure a safe discharge. Columns cue for review and demonstration of knowledge.

This form is supplemented by Just Do It! Patient Education for CHF Key Teaching Points (Fig. 7-3) from Rapides Regional Medical Center in California. This offers content, tips, and cues for involving other health care team members.

The discharge form from one hospital reinforces documentation of education by including a section for indicating what teaching was not completed as of discharge. This form, with a copy of the education

Northwest Medical Center, Thief River Falls, MN 56701

CONGESTIVE HEART FAILURE CHECKLIST

Patient Name:_____

TEACHING CONTENT:	Date	Initials	Teaching Method	Date Review	Demo	Comments
View CHF Video						
Krames "CHF"						
CHF Handout Reviewed						
Patient will state simple explanation of CHF:						
CHF is a condition which the heart does not pump blood efficiently causing fluids to collect in the lungs and other tissue.						
Patient will be able to list the symptoms of CHF:						
Sudden weight gain (2-5 pounds in 1-4 days)						
Swelling in the ankles, legs or abdomen						
Shortness of breath						
Frequent dry cough						
Feeling of extreme muscle fatigue						
Patient will implement treatment plan:						
Medications by name, dose, and indication. Be able to state schedule and side effects.						
Diet - Decrease sodium intake						
Daily Weight Record						
Rest and Exercise						
Patient will identify importance of follow-up care:						
Patient understands the need for doctor visits and when to report symptoms.						

Teaching Methods:
A = Audiovisual
D = Demonstration
E = Explanation
H = Handout

Source: Northwest Medical Center, Thief River Falls, MN. Reprinted with permission.

Figure 7-2

JUST DO IT!!
PATIENT EDUCATION FOR CHF

KEY TEACHING POINTS

CHF - simple definition
Condition in which the heart doesn't pump as well as it should. Although this condition doesn't go away completely, it can be treated.

Signs and symptoms

➼ Shortness of breath or a cough
➼ Weight gain of 2-3 pounds in 1-2 days
➼ Fatigue
➼ Swelling of feet, ankles or abdomen
➼ Using more pillows at night when sleeping

Before discharge, patients should understand:
➼ Their medications and the importance of taking them as prescribed. Ask pharmacists to assist, if necessary.
➼ A low-salt diet. Ask Food and Nutrition to assist, if necessary.(Note: patients on lithium may have increased or toxic lithium levels when sodium is reduced.)
➼ Importance of daily weights. Teach them to keep a record and report a gain of 2-3 lbs over 1-2 days immediately. Have them weigh at the same time everyday with the same amount of clothing.
➼ Importance of the balance between rest and   activity. (Can PT or RT help the patient? SCC or H/H?)
➼ When to call their doctor or home health nurse. (With onset of any of the signs or symptoms.)

    Reminders: ➼Show CHF video to patient and/or family.
                ➼ Review CHF packet with patient/family.
                   (Available on unit or in Patient Ed.)
                ➼ Ask for questions to assure understanding.
                ➼ DOCUMENT your good job!
                ➼ Use the Education Care Path as a *possible* timetable (in packet).
                ➼ Include other disciplines when applicable.

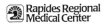
Rapides Regional
Medical Center

Figure 7-3

record, is forwarded to the health care providers who will follow the patient after hospitalization. In addition, patients and families get copies of both the discharge form and the education records. This communicates to everyone involved that teaching is an ongoing team effort.

> *"Another serious obstacle to integration is the time constraints many nurses feel. Higher patient acuities and highly demanding tasks mean that the physical needs of patients take priority over patient education and discharge planning. As already stated, standardized teaching tools can help in overcoming that obstacle. Additionally, they can help nursing staff overcome that relatively common obstacle of not knowing what to teach. If standardized plans highlight or include only the information that must be taught, the nurse is much more likely to be successful in accomplishing the necessary education with the patient."*
>
> —Menke, 1993, page 158

The best documentation forms communicate to caregivers across the continuum. When the learner leaves your care, make sure documentation communicates to the next care provider your evaluations of knowledge and what the learner still needs to know.

Professional Development

> *"Who can teach me how to do patient education better?"*
>
> —an RN

How does your organization support continuing education relating to patient and family education? Are these skills reviewed only at orientation, annually, or not at all? Are your preceptors taught to review skills in patient and family education with orientees? Do you offer inservices on topics in patient and family education? Are patient and family teaching skills taught or reinforced with health care providers who are not nurses?

> *"No matter what kind of form you have, it is hard to get staff to document. I believe this is because they don't know the 'language of education' and need to learn how to describe patient response to teaching. For example, they learn how to chart on an infiltrated IV because they have been taught that, and they need to be taught how to describe the educational process."*
>
> —an RN

One hospital used a performance-based development system during orientation to evaluate a nurse's ability to teach planned sessions. The nurse was asked to identify a teaching need, assess the learner, then prepare, teach, and evaluate the session. This is nice but not relevant to actual practice. Staff nurses in this organization rarely, if ever, had an opportunity to apply formal teaching in practice. There was no time for a nurse to plan, prepare, and implement an hour teaching session with a patient and family. This system measured a skill that wasn't used.

The hospital then changed its orientation. It shifted the focus of the evaluation from formal to informal teaching skills. In the new system, the nurse was observed during nursing practice and was evaluated on skills in listening, assessment, team involvement, teaching, evaluation, and documentation of teaching. This approach evaluated teaching skills that were actually used.

This new approach also clearly communicated to staff nurses the level and degree of patient and family education expected. In addition to orientation, the annual evaluations of performance considered continuing commitment to teaching.

Do you want more information on how to keep your staff up to date? Box 7-2 offers two resources that address continuing professional education in patient and family education skills.

BOX 7-2   **Professional Resources**

Patient Education Management Newsletter
American Health Consultants
3525 Piedmont Road, NE
Building Six
Suite 400
Atlanta, GA 30305
800-668-2421
fax: 800-284-3291
e-mail: custserv@ahcpub.com
http://www.ahcpub.com

The Exchange: A forum for patient and family educators
Krames Communications free newsletter
1100 Grundy Lane
San Bruno, CA 94066-9820
650-742-0400

Storing Your Teaching Tools

"We are not living in the best of all possible worlds. Not only are we overwhelmed by the sheer amount of information, most of us are also hampered by an education that inadequately trains us to process it."
—Wurman, 1989, page 15

"Where do I find the doll to do trach teaching?"
—an RN

As described in Chapter 3, an organized teaching environment can significantly help facilitate teaching. Someone or some group of people needs to be responsible and held accountable for storing and maintaining teaching tools, or they will fall into disarray in no time.

How do you organize teaching tools so you can find them? It depends on your patient population, your collection of tools, and your space. Here are three ways you may consider:

1. Location. Keep all teaching tools in one space, or keep teaching tools near related items, such as handouts on managing fever near thermometers and medication handouts in the medication room.
2. Alphabet. File handouts and other teaching materials alphabetically by title.
3. Category. Keep items in a similar category together. For example, organize items by disease, with all the asthma teaching tools together and all the nutrition tools in another place. Instead, you could organize teaching materials by the five-category system (1. diagnosis, disease, illness; 2. diagnostic test, examination; 3. medication; 4. procedure, treatment, home care; and 5. health promotion).

Individualizing Your Teaching Tools

Conversations are the Swiss Army Knife of patient and family education. Use them to assess, individualize, teach, and evaluate. Doak and Doak (1998) suggest you ask the learner questions. When learners paraphrase key information in their own words, they understand it better. They also suggest that you add relevant examples. For example, when a patient had trouble understanding her degenerative disc disease, a physician told her to, "think of your spine as a stack of soup cans, and one of the kids moved one a little out of place." Then she understood.

Define jargon, and use measurable terms when possible. Your definition of "excessive bleeding" or "regular bowel movements" may be different than the learner's.

If you don't speak the same language as your learner, get an interpreter. Conversations are too important a teaching tool to miss. How to use an interpreter is detailed in Chapter 10.

"Men have become the tools of their tools."
—Henry David Thoreau
(Aphorisms Galore! [On-line])

Our tools mold our behaviors. Good, readily available teaching tools will inspire health care providers to teach. Tools that lend themselves to interaction will promote active involvement of the learner.

"There are two parts to solving any problem: what you want to accomplish and how you want to do it. . . . You must always ask the question 'What is?' before you ask the question 'How to?'"
—Wurman, 1989, page 81

Assess the learning need, and then individualize your choice of tool to the learner. The quickest way to determine a person's style of learning is to ask, "The last time you wanted to learn something, how did you do it?" Did the person choose a book, a video, or ask an expert? Learners may not be able to tell you what they prefer, but they can tell you what they have chosen in the past. That answer may give you an indication about what sorts of tools might be useful now.

"The channels by which we get information affect not only the form of the information, but our perception of its importance."
—Wurman, 1989, page 312

How formal or informal is your learner? More playful teaching tools, like crossword puzzles or games, are not appropriate for everyone.

"Follow three steps when using media in instruction: preparation, presentation, and review."
—Rankin & Stallings, 1996, page 185

Preparation

Preview and evaluate all teaching materials before you use them. Know the content, and use only materials with correct, accurate information you want to communicate. Tools must communicate clearly to specific learners, with appropriate vocabulary. The more closely the images reflect your learners, the more your learners will identify with the messages.

Presentation

Have the presentation materials you need. Your learner will need a pen, paper, and something on which to lean to take notes. If you're showing a video, you'll need a quiet space and a working VCR.

Review

Review the content that was presented and evaluate whether the learner understands and can apply the information. Some tools may work with your patient population, others may not. One way to evaluate your tools is to look at how well they facilitate teaching. Does the tool help or complicate and confuse? Another way to evaluate teaching tools is to ask your learners what they think of them. Chapter 13 gives more detail about how to evaluate outcomes.

Some Retail Sources for Teaching Tools

Box 7-3 lists some general sources for teaching tools. Putting a list like this in a book is risky; companies move, merge, and go out of business.

Remember, you are responsible for the quality and accuracy of tools with which you choose to teach. Well-made materials may still be written at too high a reading level or have content that is too general to be useful.

You can create your own updated, individualized list of resources for teaching tools if you have computer access to the world wide web. Consult advocacy groups, consumer health groups, and professional organizations for teaching tools on specific diseases and conditions. See Chapter 9 for details on how to search for information. You can also consult professional colleagues across the country to find out what they use.

BOX 7-3 General Sources for Teaching Tools

Anatomical Chart Company
8221 Kimball Avenue
Skokie, IL 60076-2956
1-800-621-7500
fax: 814-674-0211, 847-679-9155
http://www.anatomical.com
Anatomical products, models, CD-ROMs, books, gift items, charts,
   posters, references, chart and poster mountings, T-shirts, mugs
Check Med Patient Education
200 Grandview Avenue
Camp Hill, PA 17011-1706
1-800-451-5797, 717-761-1170
fax: 717-761-0216
Pamphlets, handouts, booklets, drug cards, videos, kits, display cases,
   Spanish teaching materials
Health EDCO
PO Box 21207
Waco, TX 76702-1207
1-800-299-3366 extension 295
fax: 1-888-977-7653
e-mail: sales@wrsgroup.com
http://www.wrsgroup.com
Models, graphics, posters, teaching materials, videos, slides, booklets
Krames Communications
1100 Grundy Lane
San Bruno, CA 94066-3030
1-800-333-3032
fax: 1-650-244-4512
http://www.krames.com
Pamphlets, booklets and handouts, display cases, imprinting
   available, Spanish teaching materials
Milner-Fenwick, Inc.
2125 Greenspring Drive
Timmonium, MD 21093
1-800-432-8433, 410-252-1700
fax: 410-252-6316
e-mail: patiented@milner-fenwick.com
http://www.milner-fenwick.com
Videos, booklets, books, catalog, preview, closed captioning,
   imprinting and customization available, Spanish teaching materials

Box 7-3 *(Continued)*

Wellness Reproductions & Publishing Inc.
  23945 Mercantile Road
  Suite W9
  Beachwood, OH 44122-5924
  1-800-669-9208
  fax: 1-800-501-8120
  e-mail: WRI@wellness-resources.com
  http://www.wellness-resources.com
  Posters, card games, activities, books, activity worksheets, journals,
    note pads
Maxishare
  PO Box 2041
  Milwaukee, WI 53201
  1-800-444-7747, 1-414-266-2205
  fax: 1-414-266-3443
  e-mail: maxishare@chw.org
  Brochures, videos, handouts
Mosby's Patient Teaching Guides
  11830 Westline Industrial Drive
  PO Box 46908
  St. Louis, MO 63146-9934
  Handouts, disk, software, binder, illustrated
United Ad Label Company, Inc.
  650 Columbia Street
  PO Box 2216
  Brea, CA 92822-2216
  1-800-423-4643
  fax: 1-800-962-0658
  e-mail: c_s@ualco.com
  http://www.ualco.com
  Brochures, handouts, labels, signs, badges, pediatric, bandages,
    teaching materials, videos
Parlay International
  Box 8817
  Emeryville, CA 94662-0817
  1-800-457-2752, 510-601-1000
  fax: 510-601-1008
  http://www.parlay.com
  Kopy Kit, handouts, posters, displays, graphics, brochures, imprinting
    available, displays

Box 7-3 *(Continued)*

Pritchett & Hull Associates, Inc.
3440 Oakcliff Road NE, Suite 110
Atlanta, GA 30340-3079
1-800-218-0781
fax: 1-800-774-4315
Flip cards, teaching sheets, handouts, CD-ROM, slides, booklets,
Spanish teaching materials

If you want to learn more:

(1998). Integrating patient education into the continuum of care. *The Exchange: A Forum for Patient and Family Educators, 1*(2), 1–2.

(1998). Streamline CHF education to cover all points. *Patient Education Management, 5*(1), 6.

(1998). *Patient education.* Springhouse, PA: Springhouse Corporation.

Aphorisms Galore! (1998). [On-line] www.aphorismsgalore.com

Borzo, G. (1994). CIGNA gives new life to patient empowerment initiative. *American Medical News, 37*(35), 1–3.

Brass Tacks Quotations, [On-line] www.brasstacks.org/quotes.html

Breckon, D.J. (1982). *Hospital health education: A guide to program development.* Rockville, MD: Aspen.

Casey, F.S. (1995). Documenting patient education: A literature review. *The Journal of Continuing Education in Nursing, 26*(6), 257–260.

Charney, C., & Conway, K. (1998). *The trainer's tool kit.* New York City: AMACOM, American Management Association.

Clabots, R.B., & Dolphin, D. (1992). The multilingual videotape project: Community involvement in a unique health education program. *Public Health Reports, 107*(1), 75–80.

De Long, R.L. (1995). This path has pictures. *RN, 58*(9), 44–46.

Deck, M.L. (1995). *Instant teaching tools for health care educators.* St. Louis, MO: Mosby Year-Book, Inc.

Deck, M.L. (1997). *More instant teaching tools for health care educators.* St. Louis, MO: Mosby Year-Book, Inc.

Dickstein, R., Greenfield, L., & Rosen, J. (1997). Using the world wide web at the reference desk. *Computers in Libraries, 17*(8), 61–65.

Doak, C.C., & Doak, L.G. (1998). *Tailoring instructions for patients: Benefits and methods.* San Bruno, CA: Krames.

Doak, C.C., Doak, L.G., & Root, J.H. (1996). *Teaching patients with low literacy skills* (2nd ed.). Philadelphia: Lippincott-Raven.

Falvo, D.R. (1994). *Effective patient education: A guide to increased compliance* (2nd ed.). Gaithersburg, MD: Aspen Publishers, Inc.

Foltz, A., & Sullivan, J. (1996). Reading level, learning presentation preference, and desire for information among cancer patients. *Journal of Cancer Education, 11*(1), 32–38.

Giloth, B.E. (Ed.) (1993). *Managing hospital-based patient education.* American Hospital Publishing.

Grandinetti, D. (1996). Teaching patients to take care of themselves. *Medical Economics, 73*(22), 83–91.

Hussey, L.C. (1994). Minimizing effects of low literacy on medication knowledge and compliance among the elderly. *Clinical Nursing Research, 3*(2), 132–146.

Joint Commission on Accreditation of Healthcare Organizations (1998). *1998 Hospital Accreditation Standards.* Oakbrook Terrace, IL: Joint Commission on Accreditation of Healthcare Organizations.

Kantz, B., Wandel, J., Fladger, A., Folcarelli, P., Burger, S., & Clifford, J.C. (1998). Developing patient and family education services. *Journal of Nursing Administration, 28*(2), 11–18.

Kennis, N. (1996). Maximize your patient teaching potential. *RN, 59*(2), 21–23.

London, F. (1995). Getting the most out of patient teaching videos. *Nursing95, 25*(10), 31J.

Lorig, K. (1996). *Patient education: A practical approach.* Thousand Oaks, CA: Sage Publications.

Maller, C.E., Twitty, V.J., & Sauve, A. (1997). A video approach to interactive patient education. *Journal of PeriAnesthesia Nursing, 12*(2), 82–88.

Menke, K.L. (1993). Linking patient education with discharge planning. In B. E. Giloth (Eds.), *Managing hospital-based patient education* (pp. 153–164). Chicago, IL: American Hospital Publishing.

Moeller, K.A. (1997). Consumer health libraries: A new diagnosis. *Library Journal, July*, 36–38.

Piskurich, G.M. (1994). Developing self-directed learning. *Training and Development, March*, 31–36.

Rankin, S.H., & Stallings, K.D. (1996). *Patient education: Issues, principles, practices* (3rd ed.). Philadelphia: Lippincott-Raven.

Redman, B.K. (1997). *The practice of patient education* (8th ed.). St. Louis, MO: Mosby-Year Book, Inc.

Rees, A.M. (1998). *The consumer health information source book* (5th ed.). Phoenix, AZ: Oryx Press.

Senge, P.M., Kleiner, A., Roberts, C., Ross, R.B., & Smith, B.J. (1994). *The fifth discipline fieldbook: strategies and tools for building a learning organization.* New York: Currency.

Soet, J.E., & Basch, C.E. (1997). The telephone as a communication medium for health education. *Health Education & Behavior, 24*(6), 759–773.

Stallings, K.D. (1996). *Integrating patient education in your nursing practice.* Horizon Video Productions.

Symons, A. (1996). Making health info accessible in drug stores. *Drug Store News, 18*(11), 31.

Theis, S.L., & Johnson, J.H. (1995). Strategies for teaching patients: A meta-analysis. *Clinical Nurse Specialist, 9*(2), 100–104.

Tripp, K.R. (1987). *Perspectives on adult learning: Maternal coping with a monitored child in the home.* Unpublished doctoral dissertation, Arizona State University.

Weil, A.J. (1996). *State-of-the-art patient education center opens.* [On-line]. Available: http://www.lowbackpain.com/article2.html.

Whitman, N.I., Graham, B.A., Gleit, C.J., & Boyd, M.D. (1992). *Teaching in nursing practice: A professional model* (2nd ed.). Norwalk, CT: Appleton & Lange.

Winthrop, E. (1995). *Mosby's patient teaching tips.* St. Louis, MO: Mosby-Year Book.

Wurman, R.S. (1989). *Information anxiety: What to do when information doesn't tell you what you need to know* (p. 312). New York: Bantam Books.

Say it in Writing

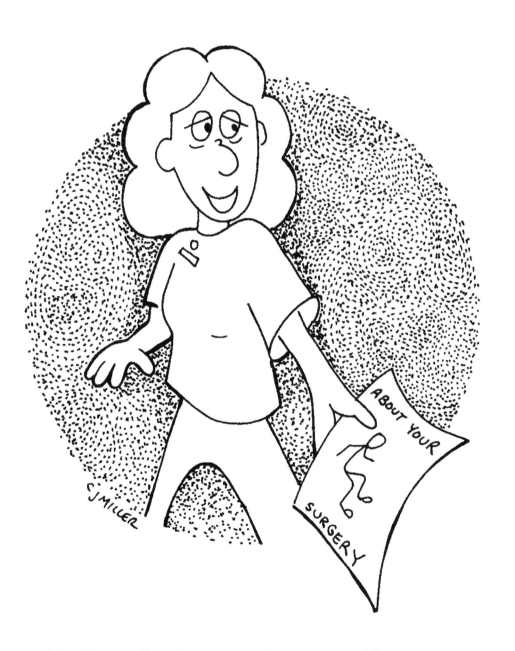

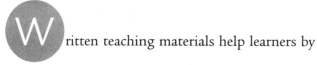

ritten teaching materials help learners by

"improving patient retention of information, [and] they can be invaluable resources for family caregivers."
—"A primer for," 1996, page 4

• •

What are the most common teaching tools? Written materials, such as handouts, booklets, and discharge instructions.
Why are they so common? They work!

"Patients discharged from a medical ward had poor recall of information on their diagnosis but this was improved by simple written information. Patient information on drugs on discharge has been shown to be of value."
—Patterson & Teale, 1997

Written teaching materials work so well, we expect to receive them:

When my son broke his arm, all the orthopedic surgeon told us to look out for was numb, blue fingers. He didn't give us any handouts or discharge instructions.
   After a few days my son was comfortable enough to stop wearing the cheap little sling made of gauze. I didn't see any problem with that. When we went back, the doctor told us the bones were out of alignment and he may need to break my son's arm again!
   Then the doctor gave him a real sling to wear all the time. When my son got the cast the doctor didn't say anything about wearing the sling! If the doctor had given us a handout about cast care, at least it might have mentioned it.
                                        —a mom who is also an RN

Written teaching materials reinforce teaching. They also provide structure and consistency to teaching. As you review the contents with the learner, they remind you of key points to address. This story also points out that sometimes we assume learners know certain things, especially if they have no questions. Sometimes we neglect to evaluate understanding of all essential information.

How to Use Written Teaching Tools

Let's start with how *not* to use teaching tools. Here's an excerpt from an article that encouraged the use of written teaching materials:

> *"But educating patients in the usual way—face-to-face at the end of a direct encounter in a physician's office—is, for the most part, a waste of time. Even when physicians spend a lot of time talking to patients, patients can't digest all the information they're getting. . . . The most important questions for patients come up after the encounter."*
> —Sandrick, 1998

This encourages the use of written teaching materials but in the context of poor teaching skills. If face-to-face education is "a waste of time," it is probably not done well. The teaching is being done at the end, so it isn't well integrated into the encounter. Learners can't digest all the information they're getting, even when the health care provider spends "a lot of time talking." Perhaps the health care provider isn't listening and assessing needs enough. The learner's most important questions may come up after the encounter because the assessment was incomplete, and the health care provider did not evaluate understanding or anticipate the questions that might arise. Handouts are not the solution to these problems. Teaching skills are the solution.

> *"Printed material serves primarily as backup and reference; it does not replace face-to-face education."*
> —Menke, 1993, page 159

So what is the best way to use written teaching tools?

Assess the Learner

Before you give a learner a handout, assess readiness to learn, learning needs, and ability to read. Specifics on how to assess ability to read are identified later in this chapter.

> *"A necessary component of the nursing history and assessment should include the evaluation of the patient's ability to read and comprehend. Simply asking the patient's grade achievement will not provide sufficient information."*
> —Wilson, 1996, page 203

Actively Involve Learner

When you've identified the informational need and the learner is ready and you know the learner can read, see if there's an appropriate handout available. If so, get it, and pick up a pen and a highlighting marker.

"To educate effectively, health care providers should use both oral and written communication. While oral communication is best for teaching patients, simple written materials can help reinforce the information given orally."
— Mayeaux, Murphy, Arnold, Davis, & Jackson, 1996

Write the learner's name on the handout, and give it to the learner with a pen. Tell the learner the pen is for taking notes. You may then go through the handout with the learner, or you may ask the learner to read it and say you'll come back to discuss it.

"Clinicians can . . . make their messages more understandable by applying techniques to enhance patient recall of the message and by encouraging patient feedback and interaction."
— Doak, Doak, Friedell, & Meade, 1998

Review the contents of the handout with the learner. Discuss and highlight or underline the key points. Encourage the learner to take notes, as appropriate.

Have the learner interact with the new information to enhance recall and application of the new information. Then document your teaching, the learner's understanding, and needed follow-up. This will help the next caregiver continue the process.

Watch Your Language

Our patients may live in different environments with which we are not familiar. One comment from a focus group participant indicates we may not realize how much more we know than many of our patients:

"Doctors use words that are very long and stuff, and you don't understand what those people are saying. They are looking at you like, weren't you sitting next to me in medical school or something? I don't know. I really don't know why they do that. Maybe they get carried away and just forget."
— Hartman, McCarthy, Park, Schuster, & Kushi, 1994, page 744

Watch and listen for this potential discrepancy. Tie new information into the learner's knowledge and lifestyle; use the same vocabulary as the learner. Evaluate your learner's understanding often.

"Asking whether a patient has questions is not enough. Patients may not understand something yet be unable to frame questions because they lack the necessary analytical skills"

—Lasater & Mehler, 1998, page 169

Remember Goals

Do you think this active involvement is too much work? How does taking time to involve your learner actively make teaching go faster?

If you teach only information the learner needs to know, then note taking, highlighting, discussing, and evaluating understanding are not too much work. They are essential. If the learner doesn't absolutely need to know specific information and does not ask for it, don't bring it up. Save your time for teaching that must be done.

If you teach necessary information well, you may only need to teach it once. If you do not teach necessary information well, it will eat up more of your time later. You and your colleagues will find yourselves repeating instructions. Haphazard teaching means the learner's understanding will not deepen, skills will not be acquired, behaviors will not change, and health outcomes will not be improved.

The teaching is done not by the piece of paper, but in the conversation. A handout is a guide, backup, and reference. Apply good teaching skills, and you will not be wasting your time.

Poor Reading Skills

What if you assess your learner's ability to read and find reading skills are present but poor?

"Even for a patient who is a poor reader, the printed material gives importance to the message, especially if the patient's name is written on the cover."

—Doak et al., 1998

Remember, teaching is done in conversation. The handout is just a tool. By making the message important, it motivates your learner to pay attention to the teaching. When the learner is a poor reader, the handout may be more useful as a backup and reference for a friend or family member who acts as a surrogate reader for the learner.

What about learners who can hardly read at all?

While working in the emergency department, I cared for a patient with an eye injury. As I explained his home care, I told him not to read because the movement of one eye would cause the other to move also and may be painful. He said, "Oh, I can't read." I proceeded to repeat the instructions, and again he told me he could not read. I told the patient that in 2 days, when the bandage was removed, he would be able to read. He laughed and said, "Wow, I've been wanting to be able to do that for years!" Then I finally realized it wasn't his eyesight problem that kept him from reading.

Most people with poor literacy skills would not admit it as freely as this patient did. When his nurse heard but didn't understand, this patient was even willing to repeat himself.

> *"Since there is a strong social stigma attached to illiteracy, nearly all nonreaders or poor readers will seek to conceal this fact. They will use ruses such as, 'I forgot my glasses,' or 'I'll have to take this home for my husband (wife) to see first,' or 'My eyes are tired.'"*
> —Doak, Doak, & Root, 1996, page 6

We who are literate can barely imagine how different life would be if we could not read. How would we deal with airports, road signs, bus schedules, telephone books, consent forms, appointment slips, and labels on medicine bottles? It must be very difficult to function under those conditions.

> *"Even though they may not be aware of it, clinicians probably encounter patients with limited literacy on a daily basis; the literacy limitations of such patients are rarely obvious."*
> —Doak et al., 1998

> *"Many well-groomed, articulate, and apparently bright parents were reading at very low levels. Reading ability cannot be accurately assessed without direct testing."*
> —Davis et al., 1994, page 464

"In terms of the U.S. population, most [poor readers] are white native-born Americans, and are found in every walk of life."
—Doak et al., 1996, page 6

In fact, even a college degree does not guarantee literacy skills. To understand the following statistic, keep in mind the U.S. Department of Education defines the lowest proficiency level of literacy as Level 1.

"Some 75 to 80 percent of adults with 0 to 8 years of education are in Level 1. . . . Only 4 percent of adults with four year college degrees are in Level 1; 44 to 50 percent are in the two highest levels [4 and 5]."
—1992 National Adult Literacy Survey

Only 4 percent of adults with 4-year college degrees fall into the lowest level of literacy skills. Therefore, even if your learner is a college graduate, he or she may not be able to read.

The health history form you use at work may ask for last grade of school the patient completed, but this is not an indication of that person's reading skills.

"Research indicates that many people read below the level of their completed formal education."
—Ott & Hardie, 1997, page 54

"Most people read at least two grade levels lower than the number of years they spent in school. And unless they read avidly, their reading level drops each year they are out of school. If you base what you write on statistics about the education level of your audience, you may still be writing over their heads."
—Clarity Associates, Inc.

Low literacy skills do not impact only the ability to read. When we learn to read and learn to understand what we are reading, we also acquire thinking and reasoning skills. Doak et al. (1996) also found the following characteristics among poor readers:

- Often read one word at a time
- Skip over uncommon words and those they don't understand
- Don't think in terms of classes or categories of information
- Take instructions literally without interpreting them differently for new situations
- May miss the context
- May not make inferences from facts

These deficiencies clearly interfere with learning and the effective application of information that is learned.

"Low literacy affects all types of communication—written oral and visual. . . . Those with low literacy skills may guess their way through an instruction. They may read so slowly that they miss the context and reach an incorrect conclusion. . . . Combined with fear that their low literacy may be found out, these communication differences become significant barriers to comprehension."

—Doak et al., 1998

Who Are These People With Poor Reading Skills?

"Persons with low literacy skills vary greatly. Many are older; others are immigrants who speak English only as a second language. Although more white Americans have limited literacy skills, a disproportionate number of those with low literacy skills are members of minority groups."

—Doak et al., 1998

In addition, it's not only our patients whose literacy skills are limited. After all, some people with low literacy skills are employed. For example, this conversation indicates the need for a literacy assessment:

Clerk in a doctor's office: *What is your date of birth?*
Patient: *April 21, 1923.*
Clerk: *I need your date of birth.*
Patient: *April 21, 1923.*
Clerk: *No, I need the exact date. You know. Like my date is 2/2/74.*
    —This conversation was reported by a family member.

Low literacy skills are a big problem in the United States. One in every five adults has poor reading skills.

"About 21 percent of the adult population—more than 40 million Americans over the age of 16—had only rudimentary reading and writing skills. . . . A subgroup of this category—representing roughly 4 percent of the total adult population or about 8 million people—was unable to perform even the simplest literacy tasks."

—1992 National Adult Literacy Survey

Did you ever deal with a patient who didn't follow directions? When your teaching becomes frustrating, it may not mean your learner is uncooperative or unintelligent. Your learner may have poor literacy skills.

"Poor reading abilities seem not only to influence understanding and interpretation of meaning but also a person's organization of perceptions and vocabulary development. A person with poor reading skills usually has difficulty analyzing instructions, which can also inhibit the person's ability to ask questions. For fear of appearing ignorant, people with poor reading skills might never ask questions."

—Wilson & McLemore, 1997, page 312

"Those with low literacy skills nearly always have adequate intelligence."

—Doak et al., 1998

We are quick to suspect alcohol or drug abuse but slower to recognize how low literacy skills interfere with the progress of our therapeutic interventions. We generally assume that everyone who has graduated or holds a well-paying job reads well.

"The physical therapist said she got John to almost write his name today. I just told her that was very nice. I didn't have the heart to tell her he couldn't write his name before the accident."

—A construction worker's wife

So appearance, occupation, and last grade completed are not necessarily indicators of literacy or comprehension skills. Isn't this an issue for educational systems and not health care professionals? No. Literacy limitations impact health care, including understanding of informed consent; medication administration, both over-the-counter and prescription; recognition and follow-up of problems; and self-care activities.

In addition, under the stress of illness, sleep deprivation, and personal crisis, functional literacy falls. Even if the learner can read the words, can he or she understand and apply them? Feeling overwhelmed impairs functioning.

What Does This Mean to Us?

What implications does this have for patient and family education?

"Health care is a technical field and most patients are not familiar with the terminology or many of the concepts. Therefore, the need for readable materials is even more pressing in our field."

—Kingbeil, Speece, & Schubiner, 1995, page 101

We need to know how to identify poor readers. We need to know how to individualize teaching so they understand what we are doing for them and so they can take good care of themselves. The written teaching materials we give our learners need to be clear and useful.

How Do You Assess Your Learner's Reading Skills?

"Literacy status is a sensitive subject to people with low literacy; therefore, they try to hide their deficiencies at all costs."
—Hanson-Divers, 1997

Perform an Informal Assessment

You can tell how well your learner can read indirectly, by doing an informal assessment. Ask your learner to read a page or two of instructions or information with a known graded reading level. Then ask the learner to tell you what was just read in his or her own words, or ask the learner a few detailed questions about the content. If the learner explains the content or answers your questions correctly, assume he or she can read text at least at that grade level.

If the learner does not answer questions correctly or does not participate, you may choose to teach as if the learner cannot read or directly test the learner's reading ability. In either case, document your results so others on the health care team will know.

"Patients who have low literacy levels need different counseling than those with high literacy levels because they cannot depend on written patient education materials or written medication instructions."
—Hanson-Divers, 1997

Use Tests

Many studies show the discrepancy between reading level of patient education materials and the reading skills of patients (for example, Wilson & McLemore, 1997; Williams et al., 1995; Davis et al., 1994). These, obviously, involve asking patients and families to take tests that measure their reading ability. Doak et al. (1996) say the willingness of people to participate in these tests and the way they feel after taking them depend on how they are introduced. If you decide to test your learner's reading skill directly, you might consider introducing the request like this:

"We want to make our instructions easy to understand, so I need to find out how well you can read. To do this I need your help to read some words. It will only take a few minutes. Will you help me?"

—Doak et al., 1996, page 30

Two easy-to-use literacy tests are the Wide-Range Achievement Test 3 (WRAT 3) and Rapid Estimate of Adult Literacy in Medicine (REALM). They each take 3 to 10 minutes to administer. Both tests consist of lists of words that become progressively more difficult. You ask learners to read the list aloud. The more words they can pronounce correctly, the higher their reading skills. The words are correlated to a grade level or grade-level range. These tests are only useful in English for English-reading learners. Others are being developed but are not ready for use yet.

Wide-Range Achievement Test 3
To administer, you give the learner a card listing 42 words and ask him or her to read each word aloud, starting with the easiest. You listen, and on a separate checklist, make a check mark over each word pronounced incorrectly. When 10 consecutive words are mispronounced, you stop the test, thank the learner, and leave to score the test.

The WRAT 3 was copyrighted in 1993 and costs about $99 in the United States for an administration manual, test cards, and scoring sheets. For the address to obtain more information, see the section "If you want to learn more" at the end of this chapter.

Rapid Estimate of Adult Literacy in Medicine
This test is similar to the WRAT 3, but the REALM lists 66 medically related words of increasing difficulty to be pronounced. At the end of the test when the reader can't read any of the words, you ask if he or she can recognize any of the words that appear later on the list.

The REALM is more appropriate in a clinical setting because the words contained are medical terms. However, it is less accurate than WRAT in assessing degree of impairment (Lasater & Mehler, 1998).

The words in the REALM are in large type on purple paper, so the layout is not very similar to that of most teaching materials. When complete, the reader is assigned not a grade level, but a range:

- Third grade or below
- Fourth to sixth grade
- Seventh to eighth grade
- High school

Medical Terminology Achievement Test

This is a newer test that is not yet widely used. Instead of a list of words, the Medical Terminology Achievement Test is designed to resemble a prescription label with its use of small print size, glossy cover, and medical terminology (Hanson-Divers, 1997).

Use Interpreters

"Word recognition and pronunciation tests are not valid in Spanish, so little is known about the ability of Spanish-speaking patients to understand health care instructions written in Spanish."
—Williams et al., 1995, page 1678

Consequently, it is essential that you use interpreters and conversation to teach Spanish-speaking and other non-English speaking learners. If you have written materials in the learner's primary language, use them, but always evaluate understanding to the same extent you would for any other learner.

Evaluate Understanding

"The ability to read material does not guarantee that the material is understood. Reading and understanding call on different skills. A patient may be able to read all the words in a sentence but not understand its meaning."
—Doak et al., 1996, page 28

It is important to evaluate the learner's understanding of material, no matter what the reading skills are. The most direct way to evaluate comprehension is to teach the learner with materials written at the appropriate reading level. If, when you review the content and evaluate understanding, you find the learner did not understand the materials, teach this learner as if he or she cannot learn by reading. You may provide written teaching materials as reinforcers and for family members to access, but do not rely on them for teaching.

Qualities of Good Written Tools

Good tools facilitate good outcomes. You know written teaching materials of good quality will make your teaching job easier, but what makes good quality?

Content

"Parents appear to respond best to information that focuses on their specific area of concern."
                    —Glascoe, Oberklaid, Dworkin, & Trimm, 1998

- Clear purpose. Learners must understand why they are reading this. If they don't understand, they may not pay attention or miss the point.
- Focus on behaviors. The content needs to solve a problem.
- Limited scope. Stick to the purpose of the material. Limit the content to what can be learned in a short time.
- Summary or review. There should be a summary of the key points in words, examples, or visuals. This helps learners not miss the key points.

Literacy Demand

- Reading grade level.

"The readability levels of patient education materials continue to be too high."
                    —Kingbeil et al., 1995, page 96

   Measure readability using a scale. It is best if the readability is fifth grade or lower. Appendix 8-1 at the end of this chapter discusses this in detail. You can use the Fry Readability formula (Appendix 8-2, also found at the end of this chapter) to determine the reading level of any teaching material written in English.
- Writing style, active voice. The material should be written in a conversational style, in an active voice. When you see forms of "to be," the sentence is in the passive voice.
- Clear vocabulary. Use common words ("doctor" instead of "physician"). Define concepts ("15 to 70" instead of "normal range"). Explain measurements ("pain lasts more than 5 minutes" instead of "severe pain"). Use visual terms ("runny nose" instead of "excess mucus").
- Context first. For example, you may say, "To find out what's wrong with you [context] the doctor will take a sample of your blood for lab tests [new information]."
- Headers, captions, subtitles. These road signs organize the text and prepare the learner for the next topic, for example, "When to call the doctor."

Graphics (Illustrations, Lists, Tables, Charts, Graphs)

"Patients who received discharge instructions with illustrations were 1.5 times more likely to score at or above the median than patients who received instructions without illustrations. . . . Illustrations made a bigger difference in patients who had no more than a high school education."
—Austin, Matlack, Dunn, Kesler, & Brown, 1995, page 319

- Purpose of graphics. The cover image can impact the learner's interest in the instruction. It should be friendly, attract attention, and clearly show the purpose of the material.
- Type of illustrations. Simple line drawings are best. They should be simple and uncluttered. Photos have too many distracting details. Although color pictures appeal more to learners than black and white pictures, they cost more to reproduce. If your teaching materials use color, it should be accurate and realistic. Illustrations should show familiar and easily recognized images. For example, when showing a body site, show enough of the body to clarify the placement of that site.

"When using visuals, include enough of the human figure to make the physical location of the information instantly clear. Use an arrow or color highlighting to direct the reader to the main point."
—Doak et al., 1998

- Relevance of graphics. Illustrations should visually communicate the key points of the teaching materials. They illustrate the meaning of the text. Use illustrations not to decorate, but to explain and teach. There should be no nonessential details that distract the eye from the message.

"Several literacy and health projects have produced booklets . . . written by and for low literacy patients. These are in story, testimonial, or photonovella formats. These materials can reinforce and support the clinician's advice."
—Doak et al., 1998

- Captions. Captions tell the learner what to look at in the graphic. Captions should be clear and legible. If there is no caption on a graphic, you have missed a teaching opportunity.
- Explanation of every list or table. Is it clear what the learner should do with this information?

Layout and Type

"Readability formulas . . . cannot reliably predict how well individual readers will comprehend particular texts. . . . Text and reader properties that cannot be measured by formulas are emphasized as having a far greater influence on comprehension. . . . No readability formula can be a reliable guide for editing a text to reduce its difficulty."
—Anderson & Davison, 1986

- Layout. A good layout makes it easy for learner to follow the flow of information. Graphics are labeled and next to related text. Sequence needs to be consistent. Shading, boxes, and arrows can direct attention to important points.

  The learner has to be able to believe he or she can read the teaching material (self-efficacy factor). Does it look hard to read? A page of solid text may, just by its imposing appearance, discourage a reader.

  The length of text lines should be between 30 to 50 characters and spaces. There should be enough white space. The page should not look cluttered.

  Content should be broken up by short, clear headings. Lists should be separated into chunks, each with a subheading. If there are more than five items in a list, use subheadings.

  If color is used, it should not distract from the message. Do not use color codes.

  The paper should be nongloss or low gloss. The glare from glossy paper makes it hard to read. There should be a high contrast between the type and paper. It's best if the type is black or very dark and the paper is white, ivory, or yellow.
- Type. The type should be in uppercase and lowercase, not all caps. The type should be 12 to 14 points. Key points can be emphasized with underlining, a bold or bigger font, or color. Emphasis should not be made in italics or all caps, which are both hard to read. Including headings, subheadings, and captions, do not use more than six font styles (plain, bold, underline) and sizes (12, 14, 18) on a page.

  The font should be a serif font, which means it has beginning or finishing strokes (serifs) drawn across the arm or stem of a letter. Examples of serif fonts are Times, Times Roman, and Bookman.

  The font should not be a sans-serif font, which has no serifs, is more geometric, gives the page a flatter feel, and may be harder to read. Examples of sans-serif fonts are Helvetica, Universal, and Geneva.

If you are creating a written handout and expect to translate the text into a foreign language, plan for this when you design the English version so they can both look the same. French, German, and Spanish translations take up 15% to 20% more space than the same content in English. Your computer software (for example, Word, PageMaker, and Quark) has a formatting option for spacing of letters. When you lay out the English version, space letters looser than normal (2.5% more than the default spacing). When you lay out the translated text, set letter spacing tighter than normal (about 2.5% less than the default spacing). The translated text should then fit into about same space (McCarthy, 1997).

Stimulation for Learning

- Use interaction. The teaching material asks the learner to solve a problem, make a choice, or demonstrate a behavior. For example, a handout on ferrous sulfate includes the following:

  ☐ Tell your nurse or doctor where you will store this medicine. (Check when done.)

- A handout on how to use a small-volume nebulizer includes:

  ☐ Tell your nurse or doctor what you would do if you took in all the medicine in the nebulizer cup but still felt tight and short of breath. (Check when done.)

"In many print instructions, the reader does not encounter the behavioral information early enough. That is, no priority is given to behavioral information; instead the priority is given to the epidemiologic and statistical data, which creates an image of irrelevancy to many patients."
—Doak et al., 1998

- Behaviors are specific and modeled. The instructions tell how to do the behavior and give an example.

"The essential components of good directions are time (estimated time it should take), anticipation (what you can expect to see along the way), and failure (indications that you have gone too far, and should turn back)."
—Wurman, 1989, page 97

- The information provides motivation and supports self-efficacy. Complex topics should be divided into small, doable steps.

"Good instructions walk you through errors and problems. We should plan our instructions with more thought. Ask ourselves, what are the essentials of this explanation? How can I build in reassurance so the followers will know they are on the right track? What would help them understand?"
—Wurman, 1989, page 99

Cultural Appropriateness

"Although the community health nurses provided care in a setting that served more than 90 different ethnic and cultural groups, . . . the materials used to educate these groups failed to recognize cultural beliefs, values, languages, perceptions, behaviors, or attitudes held by patients and families. In essence, there were no references in texts of the materials that addressed the diverse needs of patients based on their ethnicity or cultural background."
—Wilson, 1996, page 202

- Match in logic, language, experience. Does the logic, language and experience match those of the audience? Written materials should reflect the learner's point of view.

"Mismatches in logic affect the way patients carry out the advice they receive. For example, patients without the benefits of scientific or medical training may find it logical to stop taking medicine as directed once they feel well."
—Doak et al., 1998

"Patients are sometimes advised to obtain a second opinion. Having doubts about the first doctor's opinion, however, may not seem logical to the patient."
—Doak et al., 1998

"An instruction sheet that advises 'talk with each member of your treatment team before treatment starts' can leave the patient questioning what aspects to discuss."
—Doak et al., 1998

- Cultural images and examples. Don't assume common knowledge across cultures. Words may have different meanings for different cultural groups. Images and examples should present the culture of the audience in positive ways.

"For example, the written instructions should include information that counsels African-American patients on the appropriateness of using home remedies such as ointments and creams that are believed to promote healing."
—Wilson & McLemore, 1997, page 31

When possible, use bilingual materials so translators and family members who are comfortable with English can help the learner understand the content.

"Educational materials must highlight beneficial customs, disregard the innocuous ones, and tactfully confront the harmful practices, proposing alternatives and means. For the educator to successfully incorporate traditional values and customs in educational materials he needs to elicit the participation of community members in all phases of this development."
—Rice & Valdivia, 1991, page 81

"The target audience should be intensely involved in the conceptualization and development stages of the health messages. It is preferable that some of the team belong to the target audience to more genuinely reflect the cultural characteristics of the target population. The best educational materials are produced by the community itself."
—Sabogal, Otero-Sabogal, Pasick, Jenkins, & Pérez-Stable, 1996, page S132

How to Evaluate Quality of Written Materials

A lot of variables go into determining the quality of written teaching materials. Fortunately, there is a simple way to quantify these.

Appendix 8-3, found at the end of this chapter, is the Suitability Assessment of Materials (SAM) scoring sheet, by Doak et al. (1996).

The best way to learn how to evaluate the quality of written materials is to do it. Photocopy the SAM scoring sheet. Then turn to Figure 8-1 on page 201. Evaluate this teaching material, using the SAM instrument and the Fry Readability formula.

Then evaluate some of the teaching materials you now use in your clinical practice. When you revise teaching materials, evaluate them with the SAM instrument to determine how they can be improved. Few teaching materials have a perfect score, but the higher the better.

When Your Child's Head Has Been Hurt:

Many children who hurt their heads get well and have no long-term problems. Some children have problems that may not be noticed right away. You may see changes in your child over the next several months that concern you. This card lists some common signs that your child may have a mild brain injury. If your child has any of the problems on this list — AND THEY DON'T GO AWAY — see the "What to Do" box on the back of this sheet.

HEALTH PROBLEMS

Headaches

Including:
- headache that keeps coming back
- pain in head muscle
- pain in head bone (skull)
- pain below the ear
- pain in the jaw
- pain in or around the eyes

Balance Problems

- dizziness
- trouble with balance

Sensory Changes

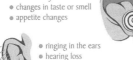

- bothered by smells
- changes in taste or smell
- appetite changes

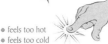

- ringing in the ears
- hearing loss
- bothered by noises
- can't handle normal background noise

- feels too hot
- feels too cold
- doesn't feel temperature at all

- blurry vision
- seeing double
- hard to see clearly (hard to focus)
- bothered by light

These problems don't happen often. If your child has any of them, see your doctor right away.

▲ severe headache that does not go away or get better
▲ seizures: eyes fluttering, body going stiff, staring into space
▲ child forgets everything, amnesia
▲ hands shake, tremors, muscles get weak, loss of muscle tone
▲ nausea or vomiting that returns

Sleep Problems

- can't sleep through the night
- sleeps too much
- days and nights get mixed up

Pain Problems

- neck and shoulder pain that happens a lot
- other unexplained body pain

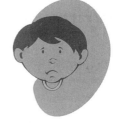

Figure 8-1.

BEHAVIOR and FEELINGS

Changes *in personality, mood or behavior*

- is irritable, anxious, restless
- gets upset or frustrated easily
- overreacts, cries or laughs too easily
- has mood swings

- wants to be alone or away from people
- is afraid of others, blames others
- wants to be taken care of
- does not know how to act with people
- takes risks without thinking first

- is sad, depressed
- doesn't want to do anything, can't "get started"
- is tired, drowsy
- is slow to respond
- trips, falls, drops things, is awkward

- eats too little, eats all the time, or eats things that aren't food
- has different sexual behavior (older children)
- starts using or has a different reaction to alcohol or drugs
- takes off clothes in public

THINKING PROBLEMS

- has trouble remembering things
- has trouble paying attention
- reacts slowly
- thinks slowly
- takes things too literally, doesn't get jokes
- understands words but not their meaning
- thinks about the same thing over and over
- has trouble learning new things

- has trouble putting things in order (desk, room, papers)
- has trouble making decisions
- has trouble planning, starting, doing, and finishing a task
- has trouble remembering to do things on time
- makes poor choices (loss of common sense)

TROUBLE COMMUNICATING

- changes the subject, has trouble staying on topic
- has trouble thinking of the right word
- has trouble listening
- has trouble paying attention, can't have long conversations
- does not say things clearly
- has trouble reading
- talks too much

WHAT TO DO:

If your child has any of the problems on this list, and they don't go away:

▲ Ask your child's doctor to have your child seen by a specialist in head injury who can help your child learn skills (rehabilitation).

▲ Ask your child's doctor to have your child seen by a Board-certified Neuropsychologist. This specialist can help you understand and deal with your child's behavior and feeling changes.

▲ Call the Brain Injury Association of Arizona for more information:

(602) 952-2449 Phoenix Headquarters
(520) 747-7140 Tucson Hotline

We have only listed the problems we see most often when a child's brain is hurt. Not every problem that could happen is on this list.

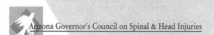 Arizona Governor's Council on Spinal & Head Injuries

 Arizona Department of Health Services

 TBI TRAUMATIC BRAIN INJURY STATE DEMONSTRATION GRANT PROGRAM

For additional copies of this publication, or to obtain this information in an alternative format, contact the Arizona Governor's Council on Spinal & Head Injuries at: **Voice** / (602) 883-0484 or through the AZ Relay Service.

Figure 8-1. (*Continued*)

Create Your Own Written Teaching Materials

The best guide for creating your own written teaching materials, is *Teaching Patients with Low Literacy Skills* by Doak et al. (1996). This book also helps you evaluate the quality of teaching materials you don't create yourself. Use it.

Consider the criteria for quality teaching materials when creating the draft of the teaching material. If you can, computerize the process. Teaching materials created on computers can be readily available to print out and are easily revised as needed.

Identify Areas in Need of Written Materials

For what topics should you create handouts?

Ask your learners what instructions they wish they had in writing. What information do they need? What must the learner do or know to manage the disease or condition?

Also ask former patients and their families what information was helpful for them. What did they learn on their own and wish they had received from their health care providers?

A good way to do this is to hold focus groups with select groups of learners. You gather a small group from your target population, ask questions, and take notes. If you want to learn how to plan, hold, and analyze the results of focus groups, read *The Focus Group Kit*, edited by Morgan and Krueger (1998). It contains six slim softcover books that walk you through the process.

The focus group will provide you with a list of actual learner questions. Turn these questions into a handout with a question and answer format.

> *"How-to information is needed by most patients, but is especially important for low literacy populations. Patients with low literacy skills need explicit information."*
>
> —Doak et al., 1998

Ask health care providers what information falls into those topics identified by learners. What behaviors do they teach many learners? What carries the greatest risk if not done correctly? What instructions do they write out for learners? What is important for the patient to learn?

Identify behavior change objectives with measurable outcomes. These may include taking a specific medication safely or performing a self-care skill correctly. Limit advice to key information the learner needs at the time.

Does this topic fall into one of the goals of patient and family education? What information is essential to achieve this?

To determine if the information is essential, ask the following questions: Does the learner need to know this information for informed consent, self-care, or to recognize problems and know how to respond? Is it worth the time of a health care professional to review and evaluate understanding of the content of proposed teaching material? If not, it's information that's nice to know but not needed. Don't create a handout for it. After all, no handout should be given to a learner without discussion and evaluation of understanding. How is this information best taught? Is a written handout appropriate? Can this topic be taught in one brief sitting?

> If the topic is too broad for a single, brief teaching material, such as "Diabetic Self-Care," or "Cardiac Rehabilitation," break the topic into sections of essential information. Create a separate handout for each section. Then give the learner a three-ring binder to keep all teaching materials together, and add topics as they are taught.

"Start with a short topic that needs immediate attention."
—Hussey, 1997, page 37

Lower the Reading Level

"I tried to lower the reading level using a thesaurus. I got so frustrated!"
—an RN

"If you use a vocabulary with which your audience is familiar, if you create a context that is relevant to their daily lives, the message in your writing will have more impact and will be more clear. This is not done by applying a word processing utility or a reading scale score. It is done by being aware of your audience and what their needs are."
—WordsWork, 1997

You know readability scales measure syllables and sentence length, so the following will help to lower reading levels:

- Use common, easily understood words.
- Keep word choices under three syllables whenever possible.
- Use short sentences with one thought.
- Use short paragraphs.

- Use a simple word or group of words instead of a fancy word.

ask or talk to	instead of	consult
drug or medicine	instead of	medication
every day	instead of	on a daily basis
expect	instead of	anticipate
heart	instead of	cardiac
help	instead of	assistance
lung	instead of	pulmonary
more	instead of	additional
must	instead of	it is essential
talk about	instead of	discuss
use	instead of	utilize

Say: "In case of overdose, get medical help right away."
Instead of: "In case of accidental overdose, seek professional assistance or contact a poison control center immediately."

- Write in a conversational style.
- Pretend you are talking to a learner who is having trouble understanding you.
- Ask a learner how to present the information best.
- If you're having trouble figuring out how to write something at a lower reading level, ask yourself:
  - What do I mean?
  - What am I trying to say?

When you answer these questions, you may hear a simpler way to say the same thing.

If this skill is difficult for you to master, consider purchasing *Just Say It! How to Write for Readers Who Don't Read Well: A Training Manual for Writers* (Baker, 1992). It is a workbook that takes you step-by-step through the process of learning how to "just say it."

Ready to try it yourself? Here's a paragraph titled "Discharge Procedures" from an actual patient information booklet from a university medical center hospital. How would you write the same message in a lower reading level?

Before leaving the hospital, you will be escorted to the Discharge Office for discharge clearance. If all arrangements concerning the payment of your bill have not been completed prior to the time of discharge, you will be interviewed by a Financial Counselor who will work with you to complete financial arrangements. When all paperwork has been completed, you will be escorted to the main lobby where your mode of transportation should be awaiting you.

It's easiest to understand the process of creating a teaching material if you see it unfold. Follow this handout through the steps of develop-

---

PHOENIX CHILDREN'S HOSPITAL
PEDIATRIC BIOBEHAVIORAL UNIT

HOME CARE INSTRUCTIONS: *FOLLOWING DIRECTIONS*

for _____
      child's name

—Get your child's attention before speaking. (If running around, he/she may not hear you.) Keep eye contact while giving the direction.
—Give simple directions in a calm, but firm voice. Give the direction only once.
—Be sure you let your child know what you expect of him/her—what the rules for following the direction are.
—Have the child repeat the direction to make sure he/she understands what you said.
—Make sure that what you ask your child to do is within his/her abilities to avoid *setting* him/her up for failure.
—Give a time frame for the task to be completed.
—If the child does not follow the direction please refer to the instructions—"what to do when your child doesn't follow directions".

Be as positive as possible with your child. Praise them, spend extra time with them, give them hugs, etc. when they do follow directions. You may want to use things such as Nintendo, special toys and activities that are enjoyable as incentives for positive behavior.

Keep the expectations and consequences as consistent as possible. It is important for your child to know what to expect.

Try to give directions as positive behaviors. (For example, "speak softer please", instead of "stop yelling")

ADDITIONAL GUIDELINES:

_____

_____

_____

Figure 8-2.

ment (editing, expert review, patient and family review). See what changes were made and what additional improvements you would make. (Hint: This handout is not perfect. It is designed to test your critical thinking skills and help you apply what you learn here.)

The handout is called "Following Directions." Parents often need help getting their children to follow directions. Figure 8-2 is a first draft of a handout that addresses this problem. Read it, and think about how you might write the same messages in simpler language.

Write Understandably

There's much more to comprehension than word choices. For example, the following sentence contains common words that you could probably define (such as "freedom," "interaction," "degrees," and even "variance"); however, is this sentence easily understandable?

> *"Under certain circumstances the within-cells and the interaction sums of squares may be added together and divided by the combined degrees of freedom to obtain an estimate of the variance based on a larger number of degrees of freedom."*
> —Doak, Doak, & Root, 1998, page 48

This one sentence has 39 words, so it would rate high on any readability test. Its difficulty lies in its length, passivity, and the ways even common words are used.

The moral is that making a passage readable is not just a question of word choices. A thesaurus may help you find simple words, but it will not help you say something simply.

> *"If you simply eradicate complex information to lower the reading level, much of the essential message is gone. If instead, you break all lengthy sentences two or more shorter ones, your writing may be so choppy that no one will bother to read it."*
> —WordsWork, 1997

When editing teaching materials, you have to find a balance. It takes practice. Here are some tips:

- Write in an active voice. Use active verbs. Whenever possible, avoid all forms of "to be" (such as "are," "is," or "been").
- Focus on skills and behaviors.
- Use short words and short sentences but only if they sound natural. This will keep your work from being choppy.
- Use headings. Let the reader know the topic of the message.
- Move from general to specific.
- Put topic sentences first.
- Describe what you mean and then give the medical term. For example, "The nurse will put in a thin plastic tube (a catheter)."
- Limit each paragraph to a single message or action.
- Break the content up into logical sections that flow in order.

- Use bullets and lists, when appropriate.
- Use personal pronouns ("you") rather than impersonal pronouns ("one").
- Be consistent. Use the same terms when referring to the same things. Don't vary nouns or verbs to avoid repeating yourself. Learners with low literacy skills get confused by this.
- Use graphics to explain and emphasize key points.
- Avoid abbreviations.
- Reword sentences to avoid "he/she" and "and/or."
- Ask the reader to solve a problem based on the information provided.
- Offer additional resources, such as a support group or the doctor's telephone number.
- Summarize and review. Present the same information in a different form at the end.
- Check your draft against the SAM instrument. How can you improve it?

Figure 8-3 is the edited version of "Following Directions," now titled "How to Help Your Child Do What You Say." Compare this to the previous version in Figure 8-2. Then compare this to the SAM instrument criteria. What other changes would you make?

Gather Expert Reviews

Involve your health care team members of all disciplines in the development of written teaching materials. Ask them to review specifically to make sure the content is accurate, current, and complete. This has many advantages:

- You get the expertise of many professional points of view. Always ask nurses and physicians to review your teaching materials, but also think beyond them into other relevant specialties. For example, a registered dietitian reviewing a handout on a potassium-depleting medication can address drug–food interactions and add a list of foods that best replenish potassium. A psychiatrist may review a disease or medication handout for information about its effects on cognitive skills or emotional lability. A pharmacist can ensure that information about drug–drug interactions is complete.
- Venture beyond your organization for expert reviews. Collaborate with community experts. This expands your resources, nurtures connections, and helps develop teaching materials that can be used across the continuum of care.
- Expert reviews not only ensure accurate and complete content, they make other team members shareholders in that teaching

Name of Child:_____ Date: _____

How To Help Your Child Do What You Say

Your child can best follow your directions when he or she knows what you want. It helps if you expect the same behavior most of the time. Each time your child does not do what you say, respond the same way. This will help your child know what to expect from you.

- Before you speak, look into your child's eyes. Get your child's attention. If your child is running, he or she may not hear you.
- Talk in a calm, but firm voice.
- Tell your child what you want only once.
- Give simple directions.
- Describe what you expect your child to do. Be very clear. Instead of saying, "be nice," say "pet the cat this way."
- When you can, tell your child what to do instead of what not to do. Say, "speak softer please," instead of "stop yelling."
- Tell your child *when* you expect it to be done.
- Have your child tell you what you said. Does your child understand what you want?
- If your child has a choice, ask your child to do it. If your child must do it, tell your child what you want and when.
- Help your child succeed. Do not ask your child to do something he or she is not able to do.
- Be positive. Expect your child to obey.
- Notice when your child is good.
- Reward your child for good behavior with praise, hugs and time together. You may also reward your child with special toys or activities.

Other tips:

_____

_____

☐ See also: **What To Do When Your Child Doesn't Do What You Say**

If you have any questions or concerns,
☎ call_____ Monday through Friday, 8:00 am to 4:30 pm.

Tuesday, October 25, 1994		DRAFT
© (1994) Phoenix Children's		written at a 3rd grade
Hospital.	#83	reading level
Submitted by Paula Pastore, RN	Independent Guideline:	Parenting: Potential for Growth

Figure 8-3. First edit. "How To Help Your Child Do What You Say".

material. When it is released for use, they will feel a part of it, because they "knew it when" and contributed to its development. They will be more likely to use it in their own practices. Expert reviews promote not just quality teaching materials, but quality teaching.

After you get written feedback from the experts, you need to edit their changes into the piece. Use your professional nursing expertise to weigh and evaluate the feedback. Use the SAM criteria to determine what changes are appropriate. For example, a physician may want to add a medical illustration with a detailed explanation of physiology. Use expert reviews as opportunities to educate other members of the health care team on the latest research in how best to educate patients and families.

Sometimes health care professionals have differing viewpoints and don't agree on the content of a handout. This may happen with topics like the administration of blood products or whether or not to circumcise. You may get a range of responses from the experts. What do you do? Use the SAM criteria and your professional expertise to determine what is essential information and what is opinion. Edit the material and then send it to the same reviewers with an explanation, until you get a consensus. Remind them that the handout is never used without discussion, and details they feel are important can be added at the time of teaching.

Again, health care team members will be more likely to use the teaching material when they are part of its creation. Consensus on the content's accuracy is essential.

Figure 8-4 is the handout "How to Help Your Child Do What You Say" after expert review. Note that the experts suggested the addition of an illustration. Compare this to the SAM instrument criteria. What other changes would you make?

Get Reviews From Your Learner

The SAM instrument is wonderful for ensuring your teaching material meets with the objective criteria, but only learners can tell you if it works. Only learners can tell you if specific content or format features are not understood or accepted. Only learners can tell you what they need and what would work.

Too many producers of written teaching materials skip this step, which is the most important step. Experts are expert at professional content, not presentation. Before you print and release the final ver-

Name of Child:_____ Date: _____

How To Help Your Child Do What You Say

Your child can best follow your directions when he or she knows what you want. It helps if you expect the same behavior most of the time. Each time your child does not do what you say, respond the same way. This will help your child know what to expect from you.

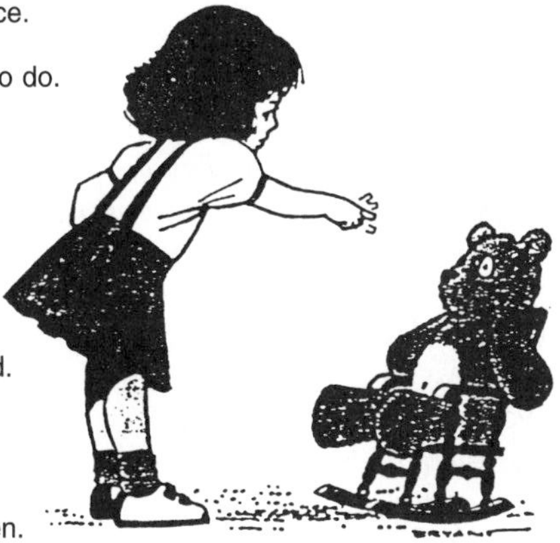

- Before you speak, look into your child's eyes. Get your child's attention. If your child is running, he or she may not hear you.
- Talk in a calm, but firm voice.
- Tell your child what you want only once.
- Give simple directions.
- Describe what you expect your child to do. Be very clear. Instead of saying, "be nice," say "pet the cat this way."
- When you can, tell your child what to do instead of what not to do. Say, "speak softer please," instead of "stop yelling."
- Tell your child *when* you expect it to be done.
- Have your child tell you what you said. Does your child understand what you want?
- *Ask* your child to do it if there is a choice. If your child must do it, *tell* your child what you want and when.
- Help your child succeed. Do not ask your child to do something he or she is not able to do.
- Be positive. Expect your child to obey.
- Notice when your child is good.
- Reward your child for good behavior with praise, hugs and time together. You may also reward your child with special toys or activities.

Other tips:

_____

_____

☐ See also: **What To Do When Your Child Doesn't Do What You Say**

If you have any questions or concerns, ☎ call your child's doctor.

Wednesday, March 22, 1995   DRAFT
© (1995) Phoenix Children's Hospital. #83   Submitted by Paula Pastore, RN

Figure 8-4. After Expert Review. "How To Help Your Child Do What You Say".

sion, find out what learners think of the teaching material; if they would add, remove, or change anything; and if it teaches as intended.

"Our handouts are so well done, they almost always breeze through patient and family review. But it's still worth doing. Every single time a patient makes a suggestion for a change I think, how could we have all missed that? Of course!"

—an RN

One way to get learner review is to hold a focus group of people chosen randomly from the target population. Offer refreshments, and invite them to read the teaching material. Then evaluate their understanding of the content, get their opinions and suggestions on the content and presentation, and record their responses.

"In focus groups conducted by our team, patients with low literacy skills thought 'fat in the diet' meant anything fattening, including potatoes, rice and bread. They often did not know what 'orally' meant, and some were unclear about what 'three times a day' meant. When administering medications to children, parents may not know the difference between a teaspoon and a tablespoon, and may not be sure if medications for an ear infection go into the mouth or in the ear."

—Mayeaux et al., 1996

Focus groups are a wonderful way to get a lot of information in a very short time. However, they may not be the best way to get critical feedback on written teaching materials. Assertiveness or cultural factors may influence the opinions expressed in a group. Your information may not be as complete or accurate as it would be if the process was more private.

A less public approach is to attach a patient and family review survey to 10 to 15 copies of the teaching material and have staff begin to use it in teaching. The learner can then evaluate its content and presentation within the actual teaching context. The health care provider can evaluate the teaching material's effectiveness as a teaching tool.

If you want to learn how to create and analyze the results of a written survey, read *The Survey Kit*, edited by Fink (1995). It contains nine slim softcover books that walk you through the process.

Get the opinions of a range of learners:

- Those who have lots of experience, who can say if the information in the handout tells patients and families what they should know and want to know
- Those who have no experience, who can say if the contents are clear and make sense
- Those who are educated
- Those who have trouble learning

If sections of the teaching material are unclear, confusing, or too difficult for the learner, the health care provider who is teaching should ask how this can be corrected and make a note of it on the review form. Then, ask the learner to fill out the review form, which asks the following:

What did you learn from this handout?
What did you like about this handout?
What didn't you like about this handout?
If a section was hard to understand, please circle it.
If you were to make this handout better, how would you change it?

Family reviews are then compiled, changes are made as necessary, and the teaching material is released. How many family reviews are necessary depends on the feedback. If family reviews indicate that significant changes are necessary, more reviews will be done to make sure the finalized handout meets learners' needs.

Handouts in Spanish go through the same review process. Even though the English version passed patient and family review, new problems could arise with translation or cultural issues. Teaching is done as usual, with an interpreter if necessary, and the health professional asks the learner to fill out the review form.

Lambert (1998) had adolescent moms review a parent manual designed to help them in their new role. The overall comments about the manual were favorable; the learners found it readable and usable. However, they needed and wanted basic child-care information. In contrast, the manual focused on development and parent–child interactions. The learners found that to be "nice to know" information rather than "need to know" information.

Even when you do a good job on design, readability, and accuracy of content, there's a chance you may not be giving the learner the most appropriate information. One way to make sure you're creating a teaching material that supports mutually defined goals is to ask learners what they need to know before you decide on the content. Involve your learners from the beginning. Base your material on actual questions from patients and family members. Include in your answers information former patients and family members have learned through experience and wish they knew at the time.

Figure 8-5 is the handout "How to Help Your Child Do What You Say" after learner review. Does this reflect some of the changes you considered making?

An interactive element was added with "Tell your child's nurse or doctor how you can help your child do what you say." Remember that illustration added after expert review? The cute kid disciplining her teddy bear? Well, one Navajo parent did not like the illustration

Name of Child:_____ **Date:** _____

How To Help Your Child Do What You Say

Your child can best follow your directions when he or she knows what you want. It helps if you expect the same behavior most of the time. Each time your child does not do what you say, respond the same way. This will help your child know what to expect from you.

- Before you speak, look into your child's eyes. Get your child's attention. If your child is running, he or she may not hear you.
- Talk in a calm, but firm voice.
- Tell your child what you want only once.
- Give simple directions.
- Describe what you expect your child to do. Be very clear. Instead of saying, "be nice," say "pet the cat this way."
- When you can, tell your child what to do instead of what not to do. Say, "speak softer please," instead of "stop yelling."
- Tell your child *when* you expect it to be done.
- Have your child tell you what you said. Does your child understand what you want?
- *Ask* your child to do it only if there is a choice. If your child must do it, *tell* your child what you want and when.
- Help your child succeed. Do not ask your child to do something he or she is not able to do.
- Be positive. Expect your child to obey.
- Notice when your child is good.
- Reward your child for good behavior with praise, hugs and time together. You may also reward your child with special toys or activities.

Other tips:

_____

_____

☐ Tell your child's nurse or doctor how you can help your child do what you say.
☐ See also: **What To Do When Your Child Doesn't Do What You Say**

If you have any questions or concerns, ☎ call your child's doctor.

© (1996) Phoenix Children's Hospital.   #83
Submitted by Paula Pastore, RN   Illustration by Dennis Swain

Figure 8-5. After Parent and Family Review. "How To Help Your Child To Do What You Say".

because "She's angry at the teddy bear." The parent's comment was very important feedback. This culturally inappropriate illustration got past the experts. It was replaced by a drawing that better illustrated the behavior the handout was meant to teach. This illustration shows how the mom gets the attention of the child and clearly communicates her expectations. This version was accepted by learners and was released.

Translate Into Foreign Languages

"When translations are required, it is essential that the material be reviewed by a diverse team of native, bilingual persons who are representative of the different ethnic groups or dialects of the target population. A community-based consulting team composed of people from different backgrounds and regions should regularly revise drafts. Consensus should be reached among translators on the best way to communicate the meaning of the original English-language document. Resolution of wording differences results in an improved translation easily understood by a wide variety of people."

—Sabogal et al., 1996, page S13

Professional translators understand concepts, and appeals for behavior change may differ by culture. They do not just say the English words in another language, they translate the meaning.

Good translations include expert translation reviewers, who refine the translation. Box 8-1, defines "Qualities to Look for in a Translation Team." When the translation is translated back into English, this English version should be reasonably close to the original, with no additions or deletions.

Teaching materials go through learner review, as with English:

"Word recognition and pronunciation tests are not valid in Spanish, so little is known about the ability of Spanish-speaking patients to understand health care instructions written in Spanish."

—Williams et al., 1995, page 1678

Use interpreters when teaching and evaluating understanding of information. All your patients deserve the same excellent quality of care.

BOX 8-1 Qualities to Look for in a Translation Team

Hire a translator who can translate documents, recruit bilingual health care editors, and coordinate team translation efforts.

If you want to hire a good translator, hire a good writer. A good writer communicates clearly and concisely in a way that is interesting to read.

Hire a translator who can write formally and avoid slang.

Look for someone who can type translations in the computer format you prefer.

Translators need to use terms that are understood universally by speakers from different regions. Think of the difference between British English and American English. Spaniards and Mexicans also speak distinct versions of the same language.

Medical translators know that medical vocabulary is as technical and precise in other languages as it is in English. One way to support accuracy is to purchase a library of medical dictionaries and text books in the target language.

A team translation is translated by one person and edited by several others, who compare the English original with the version in the target language. Once the editors agree on the accuracy of the translation, it is proofread in the target language by someone who has a literacy level similar to that of the patients who will rely on it. The translator and editors change anything the proofreader doesn't understand until the translation is clear, accurate, and interesting to read. Hire a translator who is comfortable letting other people edit his or her translations. Team translation is the internationally accepted process for achieving quality. After printing the translation, let patients and families who read it offer their suggestions for improving it. One way to do this is to staple a review form and self-addressed envelope to each translation, inviting readers to tell you their opinions in their own language.

More opinions make better translations. Better translations turn confusion into communication, and clear communication is the goal of translation.

by Barbara Rayes
Spanish Translator

Learners who speak a foreign language will often repeatedly hear some key terms in English (such as "stoma" or "graft-versus-host disease"). Consider putting both the translated and the English versions of these words in the translated handout to help the learner become more comfortable with those terms in the English-speaking environment.

You Don't Need a Handout for Everything

Creating quality written teaching materials takes time and money. Carefully select your projects. Sometimes you don't need to create a handout.

"Rewriting brochures won't get us where we want to go. At the Grady general medicine clinic, if we had rewritten all the brochures at the 4th grade level, 50% of the patients still won't have been able to read them."
—Marwick, 1997, page 972

Either your patient population or the information you need to teach may require another medium for reinforcing information.

"For example, demonstrating crutch walking or showing a videotaped illustration of the correct technique may be far superior than distributing a booklet filled with text instructions to a patient. Health educators need to consider media other than discourse in which to creatively present information."
—Meade & Smith, 1991, page 157

Remember, You're not Alone

Busy nurses don't have time to create their own teaching materials. The research, editing, layout, expert and family reviews, storage, and distribution take a lot of time and energy. On the other hand, easy access to quality teaching tools will make your teaching more efficient and effective, saving you time.

You may now realize the written materials you are working with do not support your teaching as well as they could. This chapter was not meant to frustrate you. The written teaching materials you need are probably also needed by other health care providers around the country. As more health care providers learn and apply the criteria for quality teaching materials, demands will rise. Collaborate!

Who is producing quality teaching materials?

Can you trade the rights to reproduce theirs if you give them the right to reproduce yours?

Can you buy the rights to reproduce their teaching materials and adapt them to your needs?

Does your professional specialty organization facilitate the development of patient and family teaching materials?

Do publishers of teaching materials produce what you need? Have you communicated your criteria, including costs, to them?

With shared goals, criteria, and access to computers, there is no reason why we should each create our own teaching materials.

"We suggest that each State create one or more teams of health and literacy professionals organized to produce materials and educate health care providers."

—Plimpton & Root, 1994

Why not?

 ## If you want to learn more:

(1996). A primer for better patient education: Get it in writing. *Primary Care Weekly, 2*(46), 4.

Anderson, R.C., & Davison, A. (1986). *Conceptual and empirical bases of readability formulas.* Technical Report Number 392. ERIC Number: ED281180.

Austin, P.E., Matlack, R., Dunn, K.A., Kesler, C., & Brown, C.K. (1995). Discharge instructions: Do illustrations help our patients understand them? *Annals of Emergency Medicine, 25* (3), 317–320.

Baker, C. (1992). *Just say it! How to write for readers who don't read well: A training manual for writers.* Washington, DC: Plan.

Berger, D., Inkelas, M., Myhjre, S., & Mishler, A. (1994). Developing health education materials for inner-city low literacy patients. *Public Health Reports, 109*(2), 168–172.

Christopher, M., & Lajkowicz, C. (1993). Patient teaching by the book. *RN, July,* 48–50.

Clarity Associates, Inc., 35 Sprague Street, Dedham, MA 02026, 617-461-9440. [On-line]. Available: http://www.clearspros.com

Davis, T.C., Mayeaux, E.J., Fredrickson, D., Bocchini, J.A., Jackson, R.H., & Murphy, P.W. (1994). Reading ability of parents compared with reading level of pediatric patient education materials. *Pediatrics, 93*(3), 460–468.

Doak, C.C., Doak, L.G., & Root, J.H. (1996). *Teaching patients with low literacy skills* (2nd ed.). Philadelphia: Lippincott-Raven.

Doak, C.C., Doak, L.G., Friedell, G.H., & Meade, C.D. (1998). Improving comprehension for cancer patients with low literacy skills: Strategies for clinicians. *CA: Cancer Journal Clinics, 48*, 151–162. [On-line]. Available: http://www.ca-journal.org/frames/articles/articles_1998/48_151-162_frame.htm

Farley, D. (1997). Label literacy for OTC drugs. *FDA Consumer, May-June*, [On-line]. Available: http://www.fda.gov/dfac/features/1997/497_otc.html

Fink, A. (Ed.) (1995). *The survey kit.* Thousand Oaks, CA: Sage Publications.

Foltz, A., & Sullivan, J. (1996). Reading level, learning presentation preference, and desire for information among cancer patients. *Journal of Cancer Education, 11*(1), 32–38.

Glascoe, F.P., Oberklaid, F., Dworkin, P.H., & Trimm, F. (1998). Brief approaches to educating patient and parents in primary care. *Pediatrics, 101*(6), 1068–1072. [On-line]. Available: http://www.pediatrics.org/cgi/content/full/101/6/e10

Hanson-Divers, E.C. (1997). Developing a medical achievement reading test to evaluate patient literacy skills: A preliminary study. *Journal of Health Care for the Poor and Underserved, 8*(1), 56–70.

Hartman, T.J., McCarthy, P.R., Park, R.J., Schuster, E., & Kushi, L.H. (1994). Focus group responses of potential participants in a nutrition education program for individuals with limited literacy skills. *Journal of the American Dietetic Association, 94*(July), 744.

Hussey, L.C. (1997). Strategies for effective patient education material design. *Journal of Cardiovascular Nursing, 11*(2), 37–47.

Kingbeil, C., Speece, M.W., & Schubiner, H. (1995). Readability of pediatric patient education materials: Current perspectives on an old problem. *Clinical Pediatrics, February*, 96–102.

Lambert, C. (1998). Removing the mystery: Evaluation of a parent manual by adolescent parents. *Adolescence 33*(129), p. 61–73.

Lasater, L., & Mehler, P.S. (1998). The illiterate patient: screening and management. *Hospital Practice, 33*(4), 163–165, 169–170.

Lindsey, L.L., & Dey, B.H. (1995). Designing patient education materials to increase independence. *SCI Nursing, 12*(4), 124–126.

Marwick, C. (1997). Patients' lack of literacy may contribute to billions of dollars in higher hospital costs. *Journal of the American Medical Association, 278*(12), 971–973.

Mayeaux, E.J., Murphy, P.W., Arnold, C., Davis, T.C., Jackson, R.H., & Sentellion, T. (1996). Improving patient education for patients with low literacy. *American Family Physician, 53*(1), 205–212.

McCarthy, N. (1997). Prepare text for translations. 101 best electronic publishing tips (Tip 69). *Publish Magazine.*

Meade, C.D., & Smith, C.F. (1991). Readability formulas: Cautions and criteria. *Patient Education and Counseling, 17*, 153–158.

Morgan, D.L., & Krueger, R.A. (Ed.). (1998). *The focus group kit.* Thousand Oaks, CA: Sage Publications.

Murphy, P.W., Davis, T.C., et al. (1993). Rapid estimate of adult literacy in medicine (REALM): A quick reading test for patients. *Journal of Reading, 37*(2), 124–130.

National Center for Education Statistics. (1992). *1992 National Adult Literacy Survey.* Washington, DC: U.S. Department of Education. [On-line]. Available: http://www.ed.gov/NCES/nadlits/overview.html

Ott, B.B., & Hardie, T.L. (1997). Readability of advance directive documents. *Image: Journal of Nursing Scholarship, 29*(1), 53–57.

Patterson, C., & Teale, C. (1997). Influence of written information on patient's knowledge of their diagnosis. *Age and Ageing, 26*(1), 41–43.

Plimpton, S., & Root, J. (1994). Materials and strategies that work in low literacy health communication. *Public Health Reports, January/February*. [On-line]. Available: InfoTrac.

Rankin, S.H., & Stallings, K.D. (1996). *Patient education: Issues, principles, practices* (3rd ed.). Philadelphia: Lippincott-Raven.

Rice, M., & Valdivia, L. (1991). A simple guide for design, use, and evaluation of educational materials. *Health Education Quarterly, 18*(1), 79–85.

Sabogal, F., Otero-Sabogal, R., Pasick, R.J., Jenkins, C.N.H., & Pérez-Stable, E.J. (1996). Printed health education materials for diverse communities: Suggestions learned from the field. *Health Education Quarterly, 23*(Suppl.), S123–S141.

Sandrick, K. (1998). Teach your patients well. *Health Management Technology, 19*(4), 16–20. [On-line]. Available: InfoTrac.

Weiss, B.D., Blanchard, J.S., McGee, D.L., Hart, G., Warren, B., Burgoon, M., & Smith, K.J. (1994). Illiteracy among Medicaid recipients and its relationship to health care costs. *Journal of Health Care for the Poor and Underserved, 5*(2), 99–112. [On-line]. Available: InfoTrac.

Wide Range Achievement Test (WRAT 3). (1993). Wilmington, DE: Wide Range.

Williams, M.V., Parker, R.M., Baker, D.W., Parikh, N.S., Pitkin, K., Coates, W.C., & Nurss, J.R. (1995). Inadequate functional health literacy among patients at two public hospitals. *Journal of the American Medical Association, 274*(21), 1677–1682.

Wilson, F.L. (1996). Patient education materials nurses use in community health. *Western Journal of Nursing Research, 18*(2), 195–205.

Wilson, F.L., & McLemore, R. (1997). Patient literacy levels: A consideration when designing patient education programs. *Rehabilitation Nursing, 22*(6), 311–317.

WordsWork (1997) [On-line]. Available: http://www.wordswork.com/tips/audience.html

Wurman, R.S. (1989). *Information anxiety: What to do when information doesn't tell you what you need to know.* New York: Bantam Books.

Appendix 8-1. Everything You Want to Know About Readability Formulas

"Knowing how to determine the readability level of your materials is critical to you and to your patients."
—Doak, Doak, & Root, 1996, page 44

Once again, the nurse's scope of practice overlaps with that of other professions, in this case, education. There are at least 40 different readability formulas, and nearly all readability formulas are reasonably accurate (Doak et al., 1996). Some word processors and grammar check programs calculate results in one or several of the formulas. How do you know which to use? Here's a quick course in readability formulas.

Fry Readability Formula

If you only learn about one readability formula, Fry is it. The Fry Readability formula and directions for using it appear in Appendix 8-2 on page 227.

The Fry readability formula is widely accepted by reading professionals and is not copyrighted. This formula is preferred by Doak, Doak, and Root (1998) for use with health-related teaching materials. It is accurate and simple and can be done without a computer.

It calculates readability using the ratio of number of syllables per 100 words to the number of sentences per 100 words. You need to select test three samples from three different parts of the written material or if the original is a long booklet, six samples.

The calculation assigns a readability score between grade 1 to grade 17. The Fry readability formula requires that 50% of people reading at a given grade level be able to understand the text (Kingbeil, Speece, & Schubiner, 1995).

SMOG

The SMOG is a popular readability formula used by U.S. Department of Health and Human Services and American Cancer Society (Foltz & Sullivan, 1996). It is accurate and simple and can be done without a computer.

It calculates readability using the number of syllables per word in a set number of sentences. The SMOG is based on 100% comprehension. It requires that 100% of people reading at a given grade level be able to understand the text; most other formulas are based on 50% to 75% comprehension (Kingbeil et al., 1995).

Flesch Reading Score

The Flesch reading score is used by U.S. Department of Health, Education, and Welfare, which aims for seventh to eighth grade readability levels. It uses average number of words per sentence and the average syllables per word to calculate the score (Ott & Hardie, 1997).

Fog Readability Test

The Fog readability test uses average sentence length and the percentage of polysyllabic words to calculate the reading score. It requires that 75% of people reading at a given grade level be able to understand the text (Kingbeil et al., 1995).

Gunning Fog Index

The Gunning Fog index counts the difficult words of three or more syllables per words. It puts more emphasis on word length than on the number of words in a sentence (Ott & Hardie, 1997).

Flesch-Kincaid Grade Level

The Flesch-Kincaid test was developed to assess readability for adults. It evaluate readability as the average number of words per sentence and the average number of syllables per word, from which a grade-level score is assigned (Ott & Hardie, 1997).

> *"Readability measures should be used as general guidelines and the authors caution others against relying too heavily on individual readability scores."*
> —Kingbeil et al., 1995, page 101

Problems With Readability Formulas

How clear and understandable written material is depends on more than readability scores. Syllables and sentence length are not the only things that influence understandability.

"Readability scores fail to weigh the contextual meaning, obscurity of the language used, and a reader's motivation in attempting to comprehend the document—qualities that require complex analysis of both document and reader."

—Ott & Hardie, 1997, page 54

"Readability formulas . . . do not consider factors such as format, layout, complexity of the subject, word load or reader interest."

—Wilson, 1996, page 200

Some multisyllabic words may raise the grade level of the written teaching material but may not make it harder to read for a learner who has a special interest in the subject.

"In some situations, longer words may increase learnability because of the patient's familiarity with them. For example, a renal transplant recipient would be quite familiar with terms such as immunosuppressive, rejection and infection because they are emphasized often and repetitively in verbal and written interactions . . . long sentences or words may correlate with reading difficulty, but they may not cause learning difficulty."

—Meade & Smith, 1991, page 156

Remember you're ultimately evaluating teaching materials for understandability so you can teach your learner better and faster.

Using Readability Formulas

You may choose a formula, such as the Fry; calculate the score by hand; and use that score to evaluate the appropriateness of the written material for your learners. Instead, you may take advantage of features already on your computer to calculate readability scores.

"We urge the use of computer programs that will give the author several different indices to help accurately gauge reading level."

—Kingbeil et al., 1995, page 101

Some examples of software that calculates readability scores include Correct Grammar, Grammatik, RightWriter, WordPerfect, and Word. Check your software's tools for your options.

When we manually calculate readability scores, we look at several passages. When computer software calculates readability scores, it looks at the entire text. This means if one passage is more difficult than the rest, it is just averaged in to the total score. One researcher advises,

"Look at discrete sections of the text in addition to determining the average of the total text. . . . If an individual confronts a difficult section of a pamphlet, he or she is likely to stop reading the material at that point."
—Kingbeil et al., 1995, page 101

You can do this by highlighting the suspect section and checking it alone or copying and pasting it into a new file and checking it there. If the passage is significantly more difficult than the rest of the document, reword it.

How Far Down Should the Reading Level Be?

The Suitability Assessment of Materials (SAM), an instrument developed by Doak et al. (1996), can help you systematically assess the quality of health care instructions. This scale gives a score of "superior" to materials that are written at a fifth grade level or lower and "adequate" to sixth, seventh, or eighth grade levels. Ott & Hardie (1997) recommend that written materials given to patients should not be above the sixth grade level.

Given the technical content of some health instructions, it may be very difficult, if not impossible, to achieve a very low grade level while retaining meaning of content. For example, "diabetes" is three syllables, and "acetaminophen" is six. However, using these words with motivated readers may not decrease understandability of the text. So consider readability scores in context.

"Reading ability is not a sign of intelligence. You do your audience and yourself a disservice if you leave out information they need. Even complex ideas can be gotten across with simple language and with text aimed at your readers. The simpler the language, the easier it is for readers to use the information."
—Clarity Associates, Inc.

If You Get Resistance

Some people may consider it "dumbing down the text" if you lower reading levels so people understand the material. These people say they want to uphold certain standards or maintain an image of knowledgeable professionalism.

This is hogwash. After all, what is the purpose of written teaching materials?

The purpose of writiten teaching materials is to help learners make informed decisions, develop basic self-care skills, recognize problems, know what to do in response, and get questions answered. The point is to communicate specific information. If our learners don't understand the content, the materials are useless.

The purpose of written teaching materials is not to promote high educational standards in the community or prove that your health care facility's staff is smart.

Understandable teaching materials facilitate transfer of information and promote quality care. Clinicians should focus on the needs of the patients and families they serve. Indeed, every employee in the health care industry should adopt this focus. When done well, meeting the needs of our customers is our best marketing tool.

Like television programming, are health care providers aiming to the lowest common denominator by lowering reading levels? Are we lowering our standards of care? Absolutely not. Teaching materials written understandably include all the information the learner needs. The learner is not denied any data. The information is merely presented so it is clear.

> *"The same strategies that help low literacy patients will also help highly literate patients."*
> —Doak et al., 1998

> *"Our experience has been that when given a choice, at health fairs for example, even able readers choose easy-to-read materials if they have visual appeal."*
> —Plimpton & Root, 1994

> *"People with higher literacy skills, even people with a college education, learned more when information was presented in a way that was easy to read."*
> —Clarity Associates, Inc.

> *"Half the adult population needs easy-to-read materials, and the other half who do not need them wants them anyway. People under stress have limited ability to understand, and otherwise-abled readers prefer their information brief and concise."*
> —Plimpton & Root, 1994

Is the Reading Level Ever Too Low?

"Everyone loves our handouts. Except one patient. He had a PhD in Engineering and spent an hour telling us they should have had more detail."

—an RN

Does this mean the reading level of the handout was too low? No. It means this learner needed more information than was in that particular handout.

If this happens to you:

—Explain that the purpose of the handout was to summarize the most important points.
—Invite the learner to ask questions during the teaching discussion and augment the handout with notes.
—Provide the learner with additional resources so he can get detailed information.

Appendix 8-2. Fry Readability Formula

Assessing Readability Using the Fry Formula

Nearly all the 40+ readability formulas provide a reasonably accurate grade level (typically plus or minus one grade level with a 68-percent confidence factor). Among these formulas, the authors recommend the Fry formula. The Fry is widely accepted in the reading literature and among reading professionals and is not copyrighted. This formula applies from grade 1 through grade 17, and compared to some formulas, the Fry does not require as extensive a test sample.

It is not necessary to test the readability of every word and sentence. This would be especially tedious in a long booklet. Instead, test three samples from different parts of the instruction. For a very long text, such as a book of 50 pages or more, double the number to six samples.

Select a piece of material that you customarily use with your patients/clients and follow the five steps given below to determine its reading level using the Fry formula.[9]

Detailed Directions

1. **Select three 100-word passages from the material you wish to test.** Count out exactly 100 words for each passage, starting with the first word of a sentence. (Omit headings.) If you are testing a very short pamphlet that may have only a few hundred words, select a single 100-word sample to test.

   Readability levels may vary considerably from one part of your material to another. Therefore, select the three samples from different content topics, if possible. For example, if a pamphlet includes such topics as the disease process, treatment options, and actions the patient should take, select one sample from each of these topics.

   Additional information:
   • Count proper nouns. Hyphenated words count as one word.
   • A word is defined as a group of symbols with a space on either side; thus "IRA," "1994," and "&" are each one word.

2. **Count the number of** *sentences* **in each 100 words, estimating the fractional length of the last sentence to the nearest 1/10.** For example, if the 100th word occurs 5 words into a 15-word sentence, the fraction of the sentence is 5/15 or 1/3 or 0.3.

3. **Count the total number of** *syllables* **in each 100-word passage.** You can count by making a small check mark over each syllable. For initializations (e.g., IRA) and numerals (e.g., 1994), count 1 syllable for each symbol. So "IRA" = 3 syllables and "1994" = 4 syllables.

    There is a short cut to counting the syllables. Since each 100-word sample must have at least 100 syllables, skip the first syllable in each word. Don't count it; just add 100 after you finish the count. Count only the remaining syllables (that are greater than one) in the 100-word sample. Thus, you don't put check marks over any of the one-syllable words; you put only one check over each two-syllable word, two checks over three-syllable words, and so forth.

    Occasionally you may be in doubt as to the number of syllables in a word. Resolve the doubt by placing a finger under your chin, say the word aloud, and count the number of times your chin drops. Each chin drop counts as a syllable.

4. **Calculate the average number of sentences and the average number of syllables from the three passages.** This is done by dividing the totals obtained from the three samples by 3 as shown in the example below.

Example:

	NUMBER OF SENTENCES	NUMBER OF SYLLABLES
1st 100 words	5.9	124
2nd 100 words	4.8	141
3rd 100 words	6.1	158
Totals	*16.8*	*423*
Divide Totals by 3:	5.6 Average	141 Average

5. **Refer to the Fry graph.** On the horizontal axis, find the line for the *average number of syllables* (141 for above example). On the vertical axis find the line for the *average number of sentences* (5.6 for the example). The readability grade level of the material is found at the point where the two lines intersect.

    In the example above, the Fry chart shows the readability level at the 8th grade (see dot at the intersection in the figure

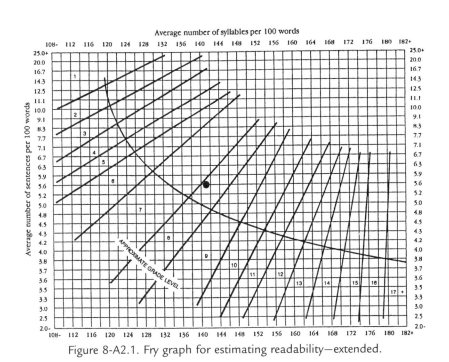

Average number of syllables per 100 words

Figure 8-A2.1. Fry graph for estimating readability—extended.

above). The curved line through the center of the Fry graph shows the locus of greatest accuracy. With a little practice, the five-step process will become much easier. You will soon be able to determine a readability level in less than 10 minutes.

Appendix 8-3. SAM, Suitability Assessment of Materials

Using SAM to Evaluate a Health Care Instruction

To use SAM for the first time, follow the six steps below:

1. Read through the SAM factor list and the evaluation criteria.
2. Read the material (or view the video) you wish to evaluate, and write brief statements as to its purpose(s) and key points.
3. For short instructions, evaluate the entire piece. For long instructions, select samples to evaluate.
4. Evaluate and score each of the 22 SAM factors.
5. Calculate total suitability score.
6. Decide on the impact of deficiencies and what action to take.

The entire process to evaluate your instructional material should take 30 to 45 minutes the first time through. For subsequent applications of SAM, you may skip the first step because the SAM factors and criteria will be already familiar to you.

For a first-time use of SAM, we suggest you test a simple, short example that has only a few illustrations.

1. **Read the SAM instrument and the evaluation criteria.**
2. **Read the material to be assessed.** Read (or view) the material you plan to evaluate. It will help if you write brief statements as to its purpose(s) and its key points. Refer to these as you evaluate each SAM factor. Use a note pad to jot down comments and observations as you read the material, view the video, or listen to the audiotape.
3. **The sampling process for SAM is somewhat similar to that described earlier for selecting samples to apply a readability formula.** If you are applying SAM to short material, such as a single-page instruction or a typical pamphlet (twofold or threefold), assess the entire instruction. Similarly, for audiotaped and videotaped instructions of less than 10 minutes, evaluate the entire instruction.

    To apply SAM to a longer text, such as a booklet, select three pages that deal with topics central to the purpose of the booklet. For booklets of more than 50 pages, increase the sample size to six pages. For videotaped or audiotaped instructions exceeding 10 minutes, select topics in 2-minute blocks from the beginning, middle, and end sections of the video or audio presentation.

4. **Evaluate material versus criteria for each factor, decide on its rating, and record it on the score sheet.** As you seek to evaluate your material against each factor, you are likely to find wide variation among different parts of your material. For any one factor, some parts may rate high (superior) while other parts of the same material rate low (unsuitable). For example, some illustrations may include captions, while others do not. Resolve this dilemma by giving most weight to the part of your material that includes the key points that you previously identified in step 2 above.

Materials that meet the superior criteria for a factor are scored 2 points for that factor; adequate receives 1 point; not suitable receives a zero. For factors that do not apply, write N/A. Use the SAM scoring sheet shown in the following figure to record your score for each of the 22 factors and to guide you in calculating the overall rating in percent.

5. **Calculate the total suitability score.** When you have evaluated all the factors and written a score for each one on the score sheet, add up the scores to obtain a total score. Spaces to do this are provided on the score sheet. The maximum possible total score is 44 points (100%)—a perfect rating, which almost never happens. A more typical example is the total score for your material being 34; your percent score is 34/44 or 77%.

For some instructional materials, one or more of the 22 SAM factors may not apply. For example, for an audiotape or a videotape, the text readability level (factor 2a) does not apply. To account for SAM factors that occasionally may not apply to a particular material, subtract 2 points for each N/A from the 44 total. Let's do that using the example from the paragraph above. If you arrived at a total score of 34 as noted above but had one N/A factor, subtract 2 points from 44 to a revised maximum score of 42. Thus, the percent rating would become 34/42, for a rating of 81 percent.

Interpretation of SAM Percentage Ratings:

70%–100%	Superior material
40%–69%	Adequate material
0%–39%	Not suitable material

2 points for superior rating
1 point for adequate rating
0 points for not suitable rating
N/A if the factor does not apply to this material

FACTOR TO BE RATED	SCORE	COMMENTS

1. CONTENT

(a) Purpose is evident
(b) Content about behaviors
(c) Scope is limited
(d) Summary or review included

2. LITERACY DEMAND

(a) Reading grade level
(b) Writing style, active voice
(c) Vocabulary uses common words
(d) Context is given first
(e) Learning aids via "road signs"

3. GRAPHICS

(a) Cover graphic shows purpose
(b) Type of graphics
(c) Relevance of illustrations
(d) Lists, tables, etc. explained
(e) Captions used for graphics

4. LAYOUT AND TYPOGRAPHY

(a) Layout factors
(b) Typography
(c) Subheads ("chunking") used

5. LEARNING STIMULATION, MOTIVATION

(a) Interaction used
(b) Behaviors are modeled and
       specific
(c) Motivation—self-efficacy

6. CULTURAL APPROPRIATENESS

(a) Match in logic, language,
       experience
(b) Cultural image and examples

Total SAM score: _____
Total possible score: _____, Percent score: _____%

SAM scoring sheet

6. **Evaluate the impact of deficiencies; decide on revisions.** A deficiency, especially an "unsuitable" rating, in any of the 22 factors is significant. Many of these can be readily overcome by revising a draft material or by adding a supplemental instruction to a material already published. However, factors in two of the groups, the readability level and cultural appropriateness, must be considered as potential go–no/go signals for suitability regardless of the overall rating.

   For example, except in the rare cases in which an instruction contains a set of illustrations that replicate the entire message given in the text, a written instruction with a very high readability level will not be understood and is unsuitable. Similarly, a material that portrays an ethnic group in an inappropriate way is almost surely unsuitable because it is likely to be rejected by members of that ethnic group.

SAM Evaluation Criteria

1. *Content*
   A. Purpose
      Explanation: It is important that readers/clients readily understand the intended purpose of the instruction for them. If they don't clearly perceive the purpose, they may not pay attention or may miss the main point.

Superior	Purpose is explicitly stated in title, or cover illustration, or introduction.
Adequate	Purpose is not explicit. It is implied, or multiple purposes are stated.
Not suitable	No purpose is stated in the title, cover illustration, or introduction.

   B. Content Topics
      Explanation: Because adult patients usually want to solve their immediate health problem rather than learn a series of medical facts (that may only *imply* a solution), the content of greatest interest and use to clients is likely to be behavior information to help solve their problem.

Superior	Thrust of the material is application of knowledge/skills aimed at desirable reader behavior rather than nonbehavior facts.
Adequate	At least 40% of content topics focus on desirable behaviors or actions.

> > Not suitable   Nearly all topics are focused on
> > nonbehavior facts.

C. Scope
Explanation: Scope is limited to purpose or objective(s).
Scope is also limited to what the patient can reasonably
learn in the time allowed.

> > *Superior*   Scope is limited to essential information
> > directly related to the purpose. Experience
> > shows it can be learned in time allowed.
> > *Adequate*   Scope is expanded beyond the purpose; no
> > more than 40% is nonessential
> > information. Key points can be learned in
> > time allowed.
> > *Not suitable*   Scope is far out of proportion to the
> > purpose and time allowed.

D. Summary and Review
Explanation: A review offers the readers/viewers a chance to
see or hear the key points of the instruction in other
words, examples, or visuals. Reviews are important; readers
often miss the key points upon first exposure.

> > *Superior*   A summary is included and retells the key
> > messages in different words and examples.
> > *Adequate*   Some key ideas are reviewed.
> > *Not suitable*   No summary or review is included.

2. *Literacy demand*

A. Reading Grade Level (Fry Formula)
Explanation: Unless the instruction presents the topics
completely without text (via visual, demonstrations, audio),
the text reading level may be a critical factor in patient
comprehension. Reading formulas can provide a
reasonably accurate measure of reading difficulty.

> > *Superior*   Fifth-grade level or lower (5 years of
> > schooling level).
> > *Adequate*   Sixth-, seventh-, or eighth-grade level (6–8
> > years of schooling level).
> > *Not suitable*   Ninth-grade level and above (9 years or
> > more of schooling level).

B. Writing Style
Explanation: Conversational style and active voice lead to
easy-to-understand text. Example: "Take your medicine
every day." Passive voice is less effective. Example: "Patients
should be advised to take their medicine every day."
Embedded information, the long or multiple phrases

included in a sentence, slows down the reading process and generally makes comprehension more difficult.

Superior   Both factors: (1) Mostly conversational style and active voice. (s) Simple sentences are used extensively; few sentences contain embedded information.

Adequate   (1) About 50% of the text uses conversational style and active voice. (2) Less than half the sentences have embedded information.

Not suitable   (1) Passive voice throughout. (2) Over half the sentences have extensive embedded information.

C. Vocabulary

Explanation: Common, explicit words are used (for example, doctor versus physician). The instruction uses few or no words that express general terms such as categories (for example, legumes versus beans), concepts (for example, normal range versus 15 to 70), and value judgments (for example, excessive pain versus pain lasts more than 5 minutes). Imagery words are used because these are words people can "see" (for example, whole wheat bread versus dietary fiber; a runny nose versus excess mucus).

Superior   All three factors: (1) Common words are used nearly all of the time. (2) Technical, concept, category, value judgment (CCVJ) words are explained by examples. (3) Imagery words are used as appropriate for content.

Adequate   (1) Common words are frequently used. (2) Technical and CCVJ words are sometimes explained by examples. (3) Some jargon or math symbols are included.

Not suitable   Two or more factors: (1) Uncommon words are frequently used in lieu of common words. (2) No examples are given for technical and CCVJ words. (3) Extensive jargon is used.

D. In Sentence Construction, The Context Is Given Before New Information

Explanation: We learn new facts/behaviors more quickly

when told the context first. Good example: "To find out what's wrong with you (the context first), the doctor will take a sample of your blood for lab tests" (new information).

Superior   Consistently provides context before presenting new information.

Adequate   Provides context before new information about 50% of the time.

Not suitable Context is provided last, or no context is provided.

E. Learning Enhancement by Advance Organizers (Road Signs)

Explanation: Headers or topic captions should be used to tell very briefly what's coming up next. These "road signs" make the text look less formidable and prepare the reader's thought process to expect the announced topic.

Superior   Nearly all topics are preceded by an advance organizer (a statement that tells what is coming next).

Adequate   About 50% of the topics are preceded by advance organizers.

Not suitable Few or no advance organizers are used.

3. *Graphics (illustrations, lists, tables, charts, graphs)*

A. Cover Graphic

Explanation: People *do* judge a booklet by its cover. The cover image often is the deciding factor in a patient's attitude toward, and interest in, the instruction.

Superior   The cover graphic is (1) friendly, (2) attracts attention, (3) clearly portrays the purpose of the material to the intended audience.

Adequate   The cover graphic has one or two of the superior criteria.

Not suitable The cover graphic has none of the superior criteria.

B. Type of Illustrations

Explanation: Simple line drawings can promote realism without including distracting details. (Photographs often include unwanted details.) Visuals are accepted and remembered better when they portray what is familiar and easily recognized. Viewers may not recognize the meaning of medical textbook drawings or abstract art/symbols.

> *Superior*   Both factors: (1) Simple, adult-appropriate, line drawings/sketches are used. (2) Illustrations are likely to be familiar to the viewers.
>
> *Adequate*   One of the superior factors is missing.
>
> *Not suitable* None of the superior factors are present.

C. Relevance of Illustrations

Explanation: Nonessential details, such as room background, elaborate borders, and unneeded color, can distract the viewer. The viewer's eyes may be "captured" by these details. The illustrations should tell the key points visually.

> *Superior*   Illustrations present key messages visually so the reader/viewer can grasp the key ideas from the illustrations alone. There are no distractions.
>
> *Adequate*   (1) Illustrations include some distractions. (2) Insufficient use of illustrations.
>
> *Not suitable* One factor: (1) Confusing or technical illustrations (nonbehavior related). (2) No illustrations or an overload of illustrations.

D. Graphics: Lists, Tables, Graphs, Charts, Geometric Forms

Explanation: Many readers do not understand the author's purpose for the lists, charts, and graphs. Explanations and directions are essential.

> *Superior*   Step-by-step directions, with an example, are provided that will build comprehension and self-efficacy.
>
> *Adequate*   "How-to" directions are too brief for reader to understand and use the graphic without additional counseling.
>
> *Not suitable* Graphics are presented without explanation.

E. Captions Are Used to "Announce"/Explain Graphics

Explanation: Captions can quickly tell the reader what the graphic is all about and where to focus within the graphic. A graphic without a caption is usually an inferior instruction and represents a missed learning opportunity.

> *Superior*   Explanatory captions with all or nearly all illustrations and graphics.
>
> *Adequate*   Brief captions used for some illustrations and graphics.
>
> *Not suitable* Captions are not used.

4. *Layout and typography*
   A. Layout
      Explanation: Layout has a substantial influence on the suitability of materials.

       Superior   At least five of the following eight factors are present:
   1. Illustrations are on the same page adjacent to the related text.
   2. Layout and sequence of information are consistent, making it easy for the patient to predict the flow of information.
   3. Visual cuing devices (shading, boxes, arrows) are used to direct attention to specific points or key content.
   4. Adequate white space is used to reduce appearance of clutter.
   5. Use of color supports and is not distracting to the message. Viewers need not learn color codes to understand and use the message.
   6. Line length is 30–50 characters and spaces.
   7. There is high contrast between type and paper.
   8. Paper has nongloss or low-gloss surface.

       Adequate   At least three of the superior factors are present.

       Not suitable   (1) Two (or less) of the superior factors are present. (2) Looks uninviting or discouragingly hard to read.

   B. Typography
      Explanation: Type size and fonts can make text easy or difficult for readers at all skill levels. For example, type in ALL CAPS slows everybody's reading comprehension. Also, when too many (six or more) type fonts and sizes are used on a page, the appearance becomes confusing and the focus uncertain.

       Superior   The following four factors are present:
   1. Text type is in uppercase and lowercase serif (best) or sans-serif.
   2. Type size is at least 12 point.
   3. Typographic cues (bold, size, color) emphasize key points.
   4. No ALL CAPS for long headers or running text.

       Adequate   Two of the superior factors are present.

       Not suitable   One or none of the superior factors are

present, or six or more type styles and sizes
are used on a page.

C. Subheadings or "Chunking"

Explanation: Few people can remember more than seven
independent items. For adults with low literacy skills, the
limit may be three- to five-item lists. Longer lists need to
be partitioned into smaller "chunks."

Superior	(1) Lists are grouped under descriptive subheadings or "chunks." (2) No more than five items are presented without a subheading.
Adequate	No more than seven items are presented without a subheading.
Not suitable	More than seven items are presented without a subheading.

5. *Learning stimulation and motivation*

A. Interaction Included in Text or Graphic

Explanation: When the patient responds to the
instruction—that is, does something to reply to a problem
or question—chemical changes take place in the brain that
enhance retention in long-term memory. Readers/viewers
should be asked to solve problems, make choices,
demonstrate, and so forth.

Superior	Problems or questions are presented for reader responses.
Adequate	Question-and-answer format is used to discuss problems and solutions (passive interaction).
Not suitable	No interactive learning stimulation provided.

B. Desired Behavior Patterns Are Modeled, Shown In
Specific Terms

Explanation: People often learn more readily by observation
and by doing it themselves rather than by reading or being
told. They also learn more readily when specific, familiar
instances are used rather than the abstract or general.

Superior	Instruction models specific behaviors or skills. (For example, for nutrition instruction, emphasis is given to changes in eating patterns or shopping or food preparation/cooking tips; tips to read labels.)

   Adequate Information is a mix of technical and common language that the reader may not easily interpret in terms of daily living (for example: *Technical:* Starches—80 calories per serving; High Fiber—1–4 grams of fiber in a serving).

   Not suitable Informatin is presented in nonspecific or category terms, such as the food groups.

 C. Motivation

  Explanation: People are more motivated to learn when they believe the tasks/behaviors are doable by them.

   Superior Complex topics are subdivided into small parts so that readers may experience small successes in understanding or problem solving, leading to self-efficacy.

   Adequate Some topics are subdivided to improve the readers' self-efficacy.

   Not suitable No partitioning is provided to create opportunities for small successes.

6. *Cultural appropriateness*

 A. Cultural Match: Logic, Language, Experience (LLE)

  Explanation: A valid measure of cultural appropriateness of an instruction is how well its logic, language, and experience (inherent in the instruction) match the LLE of the intended audience. For example, a nutrition instruction is a poor cultural match if it tells readers to eat asparagus and romaine lettuce if these vegetables are rarely eaten by people in that culture and are not sold in the readers' neighborhood markets.

   Superior Central concepts/ideas of the material appear to be culturally similar to the LLE of the target culture.

   Adequate Significant match in LLE for 50% of the central concepts.

   Not suitable Clearly a cultural mismatch in LLE.

 B. Cultural Image and Examples

  Explanation: To be accepted, an instruction must present cultural images and examples in realistic and positive ways.

   Superior Images and examples present the culture in positive ways.

   Adequate Neutral presentation of cultural images or foods.

Not suitable   Negative image, such as exaggerated or caricatured cultural characteristics, actions, or examples.

In summary, the SAM offers a systematic method to assess suitability of materials. In about 30 minutes you can obtain a numerical suitability score that you can use to decide whether or not a material is suitable for your patient population.

When making an evaluation using SAM, or using the checklist presented earlier in this chapter, you may have uncovered one or more specific deficiencies. If so, decide on how critical the deficiencies are to patient comprehension and acceptance of the key messages of your material. Guidance for making this decision may be found in Chapters 2 and 5. To overcome the deficiencies, you will find specific details related to each instructional media in the following chapters: Chapter 6 for written materials, Chapter 7 for visuals and graphics, and Chapter 8 for videotapes, audiotapes, and multimedia.

Computers as Teaching Tools

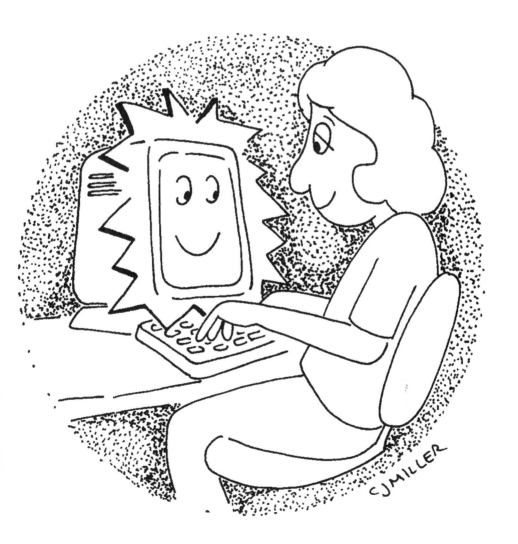

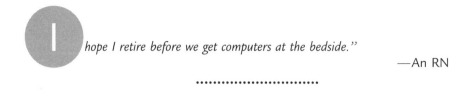

I hope I retire before we get computers at the bedside."

—An RN

....

"If we had computers, everyone could access the patient's chart. Now, we've got one chart for the nurses and one for the doctors, and the doctors don't read our notes. And I wish I could just talk my notes into a headset as I work, and have someone transcribe them and put them into a computer-generated chart. Then I'd only have to check and sign them, like the doctors do."

—An RN

....

Computers deserve their own chapter, because they are increasing in use, can be used for so many purposes, and are still misunderstood. Computers have changed how we look at information storage and gathering. The curricula of many library schools have even evolved from focusing on how to organize library materials to looking more broadly at how we access and organize information.

Computers and their applications change so fast that specific equipment, programs, and websites available as I write this may no longer exist by the time you read this. Consequently, this chapter addresses ways to use computers as teaching tools.

Computer Haves and Have-Nots

You may never use a computer, but some of your colleagues, patients, and families do. Unless you're close to retirement or working in the third world, computers may creep into your life soon, whether you want them to or not. If you don't know much about computers, skip this chapter. Find someone knowledgeable who will teach you the basics, and come back when you're ready. Glossaries of jargon will mean little to you until you see computers in action. You will learn much more and much faster if an enthusiastic fan of computers introduces you.

Even if you have no intention of ever buying a computer, they are now available for your use in libraries—public, hospital, and academic—all over the United States. Computers may be in your children's classrooms, your neighbors' dens, and your local photocopy store.

There will always be people who do not and will not use computers. Because tools change the way you think, computer haves and have-nots solve problems and communicate differently. This may cause barriers and challenges in relationships. Colleagues not on e-mail may be left out of the communication loop. Learners who won't try computers won't have access to certain teaching materials. However, this should be a problem only if computer haves and have-nots focus on the differences created by computer use. Keep your focus on shared goals and the transfer of information.

Problems With Computers

In the spirit of a good informed consent, computers have many potential problems:

- Computer hardware and software can be expensive.
- You need specific hardware and software to accomplish your tasks. You have to know how to use them.
- You need to back up what you put on your computer. If the hardware or the software fails, without a backup you will have lost your work. You need to keep a backup at some remote site, just in case there's a fire or robbery.
- Computers require electricity. You need a surge protector and a backup battery for your computer and modem to protect against lightning strikes and power surges, brownouts, and outages.
- Others could mess with your computer (hackers). They could learn your passwords or put in their own passwords so you can't get at your own data (especially if you haven't put one in yourself). Others could intercept your e-mail messages. If you don't empty the history or cache on your web browser, others could see what websites you've visited. (Your Help file or browser's documentation should tell you how to empty your history or cache.)
- Your computer could get a virus, as innocent as a runny nose or as virulent as fulminant hepatitis. Antivirus programs are slightly more effective than acyclovir. This is because new computer viruses are created and released by intelligent, mean-spirited people every day.
- Software programs can conflict with one another or develop problems over time. Hardware can break down. You could run out of hard drive space or RAM. You might buy software that is not compatible with your computer.

Aside from hardware and software, using computers could present other problems:

- The technology could overwhelm the subject matter. Computer output, on screen or printed, can look very, very good. They may look so good that you may have trouble looking beyond the neat, attractive presentation to notice the typos and blatant errors in content.
- Computers don't translate languages very well.

"It's easier to translate a document from scratch than to fix a computer translation."
                    —Barbara Rayes, a professional Spanish translator

- What you put into computers is what you get out. Forsythe (1996) said that computer programs "embody tacit assumptions held by those who build them, reflecting meanings taken for granted in particular cultural and disciplinary arenas" (page 551).

Forsythe looked at an interdisciplinary project to design and build a computerized patient education system for people with migraine. It linked a history-taking module with an explanation module. Forsythe found the design team assumed "knowledge about migraine" meant biomedical knowledge. However, migraine sufferers do not lack knowledge about migraines, it's just different knowledge from that of physicians. The information taught in the program was what the physicians knew, not necessarily what the migraine sufferers wanted to know.

In addition, the questionnaire was intended to establish the user's headache history. One multiple-choice question asked if the headaches began with illness, medication, or accident. If the headaches started after an injury from intentional violence, such as domestic violence, there was no way to report it. Violence is not an illness, medication, or accident. The correct choice was not offered.

"While intended to support migraine patients by offering useful information not given them by physicians, the system in fact offers information characterized by the same assumptions and deletions as that provided by neurologists. Thus, although intended to empower migraine patients, this system may actually reinforce rather than reduce the power differential between doctor and patient."
                    —Forsythe, 1996, page 551

Assumptions and biases are not always obvious.

Computers are only a tool. "Patient education on the web" is just information, not education. Computers merely store, sort, compute, process, and report information.

"Computers are number-crunching machines, or vehicles for gathering and storing data—not learning tools that might reshape our understanding and alter the ways we make sense out of the information we receive."
—Senge, Kleiner, Roberts, Ross, & Smith, 1994, page 529

Advantages of Computers

If you look at a limitation differently, you could see it as an advantage. Computers store, sort, compute, and process information much more quickly and accurately than your brain ever will. Because computers respond interactively, they also hold attention.

As computers get more complex and effective, they are also getting smaller and, especially if you consider computing power, less expensive. Every day, more people buy and learn how to use computers.

Applications to Patient and Family Education

"One need not have a degree in Nursing Informatics or use programs uniquely for nursing to take advantage of the many opportunities a personal computer offers to assist you in your current nursing position."
—Martin & Connor, 1996, page 76

Computers are a powerful tool for patient and family education. They have many applications.

Using the Computer to Create Teaching Materials

As indicated in the previous chapter, written materials can be created on computers. With layout software, you can add illustrations and adjust font size. Word processing and grammar software can calculate reading levels using standardized formulas. Puzzle-creating software, such as Puzzle Power, can help you create crosswords, fill-in, and other puzzles to help learners process information. If you want more details, Martin and Conner (1996) describe how they made attractive patient teaching materials using basic, inexpensive software.

If you are going to create your own teaching materials, consider copyrighting them. Copyright protection is automatically granted when an original, created work is fixed in a tangible medium of expression. This means that as I type these words, they are copyrighted. (This is true for works published after March 1, 1989.) Add "© [the year] [copyright owner's name]" to the bottom of the work to inform others of who owns the copyright.

It isn't necessary to register a copyright unless you might pursue an infringement suit. On the other hand, it costs only $20 to register materials. You can send them in large batches annually and name them "teaching materials created in [this year]." If you want to know more about how to copyright the materials you create, see Box 9-1 for details.

BOX 9-1   Learning More About Copyright

For information about copyright, rules and forms contact:

US Copyright Office
Library of Congress
Copyright Office Publication Section, LM-45
101 Independence Avenue, SE
Washington, DC 20559-6000
202-707-3000
http://lcweb.loc.gov/copyright/
$20.

If you want to use material that is copyrighted, ask the owner of the copyright for permission directly, or check to see if the item is covered by the Copyright Clearance Center (CCC). It provides users a lawful way to make photocopies from its collection of over 1.75 million titles.
Copyright Clearance Center: http://www.copyright.com/
Do you want legal information about copyrights? Check the site:
Copyright Law in the United States: http://www.bitlaw.com/copyright/
Internet copyright law is a new and developing field. If you want to find links to articles on the latest information, check the site:
Internet Copyright Law: http://www.wemsi.on.ca/netlaw.html

Internalize Information Systems

Computer networks within your organization can be used in many ways to support patient and family education. For example, a database program can be used to help you manage materials:

> *"Once the ward's articles have been cataloged into a database, if an article is needed on chest tubes, one would ask the program to search for the words 'chest tube.' It would supply the user with a list of articles the ward has obtained with those key words."*
>
> —Martin & Connor, 1996, page 78

Weaver (1995) explains how one hospital created its own teaching sheets, and the finalized versions would be "placed in the hospital's computer system, which would provide several advantages:

- Every nurse would have easy access to the teaching sheets on the nursing units.
- Sheets would be printed only as needed, reducing waste of paper.
- Teaching sheets could be updated easily to provide only current information to patients" (page 79).

Another hospital, Phoenix Children's, has taken this a step further. All of the internally created teaching materials have been converted into portable document format (PDF) files. This type of computer file is excellent for distribution of electronic documents because they keep their original look and feel, are compact, and can be read and printed on any computer with the reader software (Acrobat Readers). They can be printed but cannot be changed by the user. PDF files can be sent by e-mail, posted on the web, posted on intranets, or loaded on a CD-ROM.

In addition, this hospital uses Acrobat Catalog software to create full text indexes. Unlike title and key word indexes, these contain every word in every PDF document. Users who are looking for appropriate teaching materials can get onto any computer on the system and enter key words into Acrobat Search software. All the teaching materials that contain those words are found, and the user can review selected handouts on the screen for appropriateness and then print them out. Teaching materials print out just as they were created, with the identical fonts, illustrations, and layout. This is possible even if the software that created the document, or fonts in the document, are not on the receiving computer.

Get Information to Create Teaching Materials

When you decide to create your own teaching materials, many questions may come up. How are other nurses around the country doing this? What's the most current research on this topic? To what resources can I refer learners? Computers can help you get answers.

Use E-Mail

There are several ways computers can help you collect current research or get other information to create teaching materials. One resource is e-mail. You can send a note to clinical nurse specialists around the country with a question one morning and often get answers by the end of the day.

Plug into a network of nurses or patient education managers, and see how easy it is. They can e-mail you references, bibliographies, or whole files of information. Create a list of colleagues you meet at conferences, or tap into existing mailing lists. Externally managed mailing lists may have a moderator and may have qualifications for admission. You can find out about existing mailing lists from colleagues, or check a database of lists (such as http://www.liszt.com/, which, at the time of this writing, includes almost 300 health-related lists). The right e-mailing list could be very useful and the responses timely.

Do you want to know how other organizations solved the same problems you face? You could send an e-mail, or look at whatever is already posted on the web. For example, are you about to revise your facility's patient handbook? The patient handbook of the National Institute of Health is available online at http://www.cc.nih.gov/ccc/patient_handbook/index.html.

Search for Information

You may search for information in many places. For example, you may search on CD-ROMs, such as InfoTrac; databases on the internet; or use a search engine on the web.

Did you know there are professionals who are experts at searching? Best of all, you can consult them for free. They're called librarians, and you can find them in libraries (public, medical, academic, and industrial). They are trained in searching techniques and can save you a great deal of time and frustration. Some will even do searches for you, which, depending on the library and your relationship to it, may be done free or for a fee.

Using computers to search for information can be very rewarding or very frustrating, depending on the following variables:

- How much information actually exists on the topic you're exploring
- The database you choose
- The search engine you choose
- Your search strategy
- The phase of the moon, solar flares, or some other variable you can't identify or control (This last item has been found through subjective personal experience but has not yet been verified in the professional literature.)

If this is already sounding like gibberish to you, see Box 9-2 for definitions of some search terms.

BOX 9-2   Words to Know

browser. This program lets you read information on the world wide web. Browsers include Netscape and Explorer.

bookmark. This is a favorite site. It is the feature of browsers that lets you record a website's address so you can return to that site quickly without typing the address.

compact disc-interactive (CD-i). These look like CD-ROMs but require a CD-i player and television to use. They provide interactive, full screen, full motion digital video. They are less expensive than CD-ROMs and easy to set up, but not many programs are available.

compact disc-read-only memory (CD-ROM). This provides interactive, full screen, full motion, digitized video.

computer-assisted instruction (CAI).

computer-based teaching (CBT). These computer programs are for interactive teaching. The software may come on discs, hard drive, or CD-ROM.

cyberspace. This is the dimension you are in when you go online.

download. Copy a file from another computer onto your computer.

e-mail. Electronic mail lets you send messages and documents to anyone on the network.

hits. These are the items that are listed when you use a search engine and are often referred to as number of hits.

home page. A home page is the introduction to a website, like the contents of a book.

HTML. HTML stands for Hypertext Markup Language.

Box 9-2 *(Continued)*

Java. Computer languages are used to create websites.

internet. This worldwide system of cables links smaller computer networks together.

intranet. This organization-wide computer network is similar to the internet but is local.

laser videodisc.

interactive videodisc (IVD). This provides interactive, full screen, full motion video to a computer or television monitor and can provide better quality images than CD-ROMs and CD-is. Learners control how much and what type of data they see by touching the monitor.

link.

external link.

hypertext.

hyperlink. This lets you travel around on the web. When you are on a website, certain words and phrases will be underlined or in a different color from the rest of the text. Point to an underlined word on the screen and click on your mouse, and you will be taken (hyperlinked) to a new page.

listserv.

newsgroups.

bulletin boards.

mailing lists. Groups of computer users to carry on discussions on a particular topic. They distribute information to a large number of people at one time. If you sign up to be on a listserv on a topic of interest, you can get a lot of e-mail on that topic.

metasearch tools. Search engines combine the results of other search engines. Examples include Metacrawler and Starting Point.

navigating. This is how you find your way around the web.

online. This is the state of being connected to a computer service, bulletin board system, or public access site.

operators. These make a search more specific, like "and/+" "not/−" "next to" or "near" (like two words within 10 words of one another in a sentence).

search engine. These automated programs are used to find information. You enter a term or phrase, and the engine, according to its rules, locates and retrieves addresses for websites from its database. Search engines to search the WWW include HotBot and AltaVista. Search engines may also appear within a website to search information on that site.

search strategy. This is how you do a search or the search engine, key words or phrases, and operators you use in a search.

syntax. The order of entering words to search on a search engine is syntax.

Box 9-2 *(Continued)*

Sysop. This means system operator. It monitors and controls bulletin boards to limit profanity and inappropriate postings. Sysops may direct the discussion. Sysops may not be experts in the subject areas they monitor.

text-only browser. This browser shows only text, no pictures.

text-only option. This lets the user browse only text, and no pictures are downloaded. Because pictures can take time to download, this may speed up information gathering.

upload. Copy a file from your computer onto another computer.

URL. The Uniform Resource Locator is the address of a website, made up of letters, dots, and slashes. Websites start with "http://."

website. Computer files posted on the WWW consist of a collection of information posted on the WWW, developed by individuals, organizations, businesses, groups, and government agencies.

world wide web (WWW) (web). This part of the internet can display graphics, animations, and sound. It contains websites that use links to documents and other sites.

"The Web is not a likely source for much academic research. Scholarly journal articles, conference proceedings, statistical information, and reports on serious research initiatives are still best found in an academic or research library."
        —Dickstein, Greenfield, & Rosen, 1997, page 62

There are many databases with health information, including CINAHL, MEDLINE, CANCERLIT, and PsycLIT. Companies that market databases include SilverPlatter, InfoTrac, and EBSCO. Databases may give you citations for articles or books or full text information. The health databases of InfoTrac and EBSCO include many lay publications. The other databases listed can help you find those scholarly journal articles.

For example, you can access MEDLINE from several places on the web (one is http://igm.nlm.nih.gov). With this, you can obtain relevant bibliographic references but may not be able to access the full text of those articles without paying for them online or going to a library.

You locate information in a database with a search engine. Search engines are automated programs used to find information. How do you use them? Search engines ask for a key word or words. You type in what you are looking for (your search terms), hit the "send" key, and after a while, the results of your search appear.

They also have advanced features that let you refine your search, such as "English only" so you don't get so many irrelevant references. All search engines have search tips. Read them. For example, they explain that AltaVista, Infoseek, and Excite use quotation marks (" ") around phrases or multiple words to look for them together, as in "patient education." They also use the plus sign (+) to include and minus signs (−) to exclude specific terms.

All world wide web (WWW) search engines index web addresses (URLs) and titles of web pages. Different search engines index websites with other data, too. Other text WWW search engines may look at the following:

- Major section headers
- The first line of text on the homepage
- Frequently mentioned words
- All the text on the website

Box 9-3 lists some of the general WWW search engines.

There are also specialized search engines and search engines within websites to help you find data quicker. For example, Four11 is one of the search engines you can use to find people (http://www.four11.com). It is useful if you are looking for the e-mail address of a specific colleague. Another way to find e-mail addresses of health care providers is to look for them on the web pages of their affiliated facilities or universities.

There are also medical search engines:

Achoo: Internet Health Care Directory
    http://www.achoo.com/
HealthAtoZ
    http://www.HealthAtoZ.com/

BOX 9-3   General WWW Search Engines

AltaVista Technology	http://altavista.digital.com
HotBot	http://www.hotbot.com
Infoseek	http://guide.infoseek.com
Lycos	http://www.lycos.com
Magellan	http://www.mckinley.com
MetaCrawler	http://www.metacrawler.com
Starting Point	http://stpt.com
WebCrawler	http://www.webcrawler.com
Yahoo	http://www.yahoo.com

MEDWEB, Consumer Health
http://www.gen.emory.eduMEDWEB/keyword/
consumer_health.html

There's even a website that offers information about medical search engines, how to choose and use them: Understanding Medical Search Engines, http://www.pcs.ucdmc.ucdavis.edu/net/infomed.htm.

Search engines weigh what they find, list them in order, and present them on your screen. The logic of the order of the listings created by some search engines may not be obvious. For example, Webcrawler scans websites and counts the number of times the words you searched for appear. Therefore, some sites could get higher in your search results if they mention that key term many times in their text. Some search engines may put the websites of their advertisers higher in your search results, so sometimes the information you are looking for may be on the second or third screen.

Metasearch engines use other search engines. Metacrawler has access to AltaVista, Excite, Infoseek, Lycos, Yahoo!, and WebCrawler. It performs searches on several tools at the same time, so you don't get duplicate hits. Starting Point performs searches of specified tools, one at a time, in a sequence you choose.

Metasearch engines let you search more databases in a shorter amount of time. They let you limit your search by domain or organizational category, like "gov" or "edu." With Starting Point, you can customize searches by taking advantage of the uniqueness of each search engine or database. In general, when you use metasearch engines, you can't use the customized features of the individual search engines accessed.

To find out the latest on search engines, see the website Search Engine Watch at http://www.searchenginewatch.com. It keeps up on new and changes in existing search engines.

Tips for Searching the Web

"Persons seeking information on special medical or psychological conditions, disorders, or problems seem to use the Web very effectively to keep in touch with each other and to disseminate information."
—Dickstein et al., 1997, page 63

Imagine a spider web. That is how the web is connected, with links, or lines, from one site to another.

This is good and bad. If you follow links through different topics you could get new perspectives on a topic you would not have found if you looked up your topic in the library's Index Medicus. For example, a website discussing the treatment of cancer could link to a website on the use of marijuana to treat nausea, and that could link to the website for NORML, the organization that is working to legalize that drug. When you follow links, you could end up thinking about your topic more creatively or getting off on a tangent and wasting time.

Sparks and Rizzolo (1998) offer some tips for effectively searching the web:

- Understand your database.
- Read the frequently asked questions or help section.
- Take notes; remember the search terms and database you tried.
- Spell correctly.
- Search using the most unusual term within the topic for which you're looking (for example, "psoriatic arthritis" instead of "psoriasis").
- Search using terms that could be mentioned frequently in the site for which you're looking.
- Use appropriate operators and syntax.

If your search results are not what you hoped for, try the following:

- Try synonyms ("renal" instead of "kidney").
- Try more than one database. (You did take notes on what you tried, right?)
- Decide how your results are off, and adjust your search terms to compensate. (You did take notes on what you tried, right?) (If "nursery" comes up with too many botanical hits, add the word "infant.")
- If you still get too many hits, try advanced searching adjustments to refine your search.
- If the site you want charges an access fee, don't just resign yourself and jump on. First, use a search engine to see if you can access the same information without paying a fee. For example, MEDLINE is available on the web for a fee and for free.
- If you enter a URL and get back a message telling you that it is a dead link (such as "Not Found"), don't give up. Just like patients move and forget to give you their new whereabouts, websites are updated and their addresses change. Take the website address you are trying to access, such as http://www.phxchildrens.com/programs/emily/educationprog.html, and, starting from the right, remove one segment at a time. Next time, try accessing http://www.phxchildrens.com/programs/emily/. If that doesn't help, try accessing http://www.phxchildrens.com/programs/. You might find what you're looking for or better.
- If this method doesn't work, use a search engine to see if the information has moved elsewhere on the web. (Keep in mind that every link listed in this book is like a patient. Each is at risk for dying or moving and leaving no forwarding address.)

Don't stick with one favorite search engine. Get to know at least a few search engines well. If you do not find the information you need with one search engine, try another. If your search takes more time than usual, try another search engine. Search time will vary with the traffic on the internet, the complexity of your search, and the ability of the search engine to search quickly. Of course, it could be the moon phase or solar flares.

Sometimes it's easier to find a website with links that may help you find the topic for which you are looking. See Box 9-4 for a partial list of websites with health-related links that may help you create patient and family teaching materials.

BOX 9-4 Some Health-Related WWW Sites

The only way to find the best current websites is to do a search today. However, sometimes you just want to rely on old favorites. As websites are updated, URLs can change. Here are some sites that may have, or lead you to, the information you need.

When you find a site you expect to return to someday, you may bookmark it and keep the address in your list of favorite places. Look for this feature on your web browser. Find a balance between bookmarking a few general sites and every site on a subject.

If you create your own website, you may add links to the sources you find useful. Ask specialists in a subject to identify what they think are the best sites in their fields of expertise.

Agency for Health Care Policy Research
http://www.ahcpr.gov.80/consumer

American Academy of Family Physicians
http://www.aafp.org

American Academy of Pediatrics
http://www.aap.org/

American Medical Association
http://www.ama-assn.org

Centers for Disease Control and Prevention, CDC
http://www.cdc.gov/

Combined Health Information
http://chid.nih.gov/

FDA, Food and Drug Administration
http://www.fda.gov

Box 9-4 *(Continued)*

If you have a computer but do not have internet access, you can receive text from FDA's site (without graphics) by dialing by modem the agency's bulletin board service (BBS): 1-800-222-0185, type "bbs" and select the information you want from the menu.

FDA/Center for Food Safety
http://vm.cfsan.fda.gov

Food and Drug Administration
http://www.fda.gov

Food and Nutrition Center
http://www.nal.usda.gov/fnic/

Healthfinder
http://www.healthfinder.gov/

HealthWeb
http://www.healthweb.org/

KidsHealth
http://www.ama-assn.org/kidshealth

MEDWEB
http://www.gen.emory.eduMEDWEB/keyword/consumer_health.html

National Center for Education in Maternal and Child Health
http://www.ncemch.org

National Center for Health Statistics, NCHS
http://www.cdc.gov/nchswww/nchshome.htm/

National Highway Traffic Safety Administration
www.nhtsa.dot.gov

National Institutes of Health
http://www.nih.gov
one of the sites from which you can access free MEDLINE

National Institute for Diabetes, Digestive and Kidney Diseases
http://www.niddk.nih.gov

NIH consumer information
http://www.nih.gov/health/consumer/conicd.htm

NOAH (New York Online Access to Health)
http://noah.cuny.edu

Office of Alternative Medicine
http://altmed.od.nih.gov/

Box 9-4 *(Continued)*

OncoLink, University of Pennsylvania Cancer Center Resource
http://www.oncolink.upenn.edu/

Parents Helping Parents
http://www.php.com

Pediatric Points of Interest
http://www.med.jhu.edu/

PharmWeb
http://www.pharmweb.net/
http://www.mcc.ac.uk/pwmirror/pwi/pharmwebi.html

U.S. National Library of Medicine, NLM
http://www.nlm.nih.gov/

Tips for Evaluating the Information

"We are in an electronic environment where credibility, authority, and subject expertise are not always readily apparent."
—Dickstein et al., 1997, page 61

Academic journals go through peer review. Anyone can publish on the web. How do you know you're looking at a good website?

"Con artists and scientists have equal publishing rights on the Internet."
—Larkin, 1996

"It's your job as a searcher to evaluate what you locate, in order to determine whether it suits your needs."
—Harris, 1997

You don't want to teach your learners incorrect information. If you use the internet to obtain either teaching materials or information to put into your own teaching materials, you know anyone can have a website, and say anything on it. How do you know if your source is reliable? What are the qualities of a good website? Here's a compilation of qualities that have been identified in the literature:

- Accurate
  - Is the information on the website true?
  - Does the website indicate from where its information comes?

- Authoritative
  - Who wrote the information on the website?
  - Do the author(s) or editor(s) of the website have proper credentials to write about the topic? This includes education, training, experience, professional affiliations, certifications, and publications in a field relevant to the information.
  - Are you familiar with the reputation and professional standing of the website author(s) or editor(s)?
  - Do the author(s) or editor(s) tell you how to contact them by e-mail, postal service address, or telephone?
  - If an organization is responsible for the website, is it known and respected?
  - Is there a list of names and credentials of those who prepare and review the website's contents?
  - Who maintains the site?

The best resources are government and university websites. The websites of individuals and lay organizations may be less objective. They are more likely to publish on the web to convey a message, which may influence the contents and links they offer.

- Credible, reasonable, and responsible
  - Does the website cover all sides of the subject well? Is it objective?
  - Does the information on the website have a bibliography with scientific references from good sources?
  - If the website makes strong claims, are all sides of the issue presented fairly?
  - Does the website provide reasons, facts, and specifics?
  - What is the tone of the information offered on the website? Is it balanced? Angry, hateful, spiteful, and critical tones or extreme positiveness may indicate subjectivity.
  - Is there evidence for conflict of interest or hidden agenda?
  - Is there a slant to the information on the website? It may be political, economic, religious, or philosophical.
  - What issues does the website raise, and what issues does it ignore?
  - Does the website contain a lot of misspellings or bad grammar?

If you find a website that advocates or sells a cure to be taken instead of prescription medicine, a suspected fraudulent offering, inform the Food and Drug Administration by e-mail at otcfraud-@cder.fda.gov.

- Current
  - Is the information on the website current?
  - What is the date on the website?

  Some information, like anatomy, changes infrequently. Other information, like the latest medications, change often.
  - Is there evidence that the website is updated or maintained?
  - Is the revision date appropriate for the speed at which the field changes?
  - Is the information still valuable?
- Easy to use
  - Can you get to the information you want easily and quickly? Is the website well organized?
  - If the website has an internal search mechanism, does it help you find what you need?
  - Is the information easy to read?
  - If you need special software to access information on the website (such as an Adobe Acrobat Reader), are links available to obtain this software?
  - If there are educational graphics, do they help you understand the information?
  - If there are decorative graphics (not necessary to convey content), do they take too long to download?
  - If there are graphics, is there an option for text only?
  - If there is a text-only option, is the website still useful?
  - If there is audio or video to the website, are the contents of the website still complete if they cannot be accessed?
  - Are there options for large print or audio?
- Quality of links
  - Does the website link to other health-related websites? It should, because no reputable organization would imply it is the only source of information on the topic.
  - Does the website link only health-related websites that are reliable?
  - Do the links work?
  - Are the links relevant and appropriate?
  - Are the links current?
  - Are there links to organizations that should be represented?
- Reliability
  - Is the website accurate, authoritative, credible, and current?
  - Does the website provide sources and support for the information provided?
  - Does the website have a bibliography?
  - Is the purpose of the website clear?
  - Is the website an advertisement?

- Does the website show a bias?
- Is there evidence for quality control?
  - Does the content come from peer-reviewed journals or books?
  - Does the website have a peer review process?

Website addresses or URLs can help determine the source of the information. The URL contains a three-letter string that tells you what category of organization or individual provides this resource:

gov is a government agency, which is very reliable.

edu is an educational institution, which can be from a university department (very reliable) or a student or community member whose computer is based in the campus system (may not be so reliable).

org is a miscellaneous organization, including not-for-profits, which may or may not be reliable. Examine other indicators.

com is a commercial organization that may be promoting a product or service; it may or may not be reliable. Examine other indicators.

net is a provider of internet services. They serve as brokers for companies and organizations with websites and may or may not be reliable. Examine other indicators.

There are additional three-letter strings in website addresses outside of the United States. Examine other indicators.

- Scope and coverage
  - Is the content of the website comprehensive?
  - Is the information on the website too general or too detailed?
  - Is the information on the website too simplified or too technical?
  - Are technical terms defined?
- Stable
  - Is it a new website, or has it been on the web for several years?
- Valuable
  - Is the information on the website valuable?

See if other sources support the information you obtain from this website.

"Triangulate your findings: that is, find at least three sources that agree."
—Harris, 1997

Do you just want a check sheet for evaluating websites?

The Office of Health Promotion has developed a reliable and valid instrument to critique the credibility of health-related web sites (Fig. 9-1). The Health on the Net Foundation has created a set of principles

---

Health-Related Web Site Evaluation Form

This evaluation instrument is for health educators and clinicians to use to evaluate the appropriateness of web sites for their clients and patients for further health education. Please take a few minutes to browse the site before completing the evaluation form.

I. Web site information

Title of site: _____

Subject of site: _____

Web site address: _____

Whom do you think is the intended audience?

_____

What do you think the objective is for this site?

_____

_____

Circle the number you feel best represents the site: 1 = disagree, 2 = agree, 0 = not applicable (N/A). Add up the total points scored for each page at the bottom of each page.

II. Content

	Disagree	Agree	N/A
1. The purpose of the site is clearly stated or may be clearly inferred.	1	2	0
2. The information covered does not appear to be an "infomercial" (i.e., an advertisement disguised as health education).	1	2	0
3. There is no bias evident.	1	2	0
4. If the site is opinionated, the author discusses all sides of the issue, giving each due respect.	1	2	0
5. All aspects of the subject are covered adequately.	1	2	0
6. External links are provided to fully cover the subject (if not needed, circle 0).	1	2	0

III. Accuracy

7. The information is accurate (if not sure, circle 0).	1	2	0
8. Sources are clearly documented.	1	2	0
9. The web site states that it subscribes to HON code principles.	1	2	0

Page Score _____

Figure 9-1.

	Disagree	Agree	N/A
IV. Author			
10. The site is sponsored by or is associated with an institution or organization.	1	2	0
11. For sites created by an individual, author's/editor's credentials (educational background, professional affiliations, certifications, past writings, experience) are clearly stated.	1	2	0
12. Contact information (email, address, and/or phone number) for the author/editor or webmaster is included.	1	2	0
V. Currency			
13. The date of publication is clearly posted.	1	2	0
14. The revision date is recent enough to account for changes in the field.	1	2	0
VI. Audience			
15. The type of audience the author is addressing is evident (eg, academic, youth, minority, general).	1	2	0
16. The level of detail is appropriate for the audience.	1	2	0
17. The reading level is appropriate for the audience.	1	2	0
18. Technical terms are appropriate for the audience.	1	2	0
VII. Navigation			
19. Internal links add to the usefulness of the site.	1	2	0
20. Information can be retrieved in a timely manner.	1	2	0
21. A search mechanism is necessary to make this site useful.	1	2	0
22. A search mechanism is provided.	1	2	0
23. The site is organized in a logical manner, facilitating the location of information.	1	2	0
24. Any software necessary to use the page has links to download software from the internet.	1	2	0
VIII. External Links			
25. Links are relevant and appropriate for this site.	1	2	0
26. Links are operable.	1	2	0
27. Links are current enough to account for changes in the field.	1	2	0
28. Links are appropriate for the audience (eg, site for the general public do not include links to highly technical sites).	1	2	0
29. Links connect to reliable information from reliable sources.	1	2	0
30. Links are provided to organizations that should be represented.	1	2	0

Page Score _____

Figure 9-1. *(Continued)*

	Disagree	Agree	N/A
IX. Structure			
31. Educational graphics and art add to the usefulness of the site.	1	2	0
32. Decorative graphics do not significantly slow down-loading.	1	2	0
33. Text-only option is available for text-only Web browsers.	1	2	0
34. Usefulness of site does not suffer when using text-only option.	1	2	0
35. Options are available for disabled persons (large print, audio).	1	2	0
36. If audio and video are components of the site, and cannot be accessed, the information on the site is still complete.	1	2	0

Page Score _____
Total score _____

Total number of possible points _____
Percentage of total points _____
Total the number of points possible (the number of questions scored with either disagree or disagree multiplied by two). Divide your total score by the total number of points possible to determine the overall rating of this web site.

At least 90% of total possible points	**Excellent:** This web site is an excellent source of patient information. Patients will be able to easily access and understand the information contained in this site. Do not hesitate to recommend this site to your clientele.
At least 75% of total possible points	**Adequate:** While this web site provides relevant information and can be navigated without much trouble, it might not be the best site available. If another source cannot be located, this site will provide good information to your patient. Care should be taken to discuss with your patient what information was found on this web site and what information is still needed.
<75% of total possible points	**Poor:** This site should not be recommended to your patients. Validity and reliability of the information cannot be confirmed. All information on the site might not be accessible. Look for another web site to prevent false or partial information from being read.

Figure 9-1. *(Continued)*

to be used as guidelines to help unify the quality of medical and health information available on the web (http://www.hon.ch/HON-code/Conduct.html). The Health-Related Web Site Evaluation Form helps you evaluate websites against these principles. The form is intended for clinicians and health educators who refer their clientele to web sites for patient education.

It's easy to use and guides you through the calculation of a score for the website. This score will then fall into one of three categories: excellent, adequate, or poor. Excellent sites should be recommended to learners; adequate sites are usable, but there may be better alterna-

BOX 9-5 — If You Want to Learn More About the Quality of Websites

Ambre, J., Guard, R., Perveiler, F. M., Renner, J., & Rippen, H. (1997). Criteria for assessing the quality of health information on the Internet. [On-line]. Available: http://www.mitretek.org/hiti/showcase/documents/criteria.html.

Dickstein, R., Greenfield, L., & Rosen, J. (1997). Using the world wide web at the reference desk. *Computers in Libraries, 17*(8), 61–65.

Harris, R. (1997). Evaluating internet research sources. [On-line]. Available: http://www.sccu.edu/faculty/R_Harris/evalu8it.htm.

Health on the Net Foundation. [On-line]. Available: http://www.hon.ch/HONcode/Conduct.html.

Kelly, J.A., Anderson, P.F., Shaffer, C., & Chung, J. (1998). A Harvard graduate student seeking internet information asks: Is it a reliable source? Do I have to spend hours finding it? *Gratefully Yours, March-April,* 1–2.

Larkin, M. (1996). Health information on-line. *FDA Consumer Magazine.* [On-line]. Available: http://www.pueblo.gsa.gov/cic_text/health/on-line/on-line.txt.

tives; and poor sites should not be recommended. You can also find this Health-Related Web Site Evaluation Form at http://www.sph.emory.edu/WELLNESS/instrument.html. See Box 9-5 if you want to learn more about evaluating the quality of websites.

Download Teaching Materials

"It is reported that nearly 25% of all informational inquiries on the Web contain questions about health. As a result, thousands of health-related Web sites have already sprung up"
—American Medical Association, 1998, page 2

"The information found on the net can be passed on to [learners] in at least two ways. Hard copies can be made and handed out, or lists of helpful sites can be made available for people who have access to a computer."
—Mackenburg & Hobbie, 1997, page 91

Many websites offer teaching handouts for your learners. Search the web to find those appropriate for your patient population. Evaluate downloaded teaching materials with the same criteria you would use for those created in-house. Just because another organization uses them, it doesn't mean they're quality teaching materials. To access teaching materials on the web, see Box 9-6.

When you use teaching materials you did not create yourself, remember to evaluate them for suitability for your learners. If you have the content on disk, use your word processing software to evaluate reading level. If you only have a hard copy of the teaching material, you may use a scanner and optical character reading software (such as Omnipage) to convert the contents into text. Place this text as a file in your word processing software, and determine readability level from there.

BOX 9-6   Some WWW Sites With Teaching Handouts

To find teaching handouts or information you can print out and give your learners today, do a web search. Many health care facilities and advocacy groups post teaching materials on their sites and offer them for free.

You may also check the websites listed below for appropriate material. Some websites offer non-English materials, too.

As always, evaluate the quality and appropriateness of the material before you give it to a learner. No endorsement is stated or implied here. Websites can change significantly between the time this book is written and the time you read this page.

1-800 Numbers for Patient Support Organizations
http://infonet.welch.jhu.edu/advocacy/html

AIDS Pathfinder
http://www.nnlm.nlm.nih.gov/pnr/etc/aidspath.html

American Academy of Family Physicians
http://www.aafp.org

American Academy of Pediatrics
http://www.aap.org/

CancerNet
http://www.nci.nih.gov/hpage/cis.htm

HealthWeb
http://www.healthweb.org/

Box 9-6 *(Continued)*

KidsHealth
http://www.ama-assn.org/kidshealth

MedHelp International
http://medhlp.netusa.net/index.htm

PharmWeb
http://www.pharmweb.net/
http://www.mcc.ac.uk/pwmirror/pwi/pharmwebi.html

In addition, information for learners may be found at websites focusing on specific interests. This is, of course, a partial listing.

Alzheimer's Disease Page
http://www.biostat.wustl.edu/alzheimer

American Cancer Society
http://www.cancer.org/

American Diabetes Association
http://www.diabetes.org/

American Heart Association
http://www.amhrt.org/

Blood and Marrow Transplant Newsletter
http://www.bmtnews.org

Brain Injury Association
http://www.biausa.org

Federation for Children with Special Needs
http://www.fcsn.org

Leukemia Society of America
http://www.leukemia.org/

National Easter Seal Society
http://www.seals.com

National Parkinson's Foundation
http://www.parkinson.org

National Rehabilitation Information Center
http://www.naric.com/naric

National Spinal Cord Injury Association
http://www.spinalcord.org

You don't need access to the web to use your computer to print out teaching materials developed by others. A number of companies sell software with teaching materials, and several can be individualized for your learners. Some are also available in languages other than English. Box 9-7 lists some of your options.

If you are considering investing in this sort of software, search the web for the latest additions. Before you buy, evaluate them thoroughly and preferably with a multidisciplinary team that includes learners.

BOX 9-7   Software Options

Alpha Media
P.O. Box 1719
Maryland Heights, MO 63043-1719
314-692-2031
alphamedia@alpham.com
http://www.alpham.com

CareNotes System
Micromedex, Inc.
6200 S. Syracuse Way
Suite 300
Englewood, CO 80111-4740
1-800-525-9083; 303-486-6464
info@mdx.com
http://www.micromedex.com

Clinical Reference Systems
7100 E. Belleview Avenue
Suite 208
Greenwood Village, CO 80111-1635
1-800-237-8401
fax: 1-303-220-1685
crs-info@cliniref.com
www.patienteducation.com

E-Sheets
Krames Communications
1100 Grundy Lane
San Bruno, CA 94066-3030
1-800-955-5514, extension 4473
fax: 415-244-4568
http://www.krames.com

Box 9-7 *(Continued)*

Krames Patient Education Software
1100 Grundy Lane
San Bruno, CA 94066-3030
1-800-333-3032
fax: 1-650-244-4512
http://www.krames.com

Mosby's Patient Teaching Guides
11830 Westline Industrial Drive
PO Box 46908
St. Louis, MO 63146-9934

Patient Ed
Medifor
647 Washington Street
Port Townsend, WA 98368
1-800-366-3710, 360-385-0722
fax: 360-385-4402
info@medifor.com
http://www.medifor.com

Put Your Learner on the Computer

Another use of the computer in patient and family education is to put the learner on a computer. This tool works well when the learner seeks out information for proactive problem solving. In this way, adult learning principles support the use of computers in teaching.

Interactive teaching programs may come in the form of computer-assisted instruction, computer-based teaching, compact disc-interactive, compact disc-read-only memory, or interactive videodisc, sometimes also called laser videodisc. With each of them, the learner can set his or her own pace for learning.

Interactive teaching software may include the following:

- Information presented in text, graphics, animation, and sound
- Information presented in tutorial format so learners can choose what they want to learn
- Drills or practice to help learners learn and review
- Quizzes to evaluate understanding
- Problem solving, simulation, or games to help learners process information and learn how to apply it
- Feedback to the learner, reinforcing success and reteaching what was missed

"Rather than using the computer to replace the role of the health care provider in the educational process, the computer enhances the interaction between caregiver and consumer. Through the use of computer graphics, computer animation, and other multimedia techniques, information can be made available to the health care consumer in a more understandable fashion. Follow-up discussions between caregiver and consumer can then proceed from a similar base of conceptual knowledge."
—Sechrest & Henry, 1996, page 8

This makes the computer software a tool for teaching, like a handout or video. However, handouts and videos may be more familiar to your learners than computer programs.

"If a considerable amount of the patient's time is spent deciphering the interface, or if a staff member must spend a significant amount of time teaching the patient how to use the program, then efficiency is lost. The goal is to teach the patient about his or her disease, not about the computer."
—Sechrest & Henry, 1996, pages 11–12

When the software is user friendly, computers can be effective teaching tools. When the software is not easy for the learner to decipher, technology could rob you of valuable teaching time.

"The incorporation of a narrated sound track not only makes the program easier to follow for most people, but is critical for those patients with diminished reading skills."
—Sechrest & Henry, 1996, page 10

Like other teaching tools, test software with a few learners for feedback and for potential problems. New technologies may present new types of problems you cannot anticipate easily. For example, handouts written at a low reading level may be well tolerated by most of your learners. However, if you put the same content on a computer screen and have a narrator read it, learners with excellent reading skills may become frustrated, because they can read and absorb the information much quicker than the narrator presents it. If you purchase computer software, be sure it is a good value and that you will be able to use it with a large segment of your patient population. Again, the quality of tools in your teaching environment can facilitate or interfere with your teaching efforts.

Another advantage of computers is their ability to illustrate complex information simply, by using computer animation. These animations may also appear in some teaching videos. These are especially useful when explaining what will happen in surgery.

"The use of computer animation allows a great degree of clarity and focus without the gore. The patient is able to grasp the concepts of the material without the anxiety of encountering unpleasant visual images."
—Sechrest & Henry, 1996, page 10

Deye et al. (1997) address how to evaluate patient education software. They suggest you look for systems that are compatible with your computer's hardware, operating system, and storage capacity. Their criteria for software are similar to those for evaluation of written materials. Look for validity, value, usability, and appropriateness for your patient population. Make sure the information presented by the software is up to date and consistent with what you teach.

An alternative to purchasing software is to put your own teaching materials on a computer for learners to access. There are several ways to do this.

You can simply keep electronic files of handouts on the computer for a learner to access. You can make accessing the files easier by uploading them on your organization's intranet.

You can also upload the handouts on your organization's WWW website so learners can access them from any computer with internet access. For information on how to lay out a website that is clear, concise, and easy to read, see tips from WordsWork at http://www.wordswork.com.

In addition to handouts, you can offer learners self-learning modules to use on the computer. These can have interactive quizzes placed throughout the program so learners can review material soon after it is read.

"Computer technology is not a replacement for professional involvement in patient education, but rather offers a new arena of media to enhance and expand current teaching and learning resources."
—Chambers & Frisby, 1995, page 234

Use Kiosks

"Touchscreens seem to be the best input device for non-computer users. It is quick and easy to demonstrate how a touchscreen is used. They are durable and can be incorporated easily into a kiosk-type setting (such as a waiting area)."
—Sechrest & Henry, 1996, page 12

Health information kiosks are similar to automated bank teller machines, with a touchscreen and customized software. They can be placed in waiting rooms, lobbies, shopping malls, libraries, work sites—any secure area where potential learners might be.

The University of Michigan's Comprehensive Cancer Center has funding from proceeds from the state tobacco tax for a statewide network of about 50 interactive kiosks. Topics covered include smoking, breast cancer, prostate cancer screening, bike helmet safety, and immunization.

Phoenix Children's Hospital has kiosks with information on health promotion, first aid, diseases, tests and examinations, medications, procedures, and treatments. In addition, their kiosks have a quiz to test health-promotion knowledge. The quiz gives the correct answer immediately and computes a final score for the user. Kiosk users can read content from the screen or print it out. Information is available in English and Spanish. Contents are easily updated whenever new teaching materials are created in-house.

Teach Groups

Computers can be applied to teaching groups at many levels. Martin and Connor (1996) describe how they used a computer to create appealing transparencies. When used to teach groups, they stimulated discussion and retention of information.

With a presentation program, such as Microsoft PowerPoint, you can create a custom-made slide show on a computer, have it printed up as slides, or, with the right equipment, project it from your computer onto a screen as you teach. This system gives you more flexibility than photographic slides, because you can rearrange computerized slides as you speak.

Have Learners Use Computers at Home

"Technology assists learning by providing additional motivation and rewards at the teachable moment."
—Maricopa Center for Learning and Instruction, 1996

If learners have computers at home, you can continue patient and family education using the internet. The learner can e-mail you with questions, and you can respond with an e-mail or a telephone call.

If you know your learners use the internet at home, provide them with guidelines and resources for finding accurate health information.

"Patients may see the Internet as a vast medical encyclopedia without realizing that its entries are not edited, not filtered, and sometimes not factual."
—Baldwin, 1998, page 59

Another way to incorporate home computers into your teaching is with a system like the Comprehensive Health Enhancement Support System (CHESS) (Grandinetti, 1996). There are now CHESS programs for patients with breast cancer or acquired immunodeficiency syndrome, but others are planned, including those for patients with upper respiratory infections, recovering from heart attacks, and caregivers for those with Alzheimer's disease. CHESS is licensed to health care providers to use one module in up to six homes. It consists of a software program used by learners for 3 to 6 months and telephone training for staff to answer questions. The software helps patients weigh their treatment options, has an "ask the experts" service that lets patients ask questions anonymously, and has a discussion group that connects patients with others with the same illness. It also has full text articles, brief answers to commonly asked questions, a referral directory, and real-life accounts by others with the same illness. Up to 60 pages of text can be added by the health care providers licensing the use of the system.

Another alternative is to offer your teachings to learners beyond your immediate patient population. Apgarink (1997) created a website on cardiac arrhythmias, which included a component that took questions. Within a year, she got 55 inquiries from 20 states and nine foreign countries, plus 15 which were unidentified. Inquiries were almost always appropriate to the topic of the website. Of course, legal and security issues need to be considered when setting up such a system.

"Technology can provide focused instruction and therefore can improve the quality of learning. Technology is forcing us to re-examine how we teach and learn. It is giving us more options."
—Maricopa Center for Learning and Instruction, 1996

Document Teaching

Computers can also help us deal with the challenge of undocumented patient and family education. Weaver (1995) reported that more teaching was done than was being documented. Her organization decided to facilitate the documentation process by developing a teaching flow sheet, organized by nursing diagnoses. That flow sheet was created on a computer.

Martin and Connor (1996) describe how form-developing or word processing programs could be used to develop a form to document patient and family education effectively. They also described how they used a database program to maintain information on staff competencies. This let them determine who needed to be scheduled for recertification classes.

Use Computers Appropriately

One nurse thought it would be great to program a computer system for Joint Commission on the Accreditation of Healthcare Organizations (JCAHO)-required assessments. "Have the patient fill out a computerized survey which asks, are you in too much pain to learn now? Do you have any cultural practices that will interfere with your learning? Then, we'll not only have the learning-readiness assessment, but have it documented online for JCAHO! We don't have time to do these assessments now, anyway."

Would her proposal result in a true assessment? Imagine it from the patient's point of view. Has the patient ever used a computer before? Can the patient read? Would a learner in too much pain to learn be able to complete a computerized assessment? Because culture is a way of thinking, could a patient recognize a cultural barrier to learning?

Would it be more efficient and accurate for the nurse actually to have a conversation with the learner, make the professional assessment, and document it?

No matter how busy a nurse is, she or he would not give a patient who looks feverish acetaminophen without first assessing and documenting the body temperature. Without taking the temperature, how would the nurse know the medication was actually needed? If there were no objective data, how would the nurse be able to measure if the intervention helped?

This is no different in patient and family education. Can you say you have no time to assess learning needs but teach anyway? How do you know if the teaching you did was appropriate? How would you know if it worked?

Understand the essence of nursing and your role as a professional nurse in teaching patients and families. Computers are powerful tools. Use them wisely.

The Future

Who knows where technology will take us? Cassell, Jackson, and Cheuvront (1998) propose that the internet can also be used for public health interventions. If we are to use this medium well, however, we will need to create even broader multidisciplinary teams to tap expertise in behavioral science theory, research methods, communication technology, advertising, and promotions.

Someday you may discharge a patient from a hospital with a loan of a satellite dish. The learner hooks up the satellite dish to his or her home television. The health care provider communicates with the learner through a computer system. As mentioned in Chapter 7, this allows the learner to access teaching videos on demand. If the learner also has a computer, the learner and health care provider can be at different sites but engage in a live video and audio interaction. A home computer could also be used for an online evaluation of knowledge through puzzles, games, or multiple choice quizzes.

"The use of computers and multimedia technology in the health care field can be expected to follow the use of such technology in other fields. As costs decrease, and more programs are produced, a wider base of implementation should occur."

—Adsit, 1996, page 62

As you use computers more and become familiar with what they can do, you will think of more ways to use them.

"Don't limit yourself to only word processing or the results retrieval system your facility may have. Nurses can use easily obtained software programs to improve staff and patient education. . . . Be creative and see how far you can go. It's fun to see just what you can come up with."

—Martin & Connor, 1996, page 79

If you want to keep up with advances in technology, make friends with people who love computers or talk to children. Many children create and maintain their own websites today. Give them an opportunity to show you what computers can do. Technology changes quickly, and more options are opening up every day.

 If you want to learn more:

Adobe Acrobat, Acrobat Reader, Acrobat Catalog, Acrobat Search. [On-line]. Available: http://www.adobe.com

Ambre, J., Guard, R., Perveiler, F.M., Renner, J., & Rippen, H. (1997). *Criteria for assessing the quality of health information on the Internet.* [On-line]. Available: http://www.mitretek.org/hiti/showcase/documents/criteria.html.

Adsit, K.I. (1996). Multimedia in nursing and patient education. *Orthopaedic Nursing, 15*(4), 59–63.

American Medical Association. (1998). *KidsHealth Web Site announcement.* Chicago, IL: Author.

Apgarink, B. (1997). Medical information for patients using the Internet. *American Family Physician, 56*(2), 597–599.

Baldwin, F. (1998). Here come the web-savvy patients. *Physician's Management*, *38*(4), 59-62.

Cassell, M.M., Jackson, C., & Cheuvront, B. (1998). Health communication on the Internet: An effective channel for health benefit change? *Journal of Health Communication*, *3*(1), 71-79.

Chambers, J.K., & Frisby, A.J. (1995). Computer-based learning for ESRD patient education: Current status and future directions. *Advances in Renal Replacement Therapy*, *2*(3), 234-245.

Comprehensive Health Enhancement Support System (CHESS)
Health Companion Systems LLC
1122 Warf Building
610 Walnut Street
Madison, WI 53705
608-262-8758
fax: 608-263-4523

Deye, D.L., Kahn, G., Jimison, H.B., Renner, J.H., Wenner, A.R., & Gabello, W.J. (1997). How computers enrich patient education. *Patient Care*, *31*(3), 88-100.

Dickstein, R., Greenfield, L., & Rosen, J. (1997). Using the World Wide Web at the Reference Desk. *Computers in Libraries*, *17*(8), 61-65.

Forsythe, D.E. (1996). New bottles, old wine: Hidden cultural assumptions in a computerized explanation system for migraine sufferers. *Medical Anthropology Quarterly*, *10*(4), 551-574.

Grandinetti, D. (1996). Teaching patients to take care of themselves. *Medical Economics*, *73*(22), 83-91.

Harris, R. (1997). Evaluating Internet Research Sources. [On-line]. Available www:http://www.sccu.edu/faculty/R-Harris/evalu8it.htm.

Interactive health kiosks debut throughout Michigan. (1997). *AIDS Weekly Plus*, November 3, 16-18.

Kickstein, R., Greenfield, L., & Rosen, J. (1997). Using the world wide web at the reference desk. *Computers in Libraries*, September, 61-65.

Larkin, M. (1996). Health information on-line. *FDA Consumer Magazine*, [On-line]. Available: http://www.pueblo.gsa.gov/cic_text/health/on-line/on-line.txt.

Mackenburg, M., & Hobbie, C. (1997). Patient education on the Web. *Journal of Pediatric Health Care*, *11*(2), 89-91.

Maricopa Center for Learning and Instruction. (1996). *A dialogue on the impact of technology on learning.* [On-line]. Available: http://hakatai.mcli.dist.maricopa.edu/.ocotillo/itl/impact.html.

Martin, L.A., & Connor, F.L. (1996). Your PC can enhance staff and patient education. *Pediatric Nursing*, *22*(1), 76-79.

Peters, R., & Sikorski, R. (1997). Sharing information and interests on the Internet. *Journal of the American Medical Association*, *277*(15), 1258-1260.

Puzzle Power: The all-in-one puzzle maker. (1997). Centron Software Technologies.

Randall, T. (1993). Producers of videodisc programs strive to expand patient's role in medical decision-making process. *Journal of the American Medical Association*, *270*(2), 160-162.

Rees, A.M. (1998). *The consumer health information source book* (5th ed.). Phoenix, AZ: Oryx Press.

Rowland, R., & Kinnaman, D. (1995). *Researching on the internet: The complete guide to finding, evaluating and organizing information effectively.* Rocklin, CA: Prima Publishing.

Sechrest, R.C., & Henry, D.J. (1996). Computer-based patient education: Observations on effective communication in the clinical setting. *Journal of Biocommunication*, *23*(1), 8-12.

Senge, P.M., Kleiner, A., Roberts, C., Ross, R.B., & Smith, B.J. (1994). *The Fifth discipline fieldbook: strategies and tools for building a learning organization.* New York, NY: Currency.

Silberg, W.M., Lundberg, G.D., & Musacchio, R.A. (1997). Assessing, controlling, and assuring the quality of medical information on the internet: Caveant lector et viewor—let the reader and viewer beware. *Journal of the American Medical Association, 277*(15), 1244–1245.

Skibalp, D.J. (1997). Intellectual property issues in the digital health care public world. *Nursing Administration Quarterly, 21*(3), 11–21.

Sparks, S.M., & Rizzolo, A. (1998). World Wide Web Search Tools. *Image: Journal of Nursing Scholarship, 30*(2), 167–171.

Weaver, J. (1995). Patient education: An innovative computer approach. *Nursing Management, 26*(7), 78–79, 81, 83.

Individualizing Teaching

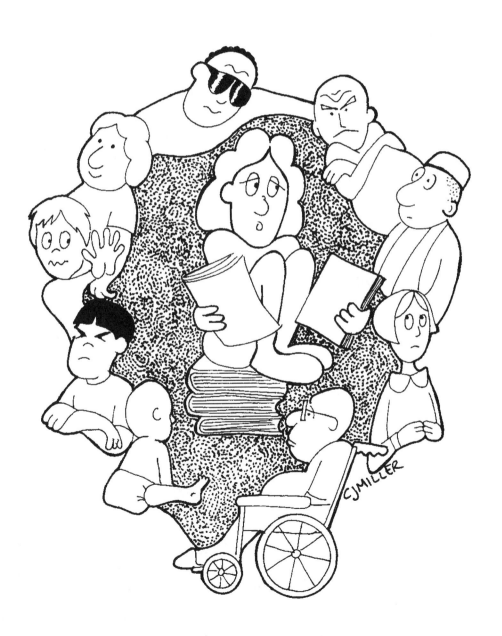

ou are lost the instant you know what the result will be."

—Juan Gris

Individualizing teaching takes effort. It's so much easier to give learners a booklet that contains everything they need to know, tell them to read the booklet, ask if they have any questions, and say you've done your teaching. How much do they learn that way, and have health outcomes been influenced at all?

When you individualize teaching, you teach faster and better. How?

- You teach only what that learner needs to learn.
- If the learner knows it already, you don't have to teach it.
- You teach only at the right time in ways the learner can learn.

When learners learn quicker, you save time teaching. You don't waste time teaching the wrong stuff, the wrong person, or the wrong way.

A good assessment will hone your intervention.

A Learned Skill

Does individualizing teaching sound too overwhelming and too time consuming?

Take a deep breath. It's not as complex as it sounds.

Individualization simply means listening to your learners, understanding who they are and what they need, and adapting your teaching accordingly.

As your skills improve, individualizing your teaching will get easier. All you have to do is practice.

Benner (1984) describes the process of developing from a novice to an expert nurse. She defines novice nurses as not just new graduates, but any nurse who is entering new clinical experience, where the goals and tools of patient care are unfamiliar. If you are unfamiliar with individualizing teaching, even if you have been a nurse for years, you may be a novice in this area.

Novices start by learning and following rules. Context-free rules guide action, such as those of the Joint Commission on the Accreditation of Healthcare Organizations (JCAHO):

"The assessment considers cultural and religious practices, emotional barriers, desire and motivation to learn, physical and cognitive limitations, language barriers, and the financial implications of care choices."

—JCAHO, 1998, page 106

However, rules don't tell you the most relevant tasks to perform in an actual situation. Time and experience do. As you gain experience, you learn *aspects,* or global characteristics that can be identified only through experience.

> *"The instructor can provide guidelines for recognizing such aspects as a patient's readiness to learn. For example, 'Notice whether or not the patient asks questions about the surgery or dressing change.' 'Observe whether or not the patient looks at or handles the wound.' But these guidelines depend on the practitioner's knowing what these aspects sound and look like in actual patient care situations. Thus, while aspects may be made explicit, they cannot be made completely objective . . . No one cue is definitive in all situations. Experience is needed before the nurse can apply the guidelines to individual patients."*
> —Benner, 1984, page 23

Books can only define the process of individualizing teaching. They can talk about it and give examples and guidelines, but written words cannot communicate the depth and breadth of the concept. You can only learn about it by doing it. With experience, awareness, and practice (active participation in the process), you can ultimately become an expert at individualizing teaching.

> *"The expert performer no longer relies on an analytic principle (rule, guideline, maxim) to connect her or his understanding of the situation to an appropriate action. The expert nurse, with an enormous background of experience, now has an intuitive grasp of each situation and zeroes in on the accurate region of the problem without wasteful consideration of a large range of unfruitful, alternative diagnoses and solutions."*
> —Benner, 1984, pages 31–32

This is a finely tuned application of knowledge that develops into expertise. It is more precise than making assumptions. As you practice individualizing your teaching, you will get better at tailoring teaching to the learner. As your teaching becomes better individualized, it will go quicker. You will develop teaching expertise.

> *"The expert always knows more than he or she can tell. The clinician's knowledge is embedded in perceptions rather than precepts."*
> —Benner, 1984, page 43

Understand the Learner's Point of View

Your point of view as a health care provider is very different from the point of view of the patient, your learner.

"I have assisted with many D and Cs in my ER career, and I think it is important to remember that even though a procedure is routine to us, as nurses, it is a unique experience to the patient. They need to know what to expect and what is happening to their bodies."

—an RN

Individualization involves understanding the learner's point of view and adapting teaching so it can be most effective. Learners don't always see things the way we do. Even if we use the same words, what we mean may not be what the learner understands. Here's an example.

I work in a busy cardiothoracic ICU where we typically transfer post-op CABG patients to our stepdown unit the day following surgery. One morning as I was getting a patient to his chair and performing the other transfer preparatory tasks, I explained that we would be transferring him to the floor as soon as possible.

After a few minutes, he looked at me bewilderedly and asked, "When you transfer me to the floor, how will I get back up?"

—an RN

We have to pay attention to correct misperceptions as they occur. This learner expressed his concerns. Many others worry in silence.

When adapting teaching methods to individual needs, you have a range of tools from which to draw, including conversation, medical supplies and equipment, written materials, videotapes, and audiotapes. Individualization involves choosing the appropriate method for the learner and using it at the right time.

Make *"teaching more effective by allowing it to be tailored to the patient's needs. An effective teacher should first be aware of the patient's learning needs, cognitive abilities, learning style, current knowledge and experience, educational level, and readiness to learn."*

—Rakel, 1992, page 398

Focus on the Patient and Family

"I can tell you about lots of times when nurses come in and start teaching. And it's about stuff I know more about than they do!"

—Parent of a chronically ill child

When we don't focus on the patient and family, we risk alienating them. When our relationship is harmed, trust is lost, and it is more difficult to be therapeutic.

There are many reasons why we might not focus on the patient and family. We may see our work as a set of tasks instead of caring for people. We may be in a hurry and thinking about our own needs and timeframes. We may put more weight on our need to help others than actually helping them. In its most extreme form,

> *"Our helping came from the source of pity rather than compassion. Pity is giving which sees the giver as in some way superior to the recipient. Compassion reduces the barriers and contains genuine respect, as equals, from one to the other . . . Compassion lies at the heart of genuine helping. Often our helping is born out of personal desperation; we go around pretending that we are not sick, nursing those who are also unwell. Helping can be a fundamental symptom of sickness, especially where it is used to conceal our own inadequacies."*
>
> —Brandon, 1976, page 102

Whatever the reasons we have failed to focus on patients and families in the past, we can make a conscious effort to correct this. Here's the story of one nurse who, with experience, gained awareness and changed her teaching to adapt better to patients and families.

Recommendations that seem very reasonable to health care providers may be completely unmanageable at home. I routinely asked parents to limit the child's salt intake while on high-dose steroids, keeping in mind normal eating habits of the child, as well as the salt cravings, huge appetites, and crankiness caused by steroids. I assumed parents were enforcing those restrictions because they never complained about them, and relatively few kids ever developed significant hypertension.

Then my best friend's son was placed on high-dose steroids, and I lived through that 3 AM begging and pleading for serving after serving of the most sodium-laden foods in existence. Thinking he was an exception to the rule, I started asking around.

I found that nearly all parents struggled with our request for a lower sodium diet in the face of starving and irrational children. Meeting the child's desperate needs always won out but caused these parents significant anguish. They didn't talk about it in clinic because they felt they had no power to comply with our recommendations yet harbored fears that they might provide less than perfect care.

I now emphasize a low-added salt diet (i.e., supplementing pizza lunches with fruits and cookies) and promise if hypertension looks like it may be an issue, we will deal with it then.

—an RN

This nurse adapted her teaching and treatments to reality, and by continuing to monitor for hypertension, she did not compromise quality of care. Indeed, the quality of life of the families probably improved. The children were not so sodium deprived that they resorted to begging in the middle of the night, and parents did not have the guilt of giving in to them.

> "The experience of helping has an internal harmony. . . . We had given up, perhaps just for a moment, our attempts at manipulating, at impressing people. We had forgotten our decisions about the 'good' and 'bad' parts of ourselves and others. It no longer seemed necessary to define the limits of our personalities and protect the boundaries of the self."
>
> —Brandon, 1976, page 13

Keeping our focus on the patient and family can be very rewarding. We actually become instruments of healing by forming a bridge between two worlds—the data-filled, analytical world of medicine and the personal world of human beings. We help people make good choices that work in the context of their lives.

> "Nurses must remember, and expert nurses do, that patients often have their own interpretations and understanding of their condition. Allowing them to express this, as well as respecting and building on their interpretations, can play an important role in the patient's illness and recovery experience."
>
> —Benner, 1984, page 84

It is easiest to individualize teaching if you shift focus from your need to teach to the learner's need to learn. This means taking a risk. When you individualize teaching, the learner may ask a question you cannot answer or may reveal some emotional conflict you feel unprepared to face. We teach to help learners best care for themselves, not to keep caregivers comfortable and safe. Develop the skills you need to face these challenging situations, and learn what resources you can access for support.

One nurse tells how she overcame a challenging situation through teaching. This teaching was motivated by her need for personal safety, but it was successful because she focused on the needs of the patient and family.

My patient had cancer, and his protocol included very high-dose steroids. They made him crazy, literally. He became psychotic. The day before he punched his nurse so hard she had to go home. This was not a psych ward. We weren't used to this sort of behavior; we were scared. We got a psych consult, and the psychiatrist prescribed Haldol. So when the man's wife came in to visit, we, of course, informed her of the events and the medication we started. Then she went bonkers. No way would she let her husband go on psych meds again. She promised him! She couldn't break her promise!

I got someone to cover my patients, and took her off the floor to a private room. I asked her to tell me about the promise. When they started dating, he had just come out of a psych admission. He hated it, and vowed he would never go on those horrible meds again. He made her promise never to let anyone give them to him. She did. And, luckily, he never had another psychotic episode. Until now.

So we talked about how this time it was different, because his steroids were making him crazy. I told her that after the steroids were done, the side effects should go away, and he could go off the Haldol. I explained how, if he kept punching nurses, they would not be able to get close enough to give him the chemo that would treat his cancer and make him well again. I asked her if she thought he wanted the chemo, and if he wanted to live.

We talked for almost an hour. She finally decided her promise was really about keeping him safe from getting drugged and locked up in psych wards, and not about getting treatment for his cancer. She agreed, with some reservations, to let him have the Haldol.

It worked. He got through the chemo without punching another nurse. After the steroids were reduced, he didn't need the Haldol any more, and the happy couple went home. Best of all, he wasn't mad at her for breaking her promise.

—an RN

"We know immediately when good helping has taken place. We have done ourselves some good as well as the other person. At the time there was a complete lack of self-consciousness or judgment. All of ourself and the other was in the actual experiencing of the contact and the merging of two or more persons."

—Brandon, 1976, page 13

Consider Your Reactions as Cues

One way to tell if you individualize care is to pay attention to your thoughts and reactions. The nurse in the story above felt good about her teaching. The learner made an informed decision, made a health-promoting choice, and the outcome was good. What sort of relationships do you have with your patients and their families? One health care provider does not like what he sees:

> *"Frequently relationships between clients and helpers are grossly unequal in a way which supports hindering and the undermining of autonomy. Genuine communication is frustrated by profuse professional jargon and crude labeling. Helpers use their own status, social position and knowledge to erect barriers rather than to establish genuine harmony and growth."*
> —Brandon, 1976, page 85

Notice your responses and the responses of those around you. Do you find yourself intolerant of certain behaviors or attitudes? Are you frustrated because a family can never get to an appointment on time? Are you considering confronting your patient, because you think she is taking herbs at home and not the prescribed medicine? Are you frustrated by the religious statue and healing dust on your patient's bedside stand, because they're always in your way? Do you just not understand where they are coming from and why they don't do what you tell them? Has a patient or family member ever accused you of being racist or not caring?

"Yes" answers to any of these questions are signs that your skills in individualizing care need work. One key to satisfying, effective, growth-producing relationships between nurses and their patients and families is a tolerance of difference. First, tolerate the difference, and then seek to understand it. If you do not tolerate the differences, you may be able to carry out tasks but will not be able to provide professional care.

The difference is in our attitudes, not in the time we have for teaching. One researcher noted,

> *"Our observation of patient visits suggested that time is not the main factor constraining explanation to patients. In fact, a great many questions are asked and answered during patient visits, but almost all of them are asked by the doctor and answered by the patient. . . . We also found that when patients attempt to bring up concerns that neurologists do not see as strictly medical, physicians often appear not to 'hear' them or attempt to pass the matter off as a joke."*
> —Forsythe, 1996, page 560

Do you ever not hear a question? Do you ever pass learners' concerns off as jokes?

How Do You Adapt to the Learner?

How do you make the transition from focusing on your job and your tasks to focusing on your learner's needs? For what do you assess when individualizing teaching? How do you adapt to the learner? The rest of this chapter shows you some ways.

Desire and Motivation to Learn

Many health care providers say a barrier they encounter is lack of motivation to learn. It's hard to teach someone who doesn't feel he or she needs any information.

The first step to overcoming this is to understand the learner's point of view of the problem.

> *"Patient perception that his or her illness was not serious was most strongly associated with lack of motivation to learn."*
> —Rakel, 1992, page 390

One of the goals of patient and family education is to help your learner make informed decisions. If the patient decides learning is not necessary, does he or she understand the problem? Many learners think surgery will make everything right and not realize that lifestyle changes are part of the treatment plan.

> *"The information the health professional believes is necessary may not be the same information believed by the patient to be necessary."*
> —Falvo, 1994, page 149

If your learner understands the problem but still does not seem interested in learning, try to understand more about the learner's story. Who is he or she?

> *"Clues to the individual motivation factors can be obtained from the client's life-style, family members, socioeconomic status, and growth and development data."*
> —Rankin & Stallings, 1996, page 300

This information will help you individualize your presentation and make the information meaningful to your learner. Once you understand the learner, you can help get him or her ready to learn. According to Rakel (1992), you can help patients prepare for learning:

- Discuss the learner's past experiences, and correct misinformation.

- Address the learner's concerns first.
- Include family members and significant others in the teaching.

Sometimes patients and family members are interested in learning but not very motivated to follow through with behaviors. Again, they may not understand the seriousness of the situation, or the reasons you give to motivate change are not meaningful to them. You may not have delivered the message in a way that makes sense to them in the context of their lives. One way to determine what motivates a learner to action is to ask, "Think back to when you last made a major change in your life. Why did you do it?"

Often, health care providers push without trying to understand the resistance, the lack of motivation. They forget that many patients come for treatments, pills, and surgery but don't want their lives changed. They just want to get fixed and get back to their activities of daily living. We have to explain that health care is more than medicine, it's also health-promoting behaviors and choices.

In other situations, we explore every avenue, and the learner is still not interested in changing.

"There are times when given all available information and after engaging in a fully participatory encounter, patients will still choose not to embrace healthy behaviors."
—Rankin & Stallings, 1996, page 112

It is good to keep trying, waiting for that teachable moment, but it is also important to accept reality.

" 'How much responsibility to learn does the patient have?' When all factors are considered, it is the patient who must ultimately decide whether he is going to accept our attempts to teach him, whether he accepts selectively, or whether he completely ignores us."
—Rankin & Stallings, 1996, page 301

Did the learner do it?

Compliance, Adherence, and Alliance

Did you expect that because a learner comes to you for advice and pays for that advice, he or she will then follow it? Have you discovered that this is not true? Does this confuse you?

We nurses have gone to school, studied, graduated, taken exams, and gotten licenses. We know stuff that can help people. Important stuff.

"I feel this powerful urge to tell people what to do. There is a great drive deep inside to manage people's lives, that only I know what really ought to happen."
—Brandon, 1976, pages 90–91

Patient and family education is a way we impose our knowledge, our information, onto other people so they choose to do the right thing.

"Many of us have justified our involvement in patient education by asserting that it would increase patient compliance, in other words, convince patients to follow our suggestions."
—Rankin & Stallings, 1996, page 101

We call ourselves caregivers. We care; we don't dictate. We believe in patient rights and even advocate for them. The patient has a right to choose not to follow our advice. We want learners to choose the behavioral changes we suggest. We want their cooperation and partnership, not compliance.

"Although the patient's understanding of illness and the proposed treatment has a beneficial impact on adherence, patient education does not guarantee it."
—Platt et al., 1994

Sometimes what you teach is understood but not applied. There are many names for this: compliance, adherence, alliance. Each has a different edge, a different slant.

"Compliance suggests a patient's unquestioning fulfillment of a physician's instructions. Adherence, which some experts prefer in this context, connotes a physician-patient partnership. Each understands the other's point of view, and both have agreed on a course of action—a treatment or life-style change—that each finds acceptable and that the patient agrees to undertake."
—Platt et al., 1994

Alliance suggests an even stronger mutuality. The health care team, patient, and family all agree on the goals and are working together to meet them. They form an alliance to fight for health.

The concept of compliance might make sense if we had only patriarchal medical care. Doctor Expert tells patient what to do, and patient does it. This is just like a child would obey a parent. However, patients and families have evolved from children into consumers, and professionals in many disciplines, not just physicians, are involved in promoting and maintaining health. Medical care has transformed into health care. Compliance isn't what it used to be.

> *"Some physicians continue to view compliance unidimensionally as patients receiving and following medical advice, but studies show that patients themselves decide whether to take their medicine as prescribed. Patients base their decisions on their personal assessments of the benefits versus the disincentives of following the therapy plan."*
>
> —National Council on Patient Information and Education, 1997

The way you define a problem influences how you solve it.

For example, if you call a behavior noncompliance, the solution is enforcement.

If you call a behavior nonadherence, the solution is legalistic agreements or contracts.

If you call a behavior nonalliance, the solution is to improve the relationship.

Mutuality

The goals of patient and family education are derived from the general goals. (Make informed decisions, develop basic self-care skills to survive, recognize problems and know what to do in response, and get questions answered.) However, actual individualized goals are created by mutual agreement between the learner and health care provider. For example, some learners may not want to know all the treatment options and fear making a wrong decision, so they choose not to hear certain information and let the physician pick the best course of action. This mutual agreement respects the learner's wishes. When the learner does not want what you want, you need to resist your urges and build the alliance.

> *"It becomes harder still to give up those ambitions for the control and changing of others; the simple desire to appear important, to have influence, to be popular and lovable."*
>
> —Brandon, 1976, page 90

The goal of compliance is to have the learner follow the plan. The key to getting compliance is to develop a mutually agreed upon plan that is medically sound and provides advice that the learner is willing and able to follow. Adaptation or individualization of the plan is the key.

> *"Problems with compliance . . . say something about our approach to health care and our knowledge of the patient, family, lifestyle and background."*
>
> —Lumsdon, 1994

When mutuality is absent, the alliance between patient and health care provider does not exist. Without an alliance, basic goals are not shared.

"Nonadherence is almost guaranteed if the patient disagrees with your diagnosis and the rationale for the treatment."
—Platt et al., 1994

It is not always easy to recognize these situations. Look to your reactions for clues.

"Patients are sometimes labeled as 'difficult.' Usually the problem is the nurse who finds it difficult to know how to treat them. Do not miss the chance to learn from such situations. These patients have much to teach us about ourselves."
—Hammerschmidt & Meador, 1993, rule number 266

Individualization is the key. If the learner does not agree with the diagnosis or treatment, have you listened to his or her thoughts on the matter? With what aspects of the diagnosis or treatment does the learner disagree? Health care providers use a different language from patients and families.

"Rehab? I'm not going to rehab! I had a heart attack. I'm not an alcoholic!"
—A patient

We need to translate words and meanings to make sure our learners understand. Otherwise, their noncompliance could be without informed consent. A patient has a right to refuse cardiac rehab, but does he or she know what cardiac rehab is?

"Clinicians are in a position . . . to influence the comprehension of their advice and instruction to patients."
—Doak, Doak, Friedell, & Meade, 1998

Working Together

The key is working together to accomplish a shared goal.

"If we focus on how the treatment would benefit the patient in terms he/ she already understands, we would accomplish more of what we want."
—Korpi, 1995, page 79

You can build an alliance by involving the learner in the process.

"A person is more likely to adhere to lifestyle and treatment plans when he feels part of the decision-making and planning process and understands that some part of the plan has been customized for him. Be clear about what you would like the patient to consider doing, and listen carefully while he explains what he will do and what he considers to be beyond his capabilities."

—Platt et al., 1994

In many situations, especially in the case of chronic illness, the behavior changes you are proposing involve the patient and family. Even if the family does not have to change, their cooperation could be a factor in the patient's commitment to change.

"Family involvement is usually helpful, even essential, when a patient faces long-term or permanent life-style changes during therapy."

—Platt et al., 1994

Compliance, then, is a collaboration. Sometimes, the question of compliance does not arise until outcomes are threatened, such as an infection that almost disappears, then returns stronger than ever. Rather than risk problems noncompliance could create, it makes sense to evaluate the learner's intent to comply at the time of teaching.

"Asking patients directly whether they plan to comply, and whether there are any problems that might stop them from following treatment, is a simple way to raise compliance issues."
—National Council on Patient Information and Education, 1997

Once you realize a learner will not follow a plan, find out what the problem is so you can address it. Figure 10-1 is a decision chart that can guide you through this process.

Notice that if early on you decide compliance is not important, ignore it. If compliance is not important, let the learner decide whether or not it's worth the trouble.

If compliance is important, then the chart identifies issues to explore with the learner. Does the learner understand the benefits from following the plan? Does the learner have the skill to follow the plan?

"Ask if the patient anticipates any trouble doing what you've asked."

—Platt et al., 1994

Teach as necessary. Many of the issues addressed in the decision tree, such as physical and cognitive limitations, belief, self-efficacy, and evaluating understanding, are described elsewhere in this book.

How to Enhance Compliance

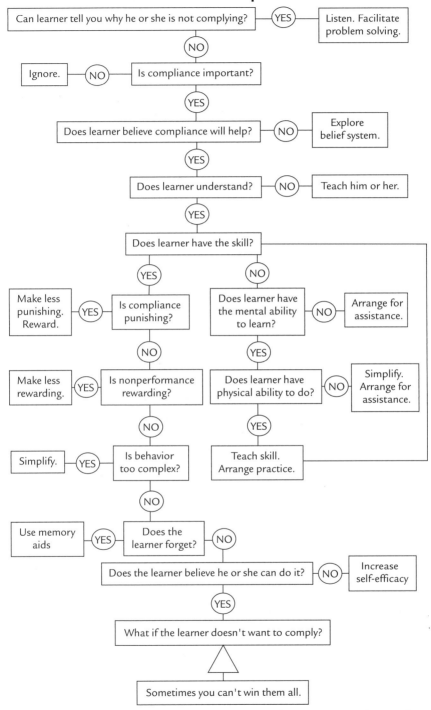

Figure 10-1. Adapted From: Lorig, K. (1996). *Patient Education: A Practical Approach.* Thousand Oaks, CA: Sage Publications. Page 185.

Rewards and punishments refer to the benefits and costs as identified by the learner. For example, the learner's diet may prescribe not eating ice cream, but to the learner, not eating ice cream is perceived as punishing, and eating ice cream is rewarding. To encourage compliance, the rewards and punishments need to be adjusted. Perhaps nonfat frozen yogurt would be an effective substitute. Perhaps an occasional ice cream needs to be used as a reward for compliance. Collaborate with the learner to determine what would and would not work. Remember, the learner agreed to the goal. Your interventions are helping the learner get there. You are not manipulating the learner into compliance with your agenda.

Some learners will not follow the plan, no matter how you try to build an alliance. After you have considered all of the contributing factors, you may recognize that the learner does not want to comply. If this is true, let go, knowing you did everything possible to encourage health-promoting behaviors. This process of coaching the learner is described in detail in Lorig (1996), *Patient Education: A Practical Approach.*

"We must also be willing to respect the patient's right to choose although we may not agree with his choice. We reserve the right to keep trying."
—Rankin & Stallings, 1996, page 101

Again, that teachable moment may occur in the future. Keep watching for it. Your understanding of the learner may deepen with time, your relationship may strengthen, and the learner may change his or her mind.

"Effective patient education requires an understanding of those factors that influence the patient in decision-making: values, beliefs, attitudes, current life stresses, religion, previous experiences with health care system, and life goals."
—Rankin & Stallings, 1996, page 101

Other Ways of Living: Culture, Religion, Lifestyle

Other people's lives may seem foreign to us for many reasons. They may come from another country, belong to another socioeconomic group than we do, or have a set of beliefs that are different from ours. They have other ways of living.

Other ways may be unfamiliar to us, and if they are unfamiliar, we may misunderstand them. If we don't understand details of what another way of living is like, we may make assumptions and generalizations from what we see. We may stereotype. If we make judgments, we may become biased or bigoted. All this would be based on too little information, and these attitudes do not promote therapeutic relationships.

After the birth of my first child, I found breast-feeding to be a bit challenging.

My son was having a lot of difficulty latching on, and I was very unsure of how to facilitate this process. I put on my call light for some assistance from the nurse.

A rather large, deep-voiced nurse walked in (she reminded me of a drill sergeant) and asked how she could help. I showed her the problem we were having with latching on. She seemed to be quite frustrated with our attempts and grabbed my breast. I was mortified. To make matters worse, she then read his wristband and saw the Irish surname. She continued to force my breast into his mouth and said, "Danaher! Danaher! I have never met an Irishman who wouldn't drink! Your baby is unbelievable!" This was not an effective teaching strategy.

—A patient and RN

The stereotyping of Irishmen was only one example of this nurse's difficulty with individualizing teaching. Can you find the others?

Where Do You Begin?

"When I ask a patient, 'Do you have any cultural or religious beliefs you want me to incorporate in my nursing care?' they look at me like I have two heads. How else do I assess for culture and religion?"

—An RN

Are culture, religion, and lifestyle too big to grasp, too vague to accommodate? You treat body, mind, and spirit, so you know they are your business, but how do you treat body, mind, and spirit? How do you consider lifestyle, culture, and religious practices in your assessment, not to mention your care?

Start by Knowing Yourself

> *"The health professional must consider more than the patient's cultural background alone. The culture of the health professional must be considered as well. Both the patient and the health professional bring their own cultural values, attitudes, and behaviors to the patient education interaction."*
>
> —Falvo, 1994, page 136

You bring to the bedside your lifestyle, culture, and religion, too. In addition to your personal attributes, you carry the culture of health care. You are also enculturated as a health care provider and as a nurse. For example, our culture of health care gives us the general goals of patient and family education.

> *"Patient education practice arises out of the belief that patients should be given information from which to make their own decisions and out of that belief that information regarding health and health care will help the individual follow medical advice, which will in turn enhance their well-being."*
>
> —Falvo, 1994, page 149

That sounds logical. Your job is to help patients and families understand so they can make informed decisions, make good choices, and live healthier lives. However, that's logical only within your context, given your assumptions. Not everyone lives in that same context. Not everyone makes the same assumptions.

> *"Although health professionals may emphasize self-determination and self-direction, other cultures may value the mystique of health professionals, believing they have healing powers, or they may expect a more authoritarian approach."*
>
> —Falvo, 1994, page 149

Your learners may not share your basic assumptions and viewpoints. How do you identify these? How do you deal with them?

Assessment

What's the problem with the nurse's question, "Do you have any cultural or religious beliefs you want me to incorporate in my nursing care?" Learners have little idea about what nursing care is. They may have trouble identifying their cultural and religious beliefs, and they probably have no idea how you would incorporate the two. This is one situation where the direct method of assessment is not very productive. It is, however, a situation that can be assessed through less direct methods. There can be many observable clues about the learner's cultural or religious beliefs. These clues tell you to assess further. They will lead you to identify information about the learner that could help you individualize your nursing care. Attend to presenting information, such as the following:

- Language spoken with family members
- Clothing
- The man of the family answering all the questions
- A Bible, Koran, or other holy book
- Talismans, charms, or crystals
- Request for a pork-free diet
- Prayer before eating
- Poor eye contact
- Comments that don't make sense to you

Focus on concrete issues, in context, as they come up. In the beginning, don't try to fit the learner into what you know about a culture, religion, or lifestyle. Pay attention to data. Find out what is, objectively.

"Discussions about culture are generalizations, individual behaviors are influenced by a variety of issues that include personality, temperament, and individual experiences. Differences between social classes within one country, which may reflect profound financial, educational, religious and cultural influences, may even be more significant."
—Chachkes & Christ, 1996, page 16

Don't make assumptions. Just as you would ask about the source of an obvious scar, ask for clarification when presented with cultural, religious, or lifestyle information.

Many journal articles and books have been written about the health beliefs and behaviors of different ethnic and religious groups. Assessment parameters have been defined by research for years. For example, the Bloch (1983, pages 63–69) Ethnic/Cultural Assessment Guide lists over 25 data categories to assess, including ethnic origin; habits, customs, values, and beliefs; language(s) or dialect(s) spoken; cultural health beliefs; cultural health practices; characteristics of food preparation and consumption; family as supportive group; institutional racism; and psychological or cultural response to stress and discomfort of illness.

Do you need to assess each of these items on every patient and family?

Think about it this way: Do you thoroughly assess every organ system on every patient? Only if you are doing a physical examination. Otherwise, you informally assess the whole body (breathing, good color, moist mucous membranes, moving well). You consider the big picture but attend to the specific systems only with presenting problems.

For example, sometimes the gastrointestinal system presents the problem. After several unsuccessful treatments, you suspect the psychological system is involved, so you assess that, too. You always look at the whole body for clues of signs and symptoms of imbalance.

It's the same with cultural and religious assessment. It would be inefficient and irrelevant to do a full ethnic/cultural assessment on every patient on admission. Not to mention, this would be impossible, given your time constraints.

However, just as you wouldn't assume, without concrete evidence, the condition of the heart of your patient who claims to exercise often, don't assume certain beliefs or behaviors because your learner speaks with an accent or has dark skin.

> *"Health professionals unfamiliar with variations within each culture may have a tendency to treat all people within a cultural group as if they were the same, not allowing for individual differences. . . . The health professional may fail to individualize patient education according to the patient's specific needs, focusing instead on beliefs about the patient's cultural group as a whole."*
>
> —Falvo, 1994, page 137

Assess. Individualize. Ask questions, such as, "Would you feel more comfortable if we used an interpreter so you could hear the doctor's diagnosis in your primary language?" "You called that a prayer wheel. It seems important to you. Is there a special place for us to put it?"

Once you start to understand the learner, you can begin to think about teaching. If the learner seems very different from you, move slowly, and assess along the way.

Keep in mind, the goals of patient and family education are general categories of information to cover. Use these categories to negotiate with the learner to determine mutual goals of patient and family education.

> *"Health professionals may assume that the major goal of patients in health care settings is to 'get better.' In some cultures, however, patients may have a stoic acceptance of poor health with little effort to change."*
>
> —Falvo, 1994, page 149

Should you study the lifestyles and beliefs of other cultures to apply to your professional practice?

There are too many cultures and too many variables to learn them all, and you would learn only generalizations. In addition, people are not in or out of a culture. There is a continuum of culture from traditional, to transplanted, to partially, and then fully acculturated. General information may be good background to help you learn about and accept variations in culture and belief. However, just as all people with appendicitis are not the same, all Jewish people are not the same.

Specific Examples

The professional literature is filled with examples of how patients with other ways of living challenge our assessment and intervention skills. Here are just a few examples of the sorts of experiences you may encounter.

> The adolescent had diabetes for 5 years. His parents brought him in because he was becoming rebellious, and they were concerned. They were a military family, and rebellion was especially difficult for them to cope with. When I assessed what was going on, I found the family still did everything literally as they had been instructed 5 years ago. They still measured every ounce of food.
>
> The boy was not allowed any food after 5 PM, ever. No wonder the kid was rebelling!
>
> —an RN

This military family did not look like they had a particularly different way of living, but clearly, they played strictly by the rules. The health care team was so used to learners not following directions, this took them by surprise. It brought to their attention that "compliance may not always be desired or even a necessary behavior" (Lorig, 1996, page 184).

Here's another example:

> A mother brought her 6-year-old son into the emergency department at three in the morning because he had ringworm of the scalp. He's had the small local infection for several days, and she wanted him treated immediately.
>
> The triage nurse and doctor considered her an abuser of the emergency department. They wondered why she got her son out of bed at three in the morning for a routine exam.
>
> But there were logical reasons. The mom works the late shift at a nursing home and got off at 11:30 at night. It took her four bus transfers to get home by two in the morning. On the table was a note from the child's teacher saying he won't be allowed back in school until his scalp was looked at by a doctor. The mom gets public assistance that is tied directly to her child's school attendance, so this was an economic emergency for the family. The mom saw herself as a good mother by bringing him to the hospital immediately.
>
> —Rickey, 1998

"The poor act according to a set of rules that are very rational in the world they live in. Those of us who take care of their health have an obligation to learn what those rules are."
—Julius Goepp, MD, in Rickey, 1998, page 11

This family lives in another context, under a different set of assumptions. The health care providers probably realized this poor family had another way of living. However, they judged the mom as an abuser of the emergency department, rather than perceiving her situation from her point of view.

In the next example, the learner was white and middle class, just like the nurse. The nurse expected the patient would share her values. She was wrong.

I said to the newly pregnant woman, "And you're going to breast-feed, right?" and she said, "Oh no, I couldn't do that! I'll pump. But I couldn't, you know, do that."

I tried to get her to talk about it. She seemed too embarrassed.

I told her about the benefits of breast-feeding for the baby and the benefits for her and how it helps bonding. She said her husband told her the same thing, but she couldn't see doing it.

"It's like being a cow," she said.

I don't understand at all. Even when I told her how much easier breast-feeding was than pumping, she wouldn't do it. Even though she understands what's best for the baby, she wouldn't do it. She's making big decisions like this based on her feelings, not on facts!

—An RN

This is a clear example of teaching without mutually agreeing to goals. The mom's goal was to give her baby healthy breast milk. The nurse's goal was to have the baby breast-feed. The nurse did not appreciate that the mom intended to nourish the baby with breast milk. The nurse could not bring herself to compromise.

The mom saw breast-feeding as animal-like and inappropriate behavior for her. She did not view it the same way as the nurse did. Their assumptions differed. In the same way, cultural groups have different ways of explaining health and illness:

"Drawing blood from a Vietnamese American may cause feelings of weakness and fatigue for weeks to months after the procedure because [sic] the belief that body fluid, once removed, cannot be replaced."
—McDermott, 1995, page 225

Here's an example of another culture's explanation of health and illness and how one health care provider worked within that framework.

Dr. Rose Jones, while working on her Southern Methodist University dissertation in St. Lucia, learned how to adapt modern medical techniques to a culture that had long ago developed a theory of disease and health based on a hot–cold dichotomy. And because diseases such as gonorrhea were viewed as 'hot' according to tradition, they need to be treated with a 'cold' remedy, the islanders believe. Because antibiotics are considered 'hot,' some islanders question their effectiveness in battling a 'hot' illness like gonorrhea. To convince patients to take their medicine, Jones began recommending that mangos, a 'cold' food, be prescribed along with the penicillin. This practice showed respect for the islanders' traditions while encouraging modern medicine's benefits.

—Martinez, 1996

Understanding the learner's point of view can help you individualize your teaching to meet their needs. Bell and Alcalay (1997) discuss a wellness guide they created in both English and Spanish. The Spanish version (Guia) was the English version (Guide) translated both in language and culture. For example,

"The Guide addresses the importance of making infants feel safe, whereas the Guia focuses upon security, warmth, and love (carino). The Guide presents exercise as something that is 'good for you' and specifically identifies walking and hiking as valuable forms of physical activity. In contrast, the Guia frames exercise as 'fun,' identifying the activities of swimming, singing, dancing, and gardening as worthwhile exemplars of it. . . . Likewise, in the section 'Death and Dying,' the Guide encourages the grieving reader to cope with his or her loss by turning to friends, clergy, grief counselors, and support groups for help. The Guia, however, notes that each culture has its own customs for dealing with loss and encourages the Hispanic reader to get together with friends and family; reliance on outside sources of support is not specifically promoted. The Guia also notes that mourning is a ritual that can help a person to deal with his or her pain."

—Bell & Alcalay, 1997

How to Adapt Your Interventions

People of all cultures respond well to the same basic characteristics of a good caregiver:

> *"Health professionals must be perceived as sincere and genuinely interested in helping patients to obtain their maximal health status. They must also be perceived as trustworthy and accepting rather than condemning, criticizing, or making light of the patients' beliefs or cultural practices."*
> —Falvo, 1994, page 139

Don't be afraid of assessment and working to individualize the care of learners whose ways of living are different from yours. The fear could make you hold back and give less than your usual quality care.

> *"Because of their fear of offending the patient in some way, health professionals may not address certain issues or may fail to obtain information that could make the patient education interaction more effective. In the same vein, health professionals may not attempt compromises or negotiation, feeling that such efforts may be misinterpreted by the patient."*
> —Falvo, 1994, pages 139–140

The same rules apply. Individualize your teaching to the patient and family. Make sure you understand before you intervene.

> *" 'Dealings between medical professionals and patients are really negotiations, a struggle for mutual respect,' Jones said. 'It helps if the clinician has respect for the patients' opinions.' "*
> —Martinez, 1996

If you find yourself pushing, trying to force understanding or cooperation, stop and step back. Are you missing something? Is your approach appropriate for this learner?

> *"Educational interventions that motivate the patient must begin with less directive approaches. Strong listening skills, respect for bicultural differences, and taking time to develop trust and a supportive relationship are helpful when providing health education and recommendations for care."*
> —Chachkes & Christ, 1996, pages 17–18

Focus on small, short-term successes first. It will help build rapport and develop your relationship with the learner. It will also give you time to gather more data about the learner's point of view. This is especially important if your learner comes from poverty.

"The patient education intervention may be more effective if the health professional first attends to the patient's perceived immediate needs and focuses on short-term, one-day-at-a-time goals rather than emphasizing long-term outcomes."

—Falvo, 1994, page 151

Some Practical Suggestions

Here are some concrete, practical suggestions for working with learners who have ways of living that are different from your own.

- Understand your own beliefs, practices, values, and traditions.
- Respect the learner's beliefs, practices, values, and traditions. Don't discredit them.
- Respecting and accepting beliefs is not the same as validating them.
- Find someone who can help you learn about the culture and community. Use this person to check your perceptions and answer your questions.
- Incorporate the learner's beliefs and practices into your recommendations.
- If beliefs or practices have potential for harm, consult your resources to identify alternatives. (Also, check to see if they really have potential for harm.)
- Make instructions clear and concrete to avoid misunderstanding.
- Find out who the learner looks to for advice and social support. Incorporate that information into your teaching.
- Consider the interaction of class, language, and cultural factors on verbal and nonverbal behavior.
- Teach in a culturally appropriate manner. Some cultures consider directives offensive; others expect a direct approach.
- Acknowledge unfamiliarity with a culture, and apologize when you make a faux pas. Say things like, "I haven't known many people from your culture, but I'd like it if you would help me learn" or "Oh, I'm sorry. I didn't mean to offend you. Please let me try again."
- Understand that learning about human variation is a lifelong process.

Actually, these suggestions for individualizing teaching apply to all learners. Culture, religion, socioeconomic status, educational status, ethnicity, and even individual eccentricity can all be approached with the same open attitude.

Creating Structured Programs

Do you teach the same topic to many people in a specific population? It may make sense to develop a teaching program that considers cultural factors, which can then be individualized to each learner. The article by Hendricson et al. ("Implementation of Individualized Patient Education for Hispanic Children With Asthma," 1996) is a detailed example of such an approach. Their article describes their four phases: baseline assessment, the educational intervention, application, and maintenance of learned behaviors. First they used questionnaires and focus groups to determine learner needs. As a result, their educational interventions focused on self-management rather than general information about asthma and its causes. Written materials were developed in both English and Spanish, simply and clearly and were illustrated. Videotapes were created to reinforce teaching. Teaching was done in a one-on-one format with nurse and family. The application phase involved the educational sessions and practice at home. Maintenance was implemented during follow-up appointments.

If you are developing a teaching program targeted to a specific population, whether the population shares a culture, ethnicity, religion, homelessness, or some other quality, involve people from that population in planning. Don't just involve leaders from that community—they may not be representative of your learners. Involve potential learners. Many researchers have found this to be essential. For example,

"The involvement of community members in the development and production of these educational tools has contributed greatly to their usefulness and acceptance within the community."
—Clabots & Dolphin, 1992, page 79

Individualizing care means adapting your interventions so they have meaning to the individual.

"It assumes that the other side has a reasonable point of view—a slice of the truth. It is opposed to people management and has no hard and delineated aims in its relations to people. It is optimistic about the nature of human beings. It holds that the organism naturally searches for both physical and mental health. . . listening carefully, trying to understand . . . listening has an open heart."
—Brandon, 1976, page 88

It's not Always Easy

In your daily encounters, you may find various barriers that prevent you from teaching your patients and families. Some of these barriers stem from differences in culture, ethnicity, and religion. Others stem from the patient's and family's physical or cognitive limitations. Still others relate to the patient's current situation or financial implications. Following is a discussion of some common limitations nurses find in their learners and suggestions of ways to accommodate to them.

Language Barriers

When English is not the primary language of the learner and it is your only language, language can be a barrier to patient and family education. Here's an example:

I was observing a student midwife teach a group of pregnant patients breathing and relaxation exercises in preparation for tightening up the pelvic floor muscles after delivery. The class included several African women, who listened politely and watched her carefully. The student-instructor asked the women to 'hold your breath, purse your lips, and pinch, pinch, pinch the lips together,' describing the act of pulling the pelvic floor muscles together in Kegel exercises. The poor student-instructor was red in the face as she tried to get the women to understand. The women pursed their lips, but not their bottoms. These women would have the tightest facial lips ever, but I am not so sure about their pelvic floor muscles.

—An RN

Foreign language skills come in a range of proficiencies. Just as functional literacy skills decrease with stress, other language skills suffer.

"Even if patients and family members are bilingual for social conversation, they may be able to communicate only in their native language under conditions of stress."

—Chachkes & Christ, 1996, page 15

What do you teach patients and families who don't speak your language? Everything you teach patients and families who speak your language. You know how stressful medical encounters can be. When their language is not the same as yours, the stress is greater. Imagine being in their situation, feeling overwhelmed and unable to understand what is happening, express feelings, or ask questions. Add to that a possible history of negative intercultural encounters. Your learners may have never had a doctor or nurse in this country even try to speak to them in their native language.

Your educational responsibilities are constant, no matter what language the patient and family speaks. Even when they speak some English, they probably understand best in their native tongue, especially when stressed by upsetting information or the demands of illness. They need to understand what the problem is. They need to know how to take the medications and prescribed diet. They need to be able to recognize signs of problems and know how to respond. They need to have their questions answered.

If you don't speak their language, how do you know they understand and will apply the information you provide?

You would evaluate learning the same way you would with other families. Ask them to demonstrate the skill while you watch. Ask them to tell you, in their own words, what they will do when they get home. Ask them how they will explain what they just learned to other family members. Give them examples of challenging situations that may come up, and ask them how they would respond. The only difference is that your conversation is being translated by an interpreter.

"Patient teaching using an interpreter takes longer. Each message must be repeated twice."
—Falvo, 1994, page 148

Yes, it takes longer, but using an interpreter conveys respect and demonstrates your care is centered on the patient and family. Interpreters help establish rapport, relay information, and explain foreign concepts. It may seem to take too much time to use an interpreter, but the enhancement of communication usually saves time by promoting trust, understanding, and compliance.

Are you uncomfortable using a language interpreter? Perhaps no one taught you how. See Box 10-1 for details.

Many organizations do not offer access to interpreters. The demand may be too infrequent to justify hiring people, or too few interpreters may be available in the community.

It is not good to use friends and family members of the patient as interpreters. You have no assurance of accuracy, and you don't know if the individuals' relationships are interfering with that accuracy. For example, a child may feel uncomfortable giving his or her mother her diagnosis.

BOX
10-1

Using a Language Interpreter

An interpreter is a professionally trained person who interprets the meaning of words and phrases from the health care provider's language to the patient's language.

Here are some tips on how best to work with an interpreter:

- Tell the interpreter the goal and purpose of the communication before speaking with the patient and family. This prepares the interpreter and helps the interpreter identify if your goals have been met.
- Communication should always be two-way. As you would in any other situation, always give the patient and family member an opportunity to respond or ask you questions. The interpreter is responsible for translating your communications, not communicating for you. You must be present for this to occur.
- You, the interpreter, and the learner or learners should sit or stand so you can all see one another. Nonverbal communication is as important as verbal communication. Observe facial expressions, tone of voice, and body movements.
- Look at and speak to the patient or family member, not the interpreter. This increases rapport and promotes trust. Don't say to the interpreter, "Tell the patient . . ." or "Ask the wife . . ." Tell the learner yourself, in English, and have the interpreter translate it.
- When using a sign language interpreter, make sure the learner can see everyone in the room, and that no light is shining into the learner's eyes. Give the learner frequent visual reassurances and demonstrations.
- Speak slowly, simply, and clearly. Avoid slang words, unnecessary technical terms, complex ideas, and long sentences without pauses.
- Repeat important information more than once. Explain the reason or purpose for a treatment or prescription, as you usually would.
- Be patient. The interpreter may need to use long explanatory phrases to be clear.
- Give the learners opportunities to ask questions.
- Evaluate understanding by asking the learner to explain what was just said in his or her own words, and use return demonstrations.

Friends and family members may not understand the meaning of what you are saying and may misinterpret it. Modesty or gender issues may also make the amateur interpreter uncomfortable and inaccurate. For the same reasons, it is not good to use other bilingual staff members, like housekeepers or secretaries, to interpret. You can only be assured of clarity and accuracy when you use those trained in medical interpretation. Clarity and accuracy are important, because you should offer the same quality of care to all of your patients and families.

Even if your organization has interpreters, you may have an occasional patient from a place like Iceland, and there is no one around who speaks Icelandic. What do you do?

Tell your manager that there are telephone interpretation services available. For example, the AT&T Language Line offers interpretation in 140 languages. If you have access to a speaker phone, the whole health care team, including patient and family, can have a bilingual meeting. AT&T Language Line's services include critical interpretation assistance (if you're in an emergency department and need to understand the patient in a hurry), personal interpretation service (one-time use), membership interpretation, and subscribed interpretation (both for frequent users). Information for further details is listed at the end of this chapter.

Whenever you teach learners who speak languages other than yours, reinforce important information in writing in the learner's primary language, using pictures whenever possible. Evaluate understanding, as you would in any other interaction. Ask that the learner repeat the information in his or her own words.

Non–English-speaking learners, like English speakers, have diverse literacy levels. For example, some Mexican adults come to this country with only a second-grade education; others went to school until they were 17 years old, which is the equivalent of achieving an Associate's degree in the United States. Often, a person may marry someone whose ability to read is very different from his or her own. Literacy levels can vary even within the same family.

If you have written materials both English and in the learner's language, give both handouts to the learner. This will help bilingual family members. One literate family member may read the primary language version aloud to others in the family. The message may be more clear and accurate if it is read rather than translated by the family member.

Another useful teaching tool for learners who don't speak your language is an audiotape of information, recorded by native speakers of the learner's primary language.

If you work in a hospital and your patient is able to listen or converse, access an interpreter at least once each shift, even if you are not intentionally teaching. After all, wouldn't you speak with each of your English-speaking learners at least once each shift? Ask how things are going and if there are any concerns or questions. Let the patient know that interpreters are available when he or she wants to be understood, as well as when health care providers have something to say.

Emotional Barriers

Lots of factors make it difficult to teach: brief emergency room, office, and clinic visits; same-day outpatient surgeries; short inpatient stays; and minimal coverage of home visits. We don't see our learners for very long, and when we see them, they are stressed, in pain, in emotional shock, or medicated.

"The patient must be ready to learn if teaching is to be effective."
—Rakel, 1992, page 390

It makes sense. If we are to individualize our teaching, we must remember,

"A patient who has just received upsetting or unexpected news should not be burdened by a nurse who wants to teach."
—Rankin & Stallings, 1996, page 317

Pay attention, and you will recognize when it is not the right time to teach. Emotional barriers can be coping mechanisms.

"Some persons cope by 'blunting,' or reducing, the input of information about their health status."
—Foltz & Sullivan, 1996, page 32

Respect your learner, understanding that everyone copes differently. Don't push your agenda. Focus on the needs of the patient and family. Some people respond to bad news with grief, others with anger.

"Do not talk to an angry patient about any other subject until you understand the source of the anger. Take as long as necessary to diffuse the anger."
—Hammerschmidt & Meador, 1993, rule number 87

Sometimes emotional barriers are created during interpersonal interactions. If your learner had been receptive, then developed an emotional barrier to communication with you, examine the situation.

"The response you get is the message you send. If a patient gets mad as you talk, you said something that angered the patient. If a patient laughs as you talk, you said something that was funny to the patient. If the patient cries as you talk, you said something that was sad or upsetting to the patient. If the patient begins to argue with you, you said something argumentative to the patient. You can be in charge of your communication."
—Hammerschmidt & Meador, 1993, rule number 127

You may not have intended your statement to upset the learner. You may think it should not have upset the learner, but if it did upset the learner, that is how this learner received that message from you. If you want the learner to change responses, change your message. You can help your learner work past the emotional barrier.

Always take the learner's concerns into account first. If you do not address them, the learner will be too distracted to hear you. For example, these lyrics from the song "Will I?" from the Broadway musical Rent (Larson, 1996) express the concerns of one patient with acquired immunodeficiency syndrome:

> *"Will I lose my dignity? Will someone care? Will I wake tomorrow from this nightmare?"*

If your learner is anxious, depressed, or worried but is willing to learn, he or she may need help focusing. Teach slowly and carefully. Engage your learner without forcing the learning. Present the context before giving new information. Make instructions interactive. Offer examples, especially visual examples. Speak in descriptive terms, draw, and point to illustrations in booklets. Evaluate and review often. Give your learner a written list of resources he or she can access when the time is right.

> *"Acknowledge each patient's support needs and his anxiety about learning new health behaviors. Patients should know that they will receive necessary help and teaching until new skills are mastered and that they will be supported by medical personnel."*
> —Rankin & Stallings, 1996, page 175

Self-Efficacy

Does your learner believe he or she can do the skill or behavior you're teaching? Does he or she believe success is possible?

> *"Some patients are discouraged by past failures to modify behavior or to follow through with a medication regimen. Discouraging, unsuccessful efforts to maintain weight loss, for example, often sabotage future attempts."*
> —Platt et al., 1994

A person must believe he or she is able to learn the skill before the skill can be learned. A person who believes he or she can accomplish a specific task has self-efficacy. Self-efficacy for future performance usually predicts actual future performance.

A person who does not believe he or she can perform a skill is less likely to be able to do it. Those with low self-efficacy on tasks they are able to perform are generally underachievers. Self-efficacy is not the same as learned helplessness, self-esteem, or locus of control. Self-efficacy is specific to behaviors; the others are personality traits or attitudes.

Self-efficacy is the perception or belief that we can do something in the future. It is behavior specific and very individual. A learner may have high self-efficacy for fixing cars but low self-efficacy for quitting smoking.

Because even your best teaching cannot work on a learner with low self-efficacy, assess for this belief. To assess self-efficacy, after describing or demonstrating a skill, ask if the learner feels he or she could do it. Ask the learner, "Using a scale of not at all confident (0%) to completely confident (100%), how confident are you that you can do this behavior?"

Self-efficacy is not always obvious. Self-efficacy is not global, but specific, so your targeted interventions can make a difference. If self-efficacy is low, stop teaching. Raise the learner's self-efficacy first. The learner needs to believe he or she can successfully perform the skill (Lorig, 1996).

The following can help to raise self-efficacy:

- Help the learner master skills. Break skills into tasks that are very small and doable. Have the learner successfully complete each small task. As a learner succeeds, he or she increases the belief that the larger goal can be accomplished.
- Use role models. Introduce the learner to others with the same problem. Match the models to the learner by age, sex, ethnicity, and socioeconomic status. Use lay instructors, and class members helping one another. Do not use super-achievers as role models.

   All teaching media (videos, tapes, books, and pamphlets) should use appropriate models who are similar to the learner in age, sex, ethnicity, and socioeconomic status.
- Help learners reinterpret signs and symptoms. If you see learners engage in behaviors you consider irrational, find out the beliefs behind those behaviors. To understand the learner's beliefs, ask questions like, "If you (change the behavior), what are you afraid might happen?" or "When you think about (disease or new behavior), what do you think of?" or "Why don't you change the behavior?"

   Then, help the learner reinterpret the information. For example, in the movie Star Wars, Luke Skywalker did not believe he could use the Force to lift the space ship out of the swamp. Yoda, who was smaller than Luke, demonstrated it was possible. Luke's beliefs changed, and he learned to accomplish this task he previously thought was impossible.

However, Yoda took a chance, because he used a super-achiever as a role model (himself). A better method would have been if Yoda showed another young man, like Luke, demonstrating the skill.

- Persuasion is a popular way to help people change behaviors, but fear arousal and social support are not very effective at changing beliefs. They may help for short-term goals.

For more information about self-efficacy and how to increase it, read Lorig's *Patient Education: A Practical Approach* (1996).

Physical and Cognitive Limitations

"How do I effectively provide education to seriously mentally ill patients at their level of understanding without missing any of the important aspects?"
—An RN

A learner with physical or cognitive limitations needs individualized teaching. However, before you begin teaching, find out what and who the learner's resources are and how the household runs. Make sure you are teaching the right person. Once again, a good assessment saves teaching time. One nurse waited until she was frustrated before she asked:

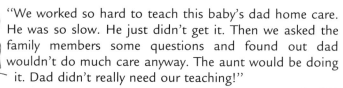

"We worked so hard to teach this baby's dad home care. He was so slow. He just didn't get it. Then we asked the family members some questions and found out dad wouldn't do much care anyway. The aunt would be doing it. Dad didn't really need our teaching!"
—An RN

Your learner has functioned with these limitations until now. Coping strategies and resources have probably been established. Perhaps someone else fills in for the patient's deficiencies. Find out what exists before you plan for the future. Involve the learner, family members, and significant others.

"If goals are mutually derived, there are fewer chances that physical limitations will hamper patient teaching."
—Rankin & Stallings, 1996, page 320

Here's an example of how one nurse tapped resources and individu-alized teaching to make a difficult situation work:

There was a baby in the CCN that needed to go home on an apnea monitor due to apnea of prematurity and periods of bradycardia. The mom and the grandmother and the aunts were all being trained to care for the baby at home. All of these dear caretakers were mentally challenged. Genetic studies were done on the infant and were definitely abnormal. The faces and other body characteristics of the baby were identical to the mom and the other family members.

The day for the classes arrived and upon looking at the family members, it was apparent to me that, indeed, this was going to be a challenge! I started off very slowly and realized that I was receiving blank looks in response to most of what I was saying, except when I was talking specifically about the baby and how she was doing. The class usually takes about one hour for each of the two segments. After 45 minutes, I was acutely aware that this was not working as planned.

I quickly decided to just emphasize the absolute essentials that, in case of emergency, would guide these loving people to do what would save the baby's life, if that became the situation. I also decided to just stop for the day and come back the next day to try again. Thankfully, the baby was not going home for a few days.

The next day, all the family was there. I began a new tactic. Today, each family member would have a part to play, should an emergency occur. We set up scenarios. Mom would check baby's color and breathing and call out what it was (good or not so good). Aunt would look at the monitor and say slow heart or no breath. Grand-mother would stand by to stimulate the baby, if necessary. Grand-mother was the most advanced in ability to respond after some judgment (i.e., color change or not), so she was chosen to know when to stimulate or not. Everyone's role was rehearsed several times. Then we play-acted out the scenarios over and over again. We had a great time, and much was accomplished.

The next day we all met again. I checked to see what each remem-bered. We reviewed and practiced a few more times. Things were looking good. Next, we had to get in the monitor that would be used at home.

I called the monitor company and filled them in on what had worked for us. The monitor company therapist, who was coming to set up, was quite interested in how we had done the training and came by my office to discuss it the next day. That afternoon the monitor was brought in. I went with the therapist to introduce him and to praise the family in front of the therapist. I felt this would increase their self-esteem and place them in a receptive frame of mind for the next challenge. The monitor company therapist took the same approach, practiced several times, and set up a time to return the next day. The next day he completed the job. Each person in the family had her own role to play and seemed to feel very good about the whole thing. Next, plans were made to have the whole family "nest in" with the baby in the hospital.

The nesting in took place the next night. The nurse caring for the baby was well aware of the whole teaching process and was excited about taking part in caring for the baby with the family that night. The report the next morning was good. The nurse worked with them closely, and they did well.

After the baby went home, a home care nurse was assigned to visit them daily for the first week. The monitor company therapist also checked in at the beginning of the week and called at the end of the week. I spoke with the family twice that first week and weekly after that. The visiting nurse said she was thrilled with this family's love and ability to care for the baby, albeit it took all of them. It was a real success story!

Each time she visited the family, the baby was well cared for and truly loved. This was a team effort that worked for all the right reasons. Great feeling for all of us who were involved.

—An RN

A good assessment of the abilities and the limitations helps you develop a teaching plan that can work.

Disorders of Integrative Processing

With disorders of integrative processing, the learner may have the following:

- Trouble sequencing visual, auditory, or tactile input
- Read words backward
- Be unable to process words
- Hear words or sentences incorrectly
- Be confused by idioms, puns, and abstract information
- Be unable to understand meanings

Do the following to best teach this learner:

- Speak simply and concretely.
- Give simple instructions, one step at a time.
- Do not use jokes or analogies.
- Ask for return demonstrations right after learning.

Memory Problems

"Every day I walked in and told her she would be in the hospital until she was placed in a nursing home. Every day she was shocked, surprised and upset by this new information. From day to day, she couldn't remember!"
—An RN

Not all learners with memory problems are as impaired as the one described above. If your learner has trouble remembering information try the following:

- Teach small amounts of information in short, frequent sessions.

"Partitioning advice also offers a natural break to obtain feedback from patients. The process of giving feedback is in itself a learning stimulus."
—Doak et al., 1998

- Use visual aids.

"Research shows memory has many more access points for visuals than for words and letters. One often can recall a person's face but not her name."
—Doak et al., 1998

- Provide reminders, such as lists, calendars, and medicine containers with timers and alarms.
- Ask the learner to explain what you taught him or her.
- Repeat information frequently.

Language Skill Deficits

Learners with language skill deficits have trouble finding the right words to say. If you ask this learner a question, he or she may not be able to answer.

There are several ways to help a learner with language skill deficits:

- Don't rush him or her.
- Don't speak for the learner.
- Give the learner enough time to organize his or her thoughts.
- After giving the learner adequate time to speak, you may prompt with a question.
- Before you teach, tell the learner what you will talk about.
- Teach a small amount in each session.
- If you need to teach a lot of information, break it down into parts.

Decreased Motor Skills

When a learner has decreased fine motor skills, he or she may be able to use a computer or paint but could have trouble writing or drawing. When a learner has decreased gross motor skills, he or she may be clumsy and have poor performance in sports.

To teach a learner with decreased motor skills, ask the learner what helps. Adapt tasks so the learner can succeed at them. Give the learner enough time to perform the tasks, and allow time for repetition. If the learner has decreased gross motor skills, make sure the environment is uncluttered to minimize falls.

Low Literacy Skills

While working as a family nurse practitioner in a country clinic, one of my clients was a 14-year-old pregnant girl. Concerned that she would not be able to attend childbirth preparation classes, I tried at each prenatal visit to do some childbirth preparation education with her and her parents. Her father took the most active part in this process.

At one visit I was attempting, with no success, to explain how to time contractions. No matter how I explained it, the father was unable to correctly time practice contractions. Getting somewhat frustrated, I finally asked the father to tell me what number I was pointing to on the clock. He was unable to answer the question. I then realized he could not read.

My demonstrations using the clock had been ineffective, because he couldn't read the numbers. Because our clinic time for that visit was exhausted (and so was I), I diverted the discussion, not wanting to cause embarrassment or make my discovery obvious. In fact, no one in the family was functionally literate. I never resolved how to effectively teach timing contractions with this family, but with subsequent teaching, I used pictures and verbal explanations that didn't require any reading of words or numbers.

—An RN

Functional health literacy is the ability to use reading, writing, and mathematical skills at a level that meets the needs of everyday situations. Functional literacy varies with context and setting. A learner's skills may be adequate at home, but when the learner is in a health care setting, skills may become marginal or inadequate.

Chapter 8 discussed how people with low literacy skills may have difficulties learning, because reading also engages other cognitive skills. What are the best ways to teach learners with low literacy skills?

"Intensive verbal counseling empowered low-literacy patients to improve their medication use and solve compliance problems."
—National Council on Patient Information and Education, 1997

"To check for understanding, ask patients to show you how they would implement instructions rather than simply have them repeat instructions."
—Lasater & Mehler, 1998, page 169

"Individuals with low literacy skills often seek their information from sources other than print materials. They have acquired information and learning skills through television and radio, personal experience, demonstration, and oral explanations. Thus, clinicians should use a variety of methods and media to meet their patients' learning needs."
—Doak et al., 1998, page 152

Hussey (1994) described a study using a picture schedule for medications. The patient crossed off the picture on a calendar as each dose was taken. The study found it helped most patients remember to take their medications better than when they took them without the chart. It also reminded them of doses already taken.

"Make sketches, use descriptive words, and point to illustrations in booklets. Cite examples of others who have successfully taken the recommended actions. Several literacy and health projects have produced booklets on cancer written by and for low literacy patients. These are in story, testimonial, or photonovella formats. These materials can reinforce and support the clinician's advice."
—Doak et al., 1998

While working as a clinical nurse specialist with an apnea monitoring program at a Children's Hospital, one of my jobs was to teach parents how to correctly measure and give oral theophylline to their newborns. One case involved a teen mother whose infant was being discharged from the neonatal intensive care nursery. Because the teen was returning to school, the grandmother would be the infant's primary caregiver. So, I met with both the young mother and grandmother at the baby's bedside to discuss and demonstrate theophylline administration. After multiple attempts, the grandmother was still unable to measure the correct dose into a syringe for oral administration. Finally, I

318 NO TIME TO TEACH

pointed to a number on the syringe and asked the grandmother to tell me the number. When she was unable to do so, I realized she could not read numbers. Fortunately, the teenage mother was able to read numbers and correctly measure the medicine. So, we worked out a system where the teenager marked the syringe with tape at the right dose level so the grandmother could correctly draw up the dose in the mother's absence. The system worked well for them.

—An RN

Here are some suggestions for overcoming the barrier of low literacy:

- Mutually agree on goals for teaching.
- Identify what the learner needs to know. Teach only the essentials.
- Teach behaviors.
- Decide how you will present the information.
- Organize your topics in a logical order, moving from general to specific. If you have trouble organizing the topics, write each topic on an index card, and sort the cards until you find a workable order.
- Minimize distractions in the environment.
- Teach in conversation.
- Teach information relevant to the learner.
- Keep tasks small and doable.
- Get and keep the learner actively involved. Give your learner something to do. (Remember, when learners interact with the material, a chemical change takes place in the brain that enables them to remember the information faster and better.)
- Speak in short sentences.
- Convey no more than one concept per sentence.
- Use short words; one or two syllables are best.
- Use the active voice; avoid all forms of "to be."
- Use illustrations and visual examples. (Remember, there are many more sites in the brain for visual stores than there are for words. All people, whether they have low literacy skills or not, remember better with a picture than with words.)
- Use repetition.
- Present important concepts first and last.
- Evaluate understanding by having the learner show you how or explain what he or she just learned.

Work with your learners to solve the problems. Use your resources. Be creative.

Sensory Deficits

Some sensory deficits can be corrected with tools like eyeglasses and hearing aids. If your learner's sensory deficits are not correctable, individualize your teaching methods to accommodate them. No matter what the sensory deficit, teach with active involvement, and evaluate learning. Identify your learner's resources, and if needed, refer your learner to additional resources.

If your learner's sensory deficit contributed to a medical problem, such as an injury or foot infection, teach preventive care.

Vision

With disorders of vision, the learner may have problems with the following:

- Visual acuity
- Ability to read
- Ability to perceive fine visual detail, like lines on a syringe
- Depth perception, judging distances
- Peripheral vision
- Ability to discriminate between blue, violet, and green

There are many ways to teach this learner best:

- Make sure the learner's glasses are clean and on or contacts are in.
- Guide the learner through unfamiliar environments.
- Use conversation and audiotapes to teach.
- Constantly describe what is happening or about to happen.
- Incorporate touch and moving objects into the teaching activities.
- Don't assume blind learners can read braille. Ask.
- Make sure teaching materials are directly in front of the learner.
- If learner has some vision, shine light from behind the learner, directly onto the point of teaching focus.
- Use printed materials with large (14- to 16-point) print and high-contrast, serif type.
- Use soft white light and yellow paper to decrease glare.
- If the learner has difficulty discriminating colors, be sure colors are not important in graphics or type.
- Use materials that are easy to read, with key words or phrases in large, black letters.
- Give the learner enough time to explore, test, and perceive depths.

- If you show a slide or transparency presentation, don't make the room completely dark. Slow down the program so the learner can accommodate to changes in light. Instead of breaks of projected white light, use black slides or transparencies.

Hearing

While I was working in the emergency room, a couple came in. The wife was in her first trimester of pregnancy with their first child, having vaginal blood flow and cramping, which signaled that she was about ready to abort. That in itself is an opportunity for many nursing skills—not only teaching, but grief management. What made this situation unique was that both the husband and wife were deaf and mute, and I wasn't versed in sign language. The patient was understandably scared and needed information about what was going on. Plus, she and her husband needed emotional support.

I took the opportunity before the procedure to communicate through writing things on paper, and drawing pictures about what was going on, what they could expect, and any discomfort she might feel. We literally walked through the procedure step by step. Then, as the doctor was doing the procedure, I stayed with the couple and shared their tears and answered more questions on paper.

It would have been easier and quicker to have just gone in and done the procedure without all of the extra time and materials it took to convey what was going on to that couple. But it was a very meaningful experience to me, and I know the couple was better able to deal with their loss and the changes in their life because of my creativity to assess the situation and adapt my teaching styles to the needs of my patient.

—An RN

With disorders of hearing, the learner may not be able to do the following:

- Discriminate sounds or hear clearly
- Hear high-frequency sounds
- Discriminate words that sound alike, like "blood" and "flood"
- Discriminate words that have a similar rhythm, like "one pill" for "windmill"
- Process sounds quickly

There are many ways to teach this learner best:

- Ask the learner how he or she prefers to learn.
- Teach in a quiet area.
- Sit close to learner's best ear.

- If your learner has a hearing aid, make sure it has a working battery.
- If your learner has a hearing aid, sit within 4 feet of him or her.
- Face your learner and don't cover your mouth so the learner can read your lips to supplement hearing.
- Speak slowly and clearly.
- Speak your normal voice or deepen your voice to a slightly lower pitch.
- Do not shout.
- Repeat information when necessary.
- Use graphics, anatomical models, videotapes, and written materials to teach.
- Assess the learner's literacy skills.
- Your learner may be able to use your stethoscope to hear better, with the bell near the source of the sound.
- Don't assume deaf learners know finger-spelling or American Sign Language. Ask.
- If your learner does use sign language, access a sign language interpreter.

Age and Development

How do you adapt your teaching to accommodate age and development of the learner? These impact the learner's ability to understand and apply information, so assess the learner, and individualize teaching, as usual.

The rules are general, and you need to determine if they fit your learner before you apply them. For example,

"Is it better to teach kids information when the parents are there, or when they aren't, or both?"

—An RN

Parents are responsible for the care of their minor children, so they, not the child patient, need to be taught how to care for the child at home. However, if a child asks if he can go swimming with the cast on his leg, answer him or her. You can tell the parents later. Occasionally the parents are so impaired or negligent that an older child has taken responsibility for the younger child's home care. If this is the case, teach both child and parents. Know your learner.

In general, normal growth and development patterns apply. As with adults, teach children honestly. You will lose their trust if you tell them a procedure will not hurt, and it does. It is better to reframe the feeling, such as "first you will feel a pinch, like a bee sting, and then you will feel a little pressure." For approaches to teaching children at various stages of development, see Table 10-1 on page 332.

TABLE 10-1. Cognitive States and Approaches to Patient Education With Children

COGNITIVE STAGE	APPROACH TO TEACHING
Ages Birth to 2 y—Sensorimotor Development	
Begins as completely undifferentiated from environment	Orient all teaching to parents.
Eventually learns to repeat actions that have effect on objects	Make infants feel as secure as possible with familiar objects in home environment.
Has rudimentary ability to make associations	Give older infants an opportunity to manipulate objects in their environments, especially if long hospitalization is expected.
Ages 2–7 y—Preoperational Development	
Has cognitive processes that are literal and concrete	Be aware of explanations that the child may interpret literally (e.g., "The doctor is going to make your heart like new" may be interpreted as "He is going to give me a new heart"); allow child to manipulate safe equipment, such as stethoscopes, tongue blades, reflex hammers; use simple drawings of the external anatomy because children have limited knowledge of organs' functions.
Lacks ability to generalize	Comparisons to other children are not helpful, nor is it meaningful to compare one diagnostic test or procedure to another.
Has egocentrism predominating	Belief that he causes events to happen may result in guilty thoughts that he caused his own pain, hospitalization, and so forth; reassure child that no one is to blame for his pain or other problems.
Has animistic thinking (thinks that all objects possess life or human characteristics of their own)	Anthropomorphize and name equipment that is especially frightening.
Ages 7–12 y—Concrete Operational Thought Development	
Has concrete, but more realistic and objective, cognitive processes	Use drawings and models; children at this age have vague understandings of internal body processes; use needle play, dolls to explain surgical techniques and facilitate learning.
Is able to compare objects and experiences because of increased ability to classify along many different dimensions	Relate his care to other children's experiences so he can learn from them; compare procedures to one another to diminish anxiety.
Views world more objectively and is able to understand another's position	Use films and group activities to add to repertoire of useful behaviors and establish role models.
Has knowledge of cause and effect that has progressed to deductive logical reasoning	Use child's interest in science to explain logically what has happened and what will happen; explain medications simply and straightforwardly (e.g., "This medicine [insulin] unlocks the door to your body's cells just as a key unlocks the door to your house. By unlocking the door to the cell, the insulin can deliver the food and energy in your blood to the cell.").

(Adapted from Petrillo, M., & Sanger, S. [1980]. *Emotional care of hospitalized children* [pp 38–50]. Philadelphia: J.B. Lippincott and Kolb, L.C. [1977]. *Modern clinical psychiatry* (9th ed, pp 90–91). Philadelphia: W.B. Saunders.)

Infants understand little, and they do best when they feel safe. Keep parents in their view, and involve parents in procedures. A familiar object from home can also be comforting. Limit the number of strangers that hold and hug the child.

Toddlers are more aware and involved than infants. Simple teaching can help you establish rapport with toddlers; prepare them shortly before procedures. Keep teaching times less than 10 minutes long. Toddlers take things literally, so watch your words. Let them know when you need their cooperation, giving one direction at a time, firmly and directly. When possible, offer appropriate choices (plain or colorful bandage, orange juice or apple juice).

Preschoolers should be involved in their own care whenever possible. They may fantasize and fear pain and physical harm. Show and explain equipment in simple terms. Use a doll to demonstrate body parts involved. Tell them what they will feel, see, and hear during the procedure. Although preschoolers may have a large vocabulary, they may not be able to see things from another point of view. Ask the child to explain to you what will be done to evaluate understanding. Correct misunderstandings right away. Encourage the child learner. Understand that age and development have an impact on ability to understand and apply information, assess the learner, and individualize teaching, as usual.

School-age children need privacy and control. Explain equipment and procedures in terms they understand. Prepare them for procedures, and encourage them to ask questions. Tell them in advance what they can expect after the procedure. A teaching session may last as long as 20 minutes. When appropriate, have children help (pulling off a dressing, choosing the color of the cast).

I was reviewing bone marrow suppressive effects of chemotherapy with a mom and daughter. The 6-year-old girl was recently diagnosed with leukemia. I met the family just the day before, but I assessed the mother as a highly intelligent woman who had already done some reading on the subject. As I spoke to the mom in fairly sophisticated terms, I stopped periodically to summarize in simpler terms for the child. Part way into the teaching, the girl asked me, in a tone of complete exasperation, if I would please use proper names when speaking to her.

She was quite aware that she had platelets rather than cells that help your blood clot, white blood cells rather than infection-fighting cells, and red blood cells rather than cells that carry oxygen to your body. After all, she was a 6-year-old!

From this experience I learned to give developmentally appropriate education, not age-appropriate!

—An RN

Adolescents need even more privacy and control than school-age children do. Seek to establish rapport with them. Listen to and guide them. Keep communication open, and maintain confidentiality, unless there is potential for harm. Involve them in planning and decision making. Expect resistance, and set limits, because they may lack self-control. Be firm and consistent in your responses. Encourage teens to talk about fears and ask questions. Talking to them at their level does not mean you should revert to behaving like an adolescent. Be a good role model.

Adults should be taught using the principles of adult learning emphasized throughout this book. By the time a learner is an adult, he or she has well established lifestyle habits. Remember this when you are trying to promote behavior changes. Midlife learners may reexamine and question their goals and values. Individualize teaching to their current needs.

Old Age

A holding room nurse was making her follow-up calls to outpatients from surgeries earlier in the week. She spoke to the wife of one of our elderly cataract patients. She asked all the usual questions and got the usual answers. Then she asked, "Do you have any questions about anything else?"

"Why yes," the woman replied, "Do you think it is safe to take those patches off of his chest now?"

The holding room nurse immediately thought of nitro patches or other transdermal medications, but a bit more discussion with the wife revealed the patient was still wearing the ECG pads which were applied by anesthesia before the cataract procedure. The nurse assured the patient's wife that it was indeed safe to remove those patches, and no, they did not have to return to the hospital to have them removed by a doctor or nurse.

—An RN

It's easy to assume that with age comes experience and knowledge. This may be true, but that experience and knowledge may not be medically or health related. Patients and families dealing with a chronic illness may know more than you or know very little. Don't make assumptions. Assess.

There are nurses who easily frustrate when teaching older learners.

"Patient education for older patients may be viewed by some as a futile task."

—Falvo, 1994, page 125

Why would older people need less teaching than anyone else? Don't they, too, have the right to understand informed consent, self-care skills, how to identify problems, and how to get their questions answered?

"That pain medicine—is that a narcotic? I don't want to become a drug addict."

—A patient

To teach older learners, make sure they can hear and understand you. Position yourself close, and speak clearly. Some older learners may prefer learning alone. If this is the case, give them teaching materials, and return later to discuss the contents. Help them problem solve.

Assess older learners well. They may have trouble following through with health maintenance activities because of physical limitations, misunderstanding, or financial barriers. Help them make optimal use of their skills and functions.

Financial Implications

A discussion of individualization of teaching would not be complete without addressing financial implications of care choices. Unlike hotels, hospitals generally do not offer our learners a menu of services with prices. In health care, we assume everyone's bottom line is getting well. We assume everyone is willing to spend whatever it takes to get well or that insurance will cover everything we do.

Expense of health care is a very real issue for many of our patients.

I'm a school nurse. A boy came into my office with a red, swollen finger. It had a gash that seemed to have been there a while, filled with oozing pus. When his dad came in to pick him up at the end of the school day, he said he knew about it and they were keeping his finger clean and soaking it every night. Dad said he had cuts like that and they healed up fine. He didn't see that it was big enough of a problem to see a doctor about. He worked construction and didn't have any health insurance.

—An RN

The treatment options we offer cost money, whether we're discussing surgery or increasing intake of fresh fruits and vegetables. We must be aware of the financial implications of care choices and assess our learners' concerns about costs.

326 NO TIME TO TEACH

When implementing the treatment plan, your learner will consider both the convenience cost and the financial cost of cooperation. If the financial cost is too high, even a committed learner will not follow the plan. Cost of transportation, medications, supplies, diet changes, medical tests, blood draws, health care visits, and interventions are all considered by your patients. Therefore, to ensure effective teaching that has an impact on health outcomes, you must consider costs when you individualize care.

Ask your learner, "If you were to have a problem doing this, what do you think it might be?" or "Do you think that you'll have any trouble doing this?" If the plan challenges the learner's finances, involve the health care team in problem solving. A plan not followed is useless and frustrating for all involved.

The Individualization Attitude

Your attitude toward the learner sets the stage for whether or not you individualize teaching. Here's an example of how a nurse behaves when she does not have the individualization attitude.

I was a diabetic educator at a VA hospital. My patients were generally in their mid 50s to 70s, with a third to eighth grade education and were often heavy smokers and drinkers. Inpatient stays for vascular compromise averaged 4 to 7 months, leading to amputation of toes, then foot, then BKA, AKA, and occasionally hip disarticulation. We usually taught in a scheduled classroom setting, with repeating classes.

One patient scheduled his first class and didn't show up. This happened several times. The head nurse talked to him several times about attending. Every class day he would get a pass to leave the unit to go to the class, but no one knew where he went.

I, being the young, idealistic nurse, ready to change my patient's health status with the knowledge I would impart, went and talked to this patient. I told him MY plan to meet his knowledge deficit and that I would meet him on class day and escort him to the classroom.

On the appointed day and time I met Harry, and started walking beside his wheelchair. We headed in the right direction, but Harry steered his wheelchair off the path and wheeled out into the crosswalk. Well, I stood there for a few minutes with a thousand thoughts going through my head. Do I go and pull him back? Call security? Ignore him and continue on my way?

No, I thought. He's not going to get away with this. He's already lost his right foot. He has to learn about diabetic care. Since the dietitian had the class for the first hour, I didn't have to go back right away.

I took off at a trot, with righteous indignation burning in my breast. I slowed down, however, and the breast burning became stomach burning as I saw him wheel into the neighborhood bar.

Would I lose my job or my license? No, I reasoned. What I was about to do was for patient education! I took a deep breath and entered the bar. After my eyes adjusted to the gloom, I saw my patient, at the end of the bar. I went over and sat down on the stool next to his chair. What do I say?

"Buy you a beer, sister?" he asked. I looked over as he began his second drink.

"No thank you," I primly stated in my very best Nancy Nurse voice, "I want to talk with you about your diabetes. You need . . ." I trailed off as I saw the look on his face and his hand raised in the "stop" gesture.

"Sister, I need a lot, but I'll decide what that might be. I'm a drinkin' man and I don't have nothin' to speak of. I have had, but it's too late for me to have again. I'm content."

With those very decisive, very final words he turned back to his beer. He never came to class and was discharged 2 weeks later. I heard from the discharge planner that the home nursing visits were not successful either. He would just nod his head and keep drinking his beer while the nurse talked.

For a while I was disconsolate about old Harry and his health care needs that I was unable to provide. I received condolences from my peers. They referred to him as a noncompliant, alcoholic, uneducated, "usual VA bum."

However, with years and experience, I look back and wonder what the outcome might have been if I had been his partner instead of The Diabetic Educator, BSN, RN.

—An RN

Might there have been a different outcome if this nurse partnered with this learner? How might she have partnered with this learner? What might she have done differently?

What would you have done? How would you individualize your teaching to this learner?

Can you think of examples in your practice when you did not individualize your teaching? Have you started with an attitude that became a barrier to effective patient and family education? How would you behave differently in those situations now?

"When the nurse is interacting with clients and their families or friends who have culturally or religiously diverse backgrounds, basic nursing rules apply: Treat everyone with dignity, respect, and compassion, and treat everyone as an individual."
—Peterson & Smith, 1996, page 76

The attitude that supports individualization of care should occur at every level of the organization. Rankin and Stallings (1996) discuss how policies sometimes work to keep patients dependent and staff in control. We give medications, treatments, and meals, even when patients can do them on their own and will be expected to do them at home. If the patient and family will do these at home, why can't they do them in the hospital?

"A learning environment should offer the patient an opportunity to try out new behaviors and receive support and instruction from the staff."
—Rankin & Stallings, 1996, page 223

Even if you have control over only your own behaviors, you do have influence over the rest, because everyone is connected. Notice organizational barriers to patient and family education, and discuss them with your colleagues. Explore what you can do to improve individualization of care and quality of service.

"If strategies for ensuring high-quality care are implemented so rigidly that they stifle the patient's development in a cooperative learning relationship, they may destroy real patient education."
—Rankin & Stallings, 1996, page 223

If you don't individualize teaching, some information may stick, and some may not, and you risk alienating the learner. Generic teaching is quick but not very effective. In time, you or someone else will have to reteach that learner the same information. It's a waste of teaching time.

The better your teaching skills, the more effective and efficient your teaching will be. When you individualize teaching, you take time to assess the learner and adapt your teaching to the individual. This personalizes the message, and learning is quicker and better. You won't need to reteach so much. Teaching goes faster.

Individualization of teaching is an attitude, an approach to the learner.

"All we have to do is listen—really listen."
—Dass & Gorman, 1985, page 69

Individualization Gets Easier With Experience

Have you ever played a computerized game? It may have been a Nintendo, computer, or arcade game. If you play any one game often enough, your skills start to improve, and you'll realize the game itself taught you how to play well. When you make a good move, whether by accident or intentionally, the game rewards you with points or sounds. When you make a bad move, you lose (or worse, get blown up or eaten). You don't learn information you can necessarily explain to other people. You learn perceptions and reactions. You start to understand the feel of the game. Through experience and attention, you learn how to play better. Your interaction with the game teaches you skills. When you get really good, you move up to the next level of difficulty.

In a sense, computer games are a metaphor for teaching. You start by following rules (push this to move forward, press that to jump); then, with practice, you stop thinking and just do it.

> *"The learning of skills begins with recipes. . . . Without practice, the concept won't be second nature; but until it's second nature, you can't practice it effectively."*
>
> —Senge et al., 1994, page 261

Be aware as you individualize teaching, and you will notice that some things you do work well, like asking questions in a certain way. Your teaching goes quicker and easier, and you're rewarded for tailoring your teaching to the learner. Soon, you'll start doing those things more frequently. Other times, when teaching takes too long or is too difficult, you'll notice where you missed an opportunity to individualize teaching. In time, you'll get really good at this skill, and you'll move up to the next level of difficulty.

> *"Past concrete experience therefore guides the expert's perceptions and actions and allows for a rapid perceptual grasp of the situation. This kind of advanced clinical knowledge is more comprehensive than any theoretical sketch can be, since the proficient clinician compares past whole situations with current whole situations."*
>
> —Benner, 1984, pages 8–9

At that point, you'll know,

> *"No expensive piece of medical equipment or technology can replace the words 'I understand.'"*
>
> —Peterson & Smith, 1996, page 79

If you want to learn more:

(1997). Tips for overcoming cultural barriers: Readiness to learn can differ from culture to culture. *Patient Education Management, July*, 91.

AT&T Language Line. Telephone interpretation in 140 languages. Services include critical interpretation assistance, Personal Interpretation service, Membership Interpretation, and Subscribed Interpretation. For information about services, call 1-800-752-0093, ext. 196; Personal Interpretation service, single use with credit card, call 1-800-528-5888; http://www.att.com/languageline.

Bell, R., & Alcalay, R. (1997). The impact of the Wellness Guide/Guia on Hispanic women's well-being-related knowledge, efficacy beliefs, and behaviors: The mediating role of acculturation. *Health Education and Behavior, 24*(3), 326–344. [On-line]. Available: InfoTrac.

Benner, P. (1984). *From novice to expert: Excellence and power in clinical nursing practice.* Menlo Park, CA: Addison-Wesley.

Bloch, B. (1983). Bloch's assessment guide for ethnic/cultural variations. In M.S. Orque, B. Bloch, L.S.A. Monrroy (Eds.), *Ethnic nursing care: A multicultural approach* (pp. 49–75). St. Louis, MO: C.V. Mosby.

Brandon, D. (1976). *Zen in the art of helping.* New York: Arkana of Viking Penguin.

Chachkes, E., & Christ, G. (1996). Cross cultural issues in patient education. *Patient Education and Counseling, 27,* 13–21.

Clabots, R.B., & Dolphin, D. (1992). The multilingual videotape project: Community involvement in a unique health education program. *Public Health Reports, 107*(1), 75–80.

Dass, R., & Gorman, P. (1985). *How can I help? Stories and reflections on service.* New York: Alfred A. Knopf.

Doak, C.C., Doak, L.G., Friedell, G.H., & Meade, C.D. (1998). Improving comprehension for cancer patients with low literacy skills: Strategies for clinicians. *CA: Cancer Journal Clinics, 48,* 151–162. [On-line]. Available: http://www.ca-journal.org/frames/articles/articles_1998/48_151-162_frame.htm.

Einhorn, C. (1998). *Steps of patient education.* [On-line]. Available: http://nisc8a.upenn.edu/psychosocial/pat_educ.html.

Ethnomed Bibliography in Cross Cultural Nursing. [On-line]. Available: http://weber.u.washington.edu/~ethnomed/resbib.htm.

Falvo, D.R. (1994). *Effective patient education: A guide to increased compliance* (2nd ed.). Gaithersburg, MD: Aspen Publishers.

Foltz, A., & Sullivan, J. (1996). Reading level, learning presentation preference, and desire for information among cancer patients. *Journal of Cancer Education, 11*(1), 32–38.

Forsythe, D.E. (1996). New bottles, old wine: Hidden cultural assumptions in a computerized explanation system for migraine sufferers. *Medical Anthropology Quarterly, 10*(4), 551–574.

Galanti, G.A. (1991). *Caring for patients from different cultures: Case studies from American hospitals.* Philadelphia: University of Pennsylvania Press.

Goldstein, N.L., Snyder, M., Edin, C., Lindgren, B., & Finkelstein, S.M. (1996). Comparison of two teaching strategies: Adherence to a home monitoring program. *Clinical Nursing Research, 5*(2), 150–177. [On-line]. Available: EBSCO.

Hammerschmidt, R., & Meador, C.K. (1993). *A little book of nurses' rules.* Philadelphia: Hanley & Belfus.

Hendricson, W.D., Wood, P.R., Hidalgo, H.A., Ramirez, A.G., Kromer, M.E., Selva, M., & Parcel, G. (1996). Implementation of individualized patient education for Hispanic children with asthma. *Patient Education and Counseling, 29,* 155–165.

Hussey, L.C. (1994). Minimizing effects of low literacy on medication knowledge and compliance among the elderly. *Clinical Nursing Research, 3*(2), 132–146. [On-line]. Available: EBSCO.

Intercultural Communication Institute
8835 SW Canyon Lane, Suite 238
Portland, Oregon 97225 USA
Phone: (503) 297-4622
Fax: (503) 297-4695
E-mail: ici@intercultural.org
Website: http://www.intercultural.org
Brief workshops each summer in various aspects of intercultural communication, and a Master of Arts degree program in Intercultural Relations.

Intercultural Press
PO Box 700
Yarmouth, ME 04096
1-800-370-2665
interculturalpress@internetmci.com
http://www.bookmasters.com/interclt.htm
Books on topics of culture, intercultural communication, and training in cultural competence.

Korpi, P.V. (1995). The myth of patient education. *Dental Economics, 85*(9), 78–81.

Larson, J. (1996)."Will I?" Lyrics from the Broadway musical *Rent.* Finster & Lucy Music LTD.

Lasater, L., & Mehler, P.S. (1998). The illiterate patient: screening and management. *Hospital Practice, 33*(4), 163–165, 169–170.

Literacy Volunteers of America. (1992). *Secret survivors: The plight of functionally illiterate adults in the health care environment.* [Video.] Syracuse, NY: Author.

Lorig, K. (1996). *Patient education: A practical approach.* Thousand Oaks, CA: Sage Publications.

Lumsdon, K. (1994). Getting real: Study finds success factors in patient education. *Hospitals and Health Networks, 68*(8), 62. [On-line]. Available: InfoTrac.

McDermott, M.K. (1995). Patient education and compliance issues associated with access devices. *Seminars in Oncology Nursing, 11*(3), 221–226.

MacDonald, D. (1998). Meeting special learning needs. *RN, April,* 33–34.

Martinez, E. (1996). *Medical anthropologist brings new perspective to treatment.* The University of Texas Southwestern Medical Center at Dallas. [On-line]. Available: http://www.swmed.edu/home_pages/news/anthrop.htm.

National Council on Patient Information and Education. (1997). Compliance: Patients need individualized approach. *Medical Practice Communicator, 4*(4). [On-line]. Available: Medscape, http://www.medscape.com/HMI/MPCommunicator/1997/v04.n04/mpc0404.02.html

Peterson, R., & Smith, J. (1996). A patient care team approach to multicultural patient care issues. *Journal of Nursing Care Quality, 10*(3), 75–79.

Platt, F.W., Tippy, P.K., & Turk, D.C. (1994). Helping patients adhere to the regimen. *Patient Care, 28*(17), 43–53. [On-line]. Available: EBSCO.

Rakel, B.A. (1992). Interventions related to patient teaching. *Nursing Clinics of North America, 27*(2), 397–423.

Rankin, S.H., & Stallings, K.D. (1996). *Patient education: Issues, principles, practices* (3rd ed.). Philadelphia: Lippincott-Raven.

Rickey, T. (1998). Bridging the cultural gulf between poverty and medicine. *Rochester Review, 61*(1), 10–11.

Senge, P.M., Kleiner, A., Roberts, C., Ross, R.B., & Smith, B.J. (1994). *The fifth discipline fieldbook: Strategies and tools for building a learning organization.* New York: Currency.

Scobey, S. (1994). *Focused listening skills: How to sharpen your concentration and hear more of what people are saying.* Boulder, CO: CareerTrack Publications.

Thiederman, S. (1996). Improving communication in a diverse healthcare environment. *Healthcare Financial Management, 50*(11), 72–74. [On-line]. Available: InfoTrac.

Tripp-Reimer, T., & Afifi, L.A. (1989). Cross-cultural perspectives on patient teaching. *Nursing Clinics of North America, 24*(3), 613–619.

CHAPTER

11

Teaching Groups

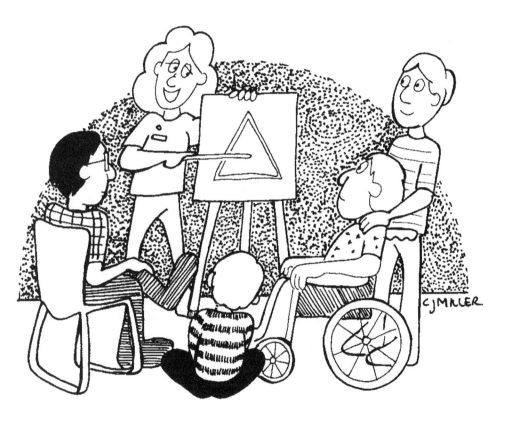

A dults have enough life experience to be in dialogue with any teacher, about any subject, and will learn new knowledge or attitudes or skills best in relation to that life experience."

—Vella, 1994, page 3

"The weather gets bad and we get filled with asthma. Instead of having every nurse doing the same asthma teaching, one patient at a time, doesn't it make sense to pay one nurse to hold a class?"

—An RN

••••••••••••••••••••••••••

If you don't have enough time to teach and several people need to be taught the same information, why not teach those people together?

Why Teach Groups?

Group teaching is common in many areas of health care, such as prenatal classes, cardiopulmonary resuscitation, and cardiac rehabilitation. We can broadly define skills to include not just physical health, but also life skills. One outpatient mental health organization offered a class titled, "Tools for Women in Early Recovery." The class was targeted to women who have been sober between 2 and 12 months and addressed ways they can integrate recovery into their day-to-day responsibilities.

However, few nurses were taught, either in school or on the job, how to teach groups.

Group teaching gives learners the opportunity to have discussions. This is a great advantage for adult learners.

"Discussion . . . differs from lecture in that it is an excellent method of actively involving patients in the learning process. This learning activity promotes understanding and application of knowledge (cognitive behaviors) as well as developing certain attitudes (affective behaviors). It is frequently directed by the teacher, who asks specific questions or proposes problem situations. Discussion facilitates learning from the experience of others, fosters a feeling of belongingness, and reinforces previous learning."
—Rankin & Stallings, 1996, page 183

Teaching groups also facilitates collaboration between members of the health care team. The content of the group teaching can be developed by a multidisciplinary team and may even be facilitated by co-leaders from different disciplines. Each team member brings to the learner a different perspective on the subject.

Because the general goals of patient and family education are universal, team members from different organizations may even choose to collaborate on developing and presenting these groups. The possibilities are endless. Through collaboration, home health care nurses and hospital nurses can help learners understand the significance of health-promoting behaviors. Community organizations and university medical centers can pool resources and reach a wider population. School nurses and doctor's office nurses can send children a coordinated message. Nursing home nurses and managed care providers can support one another's teaching efforts.

Is Group Teaching Effective?

The effectiveness of group teaching depends on how you teach the group. Lectures may work in college, where students learn concepts and theories, but they're not as effective with adults who are learning skills and behaviors. (This is good news for nurses who hate speaking in front of groups.) Even in college, skills are taught in clinicals and labs.

> *"Lectures may cause loss of attention; patients become bored, distracted, or anxious about the material presented. Learners may be eager to contribute or to try out or apply knowledge; this eagerness may be stifled by a formal lecture approach in which the teacher is the expert. Long lectures may also create the impression that the patient's problem is so complicated that he will be unable to manage it."*
> —Rankin & Stallings, 1996, page 183

Think about the research-based ways to teach well, described in Chapter 2:

- Keep focused on the goals of patient and family education.
  - Make informed decisions.
  - Develop basic self-care skills to survive.
  - Recognize problems and know what to do in response.
  - Get questions answered; find resources for answers.
- Partner with the learner to establish learning objectives.
- Assess knowledge and ability before you teach.
- Don't make assumptions.
- Focus on teaching behaviors and skills.
- Get the learner actively involved.
- Take advantage of teachable moments.
- Individualize your teaching.
- The learner must believe.

- Evaluate learning.
- Share your teaching with the rest of the health care team.

Lectures don't lend themselves to partnering, assessment, or individualization. These are more easily accomplished in one-to-one conversations. However, it is effective to teach groups with methods that encourage active involvement and discussion. Besides, it's more fun to lead a group discussion than to lecture, because you also get to interact.

How to Teach a Group

Vella (1994) describes how to apply adult learning principles with groups. She defines teachers as resources for the process and content. The job of the teacher is to design the learning and set the tasks in proper sequence. Teachers also are resources who invite and respond to questions. Learners and teachers are in dialogue.

There are 12 principles to accomplish this:

1. **Involve learners in the needs assessment.** Identify the common themes in what learners want to know, and teach from there.

   "Adult learners can decide what is to be taught. . . . They will vote with their feet if the course does not meet their needs. They will simply walk out."

   —Vella, 1994, page 5

   The assessment can be done through focus groups, telephone conversations, written surveys, or faxes.

2. **Create a safe, comfortable learning environment.** You can do this through doable objectives, an accepting atmosphere, small group work, recognizing efforts, and acknowledging success.

   "Learning . . . can only happen if there is an atmosphere of relaxation and mutual trust."

   —Lawlor & Handley, 1996, page 12

3. **Develop a sound relationship between teacher and learner.** Listen to and respect the participants. One author says the key to this is:

   "Sensory acuity. Being aware of the reaction of students to the message one is sending them."

   —Lawlor & Handley, 1996, page 88

4. **Sequence content from simple to complex; reinforce learning**. As learners build their skills, help them succeed each step of the way. Repeat facts, skills, and attitudes until they are learned.

"If the task is too difficult for most learners, it must be changed."
—Vella, 1994, page 11

5. **Alternate action with reflection; learn by doing.** Have learners practice new skills and attitudes and think about what they have just done. Give them time to reflect on its implications. Plan breaks throughout the session.

"Two types of skills are central to this work: they are reflection (slowing down our thinking processes to become more aware of how we form our mental models) and inquiry (holding conversations where we openly share views and develop knowledge about each other's assumptions)."
—Senge, Kleiner, Roberts, Ross, & Smith, 1994, page 235

6. **Respect learners.** Offer learners choices. Be clear whether you are asking learners for suggestions or offering them decision-making choices.

"All learners come with both experience and personal perceptions of the world based on that experience, and all deserve respect."
—Vella, 1994, page 23

Learners should also respect learners within the group. Encourage tolerance between learners.

7. **Involve ideas, feelings, and actions.** Involve mind, body, and spirit. Here's another way to say this:

"Make sure that the lesson contains both visual and auditory elements and opportunities for physical involvement."
—Lawlor & Handley, 1996, page 12

8. **Apply what is learned right away.** Adults want to see results. They don't want to waste time. Give them opportunities to practice.

"Don't ever do what the learner can do; don't ever decide what the learner can decide."
—Vella, 1994, page 13

9. **Make roles clear.** Introduce yourself and discuss the purpose of the group, your responsibility, and the responsibilities of the participants. Communicate clearly. Lead with humility.

"Adult students need reinforcement of the human equity between teacher and student."
—Vella, 1994, page 17

10. **Use small group work; promote teamwork.** Include everyone in the activities. Small groups promote conversations that promote learning.

"Group instruction can be effective. Group size, however, will probably be closer to six than to 30."
—Theis & Johnson, 1995, page 102

11. **Engage the learners in what they are learning.** People learn by doing.

"The body plays a vital part in learning. . . . Maintain energy in the group at an optimum level."
—Lawlor & Handley, 1996, page 12

12. **Make everyone accountable.** Everyone involved needs to be accountable. Teach what you say you will teach. Learners must demonstrate what they have learned. Find out what was useful to learners and what they suggest be changed. Use that feedback to improve your next group teaching.

"In adult learning, the accountability is mutual."
—Vella, 1994, page 10

Do these principles sound familiar? They are the same principles you used teaching one-to-one, applied to the group. In this model, the leader teaches by providing the resources and setting the environment to promote learning. You, the leader, design the activities that lead learners through the material.

Consider co-leading the group. Collaborate with another member of the health care team, from another discipline or another organization in the continuum of care. The energy created by a pair of leaders can help enliven the process. In addition, two people can support one another and share the work. Two leaders can be more aware of group responses and dynamics than one. When a group participant needs individualized attention, a leader can be made available without disrupting the process for everyone.

Find Out What to Teach

"We thought teenage mothers needed classes on parenting skills. Then we held focus groups, and discovered we were wrong. They wanted to know how they can be parents and still live normal adolescent social lives. As a result, we changed the focus of our program."

—An RN

Use focus groups to show you what your population of learners needs to know. The content should be skills and behaviors the learners feel they need to know. Ask questions such as the following:

- "When you think about _____, what do you think about?"
- "What have been your experiences with _____?"
- "What concerns you about _____?"
- "What are you afraid might happen?"

Record the responses, and analyze the answers to determine the themes that arise. Then ask other members of your target population to prioritize the themes. What is most important?

"An assessment of the target population is key to developing an effective education program. . . . Once you know the specifics of your target population, you can use the information to determine when, where, what, and how to teach."

—"Assessing your target population," 1996, page 25

Do a literature search to determine if others have created a group similar to what you are considering. If you have specific questions, call the authors of those articles and ask them what worked and did not work for them.

Plan Your Teaching

What's next? Vella (1994) also provides us with the seven steps of planning:

1. **Who.** Who are the learners? Determine the number of participants and who they are; 16 or less is good.
2. **Why.** Why do the participants need to learn these skills and behaviors; what problem makes this teaching necessary?
3. **When.** When will the group meet? This should be convenient for the participants.
4. **What.** In the needs assessment, what skills and behaviors did the learners identify they wanted to learn?

5. **Where.** Where will the group meet? Include tables and chairs for small group work; this should be convenient for the participants.
6. **For what.** What are the achievement-based objectives for the session? What behaviors and skills need to be learned?
7. **How.** How will the activities (learning tasks) help the participants learn the behaviors and skills?

Is that simpler than you thought? That's really all there is to planning. However, you do need to spend some time on each of the steps to make sure you are making the best choices. Here's more detail on each of the planning steps. Each step is illustrated with the example of the asthma class proposed in the beginning of this chapter. We follow it through the planning stages.

Who

The first step in planning is to think about qualities of your target audience.

"Demographic characteristics such as age, educational background, and socioeconomic status must be considered when patient education programs are designed because they have different impacts on patient education outcomes."

—Rankin & Stallings, 1996, page 341

Think about what your learners could be bringing to the group and how you can tap into those skills and knowledge using a group process.

If many of your learners are likely to have literacy difficulties, you may want your teaching materials to be primarily visual. If many of your learners are likely to have computers at home, the resources you provide for follow-up opportunities may include websites.

This is an example of who: Eight patients are in the hospital with asthma.

Why

Think about the problem that makes this group necessary. Why do the participants need to learn these skills? If these skills are not necessary or do not meet the goals of patient and family education, why are you considering offering this group?

This is an example of why: Participants will be discharged from the hospital and need skills to manage their asthma, recognize problems, and know what to do in response.

When and Where

The when and where of the group should be convenient for the participants. If your learners are in a hospital, avoid treatment and meal times. Retired learners may not drive at night, so a day meeting would be best. Children should be out of school, so afternoons are better. Make sure the meeting room has enough tables and chairs for small group work. Learners need to get to the meeting place. If it is an outreach program, hold it in the community you want to reach. If your target population uses wheelchairs, make sure the group meets in an accessible room.

This is an example of when and where: The group will meet at 2 PM to 3:30 PM in the conference room.

What

Go back to your assessment. What did the learners say they wanted to learn?

This is an example of what: The group will review what medications are for and how to prevent another asthma attack.

For What

Based on the above, what are your achievement-based objectives for the session? What behaviors and skills need to be learned, and how will you know that has been accomplished?

This is an example of what for: By the end of $1\frac{1}{2}$ hours, participants will report the names of the medicines they are taking and their purposes and list three things they can do to prevent another asthma attack.

How

Determine the activities, also known as learning tasks, you will use to help the participants learn the behaviors and skills. Prepare your tools and supplies.

"Be sure to include interactive teaching techniques."
— "Teach through a variety," 1998, page 65

Following are examples of how:

Activity 1: Learners will briefly share their stories of the asthma attack that brought them to the hospital.
Activity 2: Learners are each given an individualized list of the medications they will take home to treat their asthma

(provided by staff nurses caring for those patients). The group leader will hold up medication samples one by one, and learners will discuss in the group the purpose of each medication. The group leader will guide the group to define correct, complete information, as needed. At the end, the leader will summarize each medication, and learners will take notes on their lists.

Activity 3: Learners will break up into small groups and in a limited amount of time, come up with a list of ways to prevent asthma attacks. Then learners will return to the large group, and each will report to the whole group one way to prevent asthma attacks.

If correct inhaler use is mentioned in the group, the leader will review the skill in context. If correct inhaler use doesn't come up by the end of the discussion, the group leader will add this skill and ask the group to discuss and review how to use an inhaler correctly. (This is a necessary skill to review and fits in with the learners' goal of preventing future asthma attacks.)

Be Creative

Use tasks and tools to involve the audience. Can you think of ways to teach the same asthma-managing skills and behaviors with different tasks than those described previously? The possibilities are endless.

"Use a variety of teaching techniques so that everyone's individual learning needs are met."
—"Teach through a variety," 1998, page 65

Consider all the possible tools for teaching, and think about how you might use them to stimulate learning activities to accomplish your goals. The tools that involve interpersonal interaction, such as conversation, are the most effective in group work. There are many books on how to do training. They include many different sorts of interactive exercises. Look for them in your library.

You may not have attended many interactive group teachings, and it may take you time to learn how to plan the activities. Be patient with yourself. Read, think, and remember,

"Keep things simple."
—Ancheta, 1996, page 24

Activities don't have to be complex to be effective. Stick to what learners need to know and the goals of patient and family education. Like anything else, once you get used to the process, it's not difficult.

Think about what skills and behaviors you want your learners to take with them. Then think about the tools that might help them interact with the others in the group and the material to be learned. Here are some ways you might facilitate learning:

- Keep the learning session active, alternating between your brief introduction, an interactive activity for the learners, time to discuss experiences during the activity (a debriefing), and time for the participants to reflect on what they learned.
- Did you notice that each chapter in this book opens with an illustration? Do you know why? Each illustration reinforces the content. You can also use this technique when teaching groups.

"Use pictures as visual cues. Key ideas shown on slides or overheads can be included in participant materials to reinforce content."
—Backer, Deck, & McCallum, 1995, page 157

The illustration at the beginning of this chapter shows the nurse using an illustration to communicate a message to a group.

Post a "Welcome" sign in the room, inviting participants to join in and relax. If appropriate, post the learners' names around it as a personal greeting.

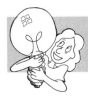

Prepare the environment for learning by posting the theme or subject in pictures around the room.

"Peripherals are visual material placed around a room to make it attractive and add to learning. They can consist of colorful posters, messages which relate to the subject being taught or affirmations or quotations."
—Lawlor & Handley, 1996, page 30

One quotation for a skills workshop may be Henry Ford's, "Whether you believe you can do a thing or not, you are right." This refers to self-efficacy and can stimulate discussion on that topic.

These environmental peripherals visually reinforce the subject, both consciously and subconsciously. They set the tone before the group begins, can create interest, and may be incorporated in the discussion. Best of all, if learners let their minds wander during the session and they explore the environment with their eyes, they are still thinking about the topic of the session. In the example of the asthma class, hang on the wall a poster showing correct inhaler use. After all, it's information you want everyone to take with them. Whether they learn it from the discussion or reading the poster does not matter.

Don't limit yourself to walls.

"The floor can be used to illustrate the steps or sequence of a procedure."
—Lawlor & Handley, 1996, page 30

You can trace your shoes and cut out as many copies as there are steps. Write each step on one of these footprints, and tape them to the floor in order. Instead, design another use for the floor, or put peripherals on the ceiling.

"Group discussion is also a good teaching method. . . . Each group is given an issue or question to discuss. A facilitator monitors and helps the groups as needed, then asks for a report from each group to be shared with the others."
—"Teach through a variety," 1998, page 65

- Write down several problem-solving situations with which learners might have to deal. Break your group into small groups, and ask each group to decide, jointly, how the person in the situation should respond. Have someone from each small group present the situation and the solution to the whole group, and discuss the solution. This is called problem-posing education.

"If, for instance, you wanted to teach eight basic rules for safety in the workplace, you could hand one of the rules to each participant or group of participants. Each of them would then have to try to convince the others that theirs was the most important. The whole group would then have the task of arranging the rules in order of importance. The group could then be asked to come up with further rules or to modify the existing ones. They might finally produce a list which was more useful and comprehensive than the original one. In this way the participants are actively involved. They think, they talk and they are listened to."
—Lawlor & Handley, 1996, page 41

- Brief videos can introduce or accent the group work but should not substitute for it.

"Provide a prefilm/prevideo worksheet for participants to use before they begin viewing the film or video. You can design the worksheet with open-ended questions about the content they observe, leaving room for note taking. Or use the form to direct their attention to certain segments of the video or film. Structure discussion time after the viewing, allowing time for reflection before you start the discussion."
—Backer et al., 1995, page 180

- Computer presentation slide shows are attractive, easy to customize, and can include sound and motion. If you use overheads or slides, handouts should include content of each slide so learners don't have to transcribe them.

"No matter how many well-prepared slides . . . [you] have to show . . . resist the temptation to allow them to become the main focus of the lesson."
—Lawlor & Handley, 1996, page 14

- Tools like overheads, slides, videos, and films can be very effective. However, they do bring the group out of interpersonal, active participation into intrapersonal, passive participation.

"Be aware that there is a price to pay in handing over her role as facilitator to a mechanical or electronic substitute. This price is the interruption of the personal rapport which has been established in her communication with the group."
—Lawlor & Handley, 1996, page 14

- Will your learners need to recall information in stressful moments, like the steps of rescue breathing? Give them tools to help them be ready.

"Provide key points of your program on pocket sized laminated cards. These will provide instant visual reminders."
—Backer et al., 1995, page 182

- When creating a written handout to supplement your group teaching, apply the same principles that work in other written teaching materials, including:

"Chunk information in small sections. This makes the information appear easier to read and absorb, not overwhelming at first glance."
—Backer et al., 1995, page 172

- Prepare the environment to include supplies that invite the learner to get involved.

"Encourage participants to 'personalize' their handout materials. Provide markers and creative materials to make this easy. Participants are more willing to take these materials home for further use when they have invested time in them."
—Backer et al., 1995, page 175

- Use the written material to encourage the learner to participate in the process of learning.

"Make your handout interactive. Involvement makes information more memorable. One way to do that is to provide blanks to fill in. Another is to provide dots for participants to mark areas of understanding (green dots), questions to be asked (yellow dots), and further study needed (red dots)."
—Backer et al., 1995, page 161

However, the dot system may be too complicated for some learners. Know your audience.

"Provide different worksheets and self-learning tools in an addendum at the end of your workbook or handout. These worksheets can be used as additional activities during the program or as follow-up activities."
—Backer et al., 1995, page 167

- Do you know what a mind map is? Mind maps are just images of connected thoughts. They describe information learned, drawn, and written in clusters, by association, not in a linear outline form. They include key words and illustrations and show connections between ideas with lines or arrows. There is no right or wrong way to draw mind maps. They are informal and right-brained (the creative side).

"The group constructs a group mind map of the contents of the lesson just presented. Alternatively they can be asked to do it before the lesson, in order to find out how much they already know about the subject. This will make apparent any gaps in the knowledge of the group and allow the facilitator to fill them in."
—Lawlor & Handley, 1996, page 51

- If your group participants are experienced, they may look forward to sharing what they know. If this is the case, consider this activity:

"Give learners Post-it notes. Ask them to write all the questions about a subject on the notes—one question per note. Post them on a board or flip chart. When all the notes are posted, ask the learners to return to the board to pick off as many of the other people's notes as they think they can answer. Then go around the room and ask everyone to answer the questions they have selected. The questions remaining on the board (there may not be any) can be answered by the facilitator."
—Lawlor & Handley, 1996, page 49

- Sometimes, a little competition can enliven learning. This activity is useful near the end of a session, where lots of information has been shared.
    Divide the group into two teams.

*"Give each team a specified time (not too long) to come up with 20
questions from the learning material. The teams ask each other questions,
one at a time and back and forth, allowing a specified time (15-30
seconds) for an answer to be given. Correct answers earn a point."*
—Lawlor & Handley, 1996, page 39

If you provide detailed handouts for follow-up after the session,
the learners may use them in this activity to come up with their
questions quicker. Consider offering prizes to all the group members,
just for participating. Prizes that are relevant to the topic, but fun,
are best. For example, for a session on asthma, carrying cases for
inhalers that can hang from belt loops are popular. (Write these items
into your budget for the group.)

- If the group topic includes many technical terms, such as
  diabetes teaching, consider this activity.

*"Distribute flashcards (of acronyms, terms, components, processes, etc.) to
each partnership. Have partner A drill partner B for a short time, say five
minutes. Then, at a signal from the facilitator reverse roles."*
—Lawlor & Handley, 1996, page 49

- If the group topic addresses major lifestyle changes, help the
  learners increase self-efficacy by visualizing themselves in this
  new role.

*"In teams ask participants to describe or draw or act out the picture of a
successful learner who is a master of the skills about to be taught. Ask the
teams to represent a detailed picture of how the learner would sound, feel
and act."*
—Lawlor & Handley, 1996, page 52

- Consider offering prizes for participants in this activity.

*"Play trivia. Collect trivia related to your content and insert questions when
energy is low and you want to stimulate thought and activity."*
—Backer et al., 1995, page 150

These are only a few of the sorts of activities you can use in your
group. Look at the tools used in teaching individuals (Chapter 7),
and think about how you might apply them for use in pairs, small
groups, or the whole group at once. Consider activities like brainstorm-
ing, acting out scenarios, puzzles, and games. Consider how you might
use props, either as peripherals or within an activity.

Let your content, the skills and behaviors the participants want to
learn, determine which activities to use. Don't be innovative for the
sake of being different. Match the teaching method to the learning objective.

Often during a group session, participants develop relationships with one another. You may observe them getting off the educational topic and sliding into social support. This is not bad.

> *"The provision of social support probably interacts with the teaching intervention to increase the efficacy of patient education."*
> —Rankin & Stallings, 1996, page 341

Just give it a little time (consider it a break), and gently pull the group back to the task.

Did you think about other ways to teach the content of the group on asthma management?

Warm up the Group

In our example of the asthma management group, the first activity was a warm up. In it, the learners, one by one, briefly shared their stories of this asthma attack that brought them to the hospital. This served as an introduction, a shared experience, and a motivator for wanting to prevent future asthma attacks.

> *"Help your students 'get set to learn' the new material. Give them a context for the new material. Help them get motivated to learn it. Tell them what new information is coming."*
> —Ancheta, 1996, page 25

Here's what can happen if your warm-up activity is not related to the topic of the group session.

As a new childbirth educator in a very small, rural community, I attempted to use a get-acquainted activity for the class. The activity involved a paper handout with criteria in boxes. Each class participant was to find someone in the class who matched the criteria in each box. The person to fill the most boxes with names won the activity. However, the activity was not well received by the men in the classes. Most of these men were farmers, ranchers, railroad or oil-field workers, or involved in some kind of blue-collar, outdoor work. Thus, this paper activity seemed frivolous and a waste of time to them. Furthermore, because the community and class size were so small, most of the men knew each other anyway. The next time I taught, I changed the get-acquainted activity to each couple sharing about their baby, plans for delivery, and concerns. This activity is more real-life and is better received by the class participants—especially the men.

—An RN

Here are some other examples of possible warm-up activities.

- Have the learners form pairs and interview each other about their expectations of the group session. Then pairs could meet as fours and compare notes. Then each foursome reports to the large group what their expectations are.
- Make two sets of cards. One set has technical terms or abbreviations relevant to the topic to be discussed. The other set has definitions or descriptions of those terms. Each term has a matching definition card. Keep an answer key for yourself. Keep the matched pairs together. When you're ready to start, count off an even number of cards, one for each learner. Shuffle them, and hand one card to each learner. Have the learners look for the person with the matching cards.

If you have an odd number of learners, the extra person can be in charge of checking matches. When a pair matches up, they call that extra person who will then check the match against the list and tell them whether they are correct or need to keep looking. If you have an even number of learners, you check the pairs.

At the end, each pair announces to the group the term and the definition they represent.

You can adapt this exercise by making the sets to be matched:

- Medication names and purposes
- Symptom and response
- Situation and response
- Question and answer
- Community resource and what services it provides

Contents of both card sets should be brief and clear, and sets should have only one possible correct match (adapted from Lawlor & Handley, 1996).

Plan Breaks

"Provide a period in which learners can be alone or away from the group to reflect, to re-energize, to formulate questions, or simply to organize their thoughts about what they are learning."
—Lawlor & Handley, 1996, page 49

Adults need to alternate action with reflection to link what they just learned to what they already know and integrate it into their lives. You do not lose teaching time when you plan breaks in your group teaching. You give learners the opportunity to process the information presented and prepare them to learn more. Besides, adults are also more likely than children to be taking diuretics and need bathroom breaks.

"To break boredom and preoccupation in the middle of the session, ask one person to roll one die. The number rolled represents the number of minutes the group gets to do absolutely nothing."
—Backer et al., 1995, page 101

Consider playing some relaxing background music before the group begins, at closing, or during breaks. Research indicates Baroque music, with around 60 beats per minute, may help learners get into a state of relaxed awareness and help them learn (Lawlor & Handley, 1996). This includes music by Bach, Vivaldi, Pachelbel, and Albinoni.

In contrast, the music of Mozart and Beethoven makes learning memorable when teaching foreign languages. If used during learning, the "voice of the teacher harmonizes with the music, and the words become memorable because of their unusual intonation and association with the music" (Lawlor & Handley, 1996, page 39).

When you offer breaks, use the time to mingle with the learners and get to know your audience. This will help you better individualize the teaching when the session resumes.

"Use breaks and informal opportunities to create rapport with individual members, particularly anyone who seems to be having difficulties with learning."
—Lawlor & Handley, 1996, page 13

Individualize to the Group Participants

"Help people personalize the material so they feel 'ownership' of it."
—Ancheta, 1996, page 26

Even though the skills and behaviors presented in the group session are determined by a needs assessment, you can further individualize group teaching. After skills are learned by participants, ask them the following:

• How would you apply this at home?
• How would you do this when you travel?

You can ask other questions that would help them make the information personally meaningful.

Here's an example of a group leader who followed her subconscious perceptions to individualize teaching to the specific participants.

I was a newcomer to a small, remote community, and a Public Health Nurse asked me to develop and teach a series of childbirth preparation classes. I had little knowledge about this rural community, except what my husband told me about his childhood and growing up there. By the time I taught my first class series, I still knew very few people. I had no personal knowledge about any of the five couples in my first series.

As part of the first class, I taught about ways to promote a healthy pregnancy. Part of the discussion involved things to avoid during pregnancy, such as smoking, alcohol, and illicit drugs. I had planned to mention these only briefly. However, as I taught the class, I found myself going into great detail about the effect of cocaine on a fetus and the dangers of cocaine use during pregnancy (not even in my notes for the class). Even during the lecture I found myself wondering why I was diverting from my notes to dwell on this information. After the class, I chastised myself mentally for focusing on information that wasn't even relevant for such a rural community. (I had moved there from a metropolitan community where such information might have been more relevant—or so I thought.)

Only later did I find out that, in fact, cocaine use truly was a problem for three of the five couples in that class. Two of the fathers were arrested, on separate occasions, for drug distribution and use 2 months after the class. One year later I found out that one of the mothers in the class (a local nurse) had been addicted to cocaine and received rehab in the year prior to her pregnancy. Thus, perhaps the information about cocaine use during pregnancy was the most important thing I taught to that particular class. I have never since felt the need to focus on that issue.

In retrospect, I still don't know why I diverted from my lesson plan to cover that information so specifically. The only visual cue I had was that the two fathers who later were arrested were young, appeared disinterested, wore "shades" even though it was dark outside, and dressed in a way that perhaps reminded me of the drug culture I had seen in the city. (They, in fact, had recently moved to this community from metropolitan areas.) I am, however, glad I let myself teach what seemed natural, though wrong, at the time. As patient educators we need to give ourselves the freedom to go with our hunches at times—even if it means diverting from our lesson plans.

—An RN

This example illustrates two important points. First, even logical assumptions can be incorrect. Illegal drugs are found in big cities, not small, remote, rural communities. Nurses know better than to use drugs. These assumptions were wrong in this case.

The second point is the value of experience and expertise in nursing. As nurses gain experience, they gain knowledge and skill. Much of that knowledge is not explicitly discussed or documented, but it is internalized. When an experienced nurse has a hunch or a feeling, it may come from the subconscious noticing a pattern that has been experienced before. This phenomenon has been discussed at length in Benner (1984). She describes the development of a novice nurse to advanced beginner to competent to proficient and finally, to an expert nurse:

> "The expert nurse perceives the situation as a whole, uses past concrete situations as paradigms, and moves to the accurate region of the problem without wasteful consideration of a large number of irrelevant opinions. In contrast, the competent or proficient nurse in a novel situation must rely on conscious, deliberate, analytic problem solving of an elemental nature."
>
> —Benner, 1984, page 3

The nurse who taught this class was an expert who saw the situation as a whole.

Example of a Creative Approach to Teaching

You may not really understand this process until you try it yourself, but here are examples of two different sorts of groups in action.

In this first group teaching, the focus was teaching skills, but it also provided a great deal of spontaneous support between learners. Lamp (1992) describes how one group of nurses approached teaching new parents what to expect in the first few weeks after delivery. In this creative approach, the group leader stimulated conversation and helped learners teach one another.

One nurse, the leader, dressed in a costume as Fredricka, a new mom taken to the extreme. The costume included prompters for the nurse to discuss common postpartum concerns. For example, she wore a robe, because new moms are never dressed. She had dark circles under her eyes for the fatigue and postpartum blues. A telephone was stuck to her shoulder, because the telephone always rings. There were birth control devices inside the robe, because breast-feeding does not protect from pregnancy.

Fredricka appeared in a group of new parents gathered for a bath demonstration. She introduced herself to the new parents as a patient who was discharged the previous week and described various complaints that developed because she was not adequately prepared for this postpartum period. Occasionally Fredricka visited a new mom alone.

"One-on-one presentations have been effective, but it is in the group forum that interaction between parents is generated. Multipara often share their previous experiences, which serve to validate Fredricka's complaints. But more importantly, the mothers with experience share solutions they found helpful. Several mothers remembered the telephone ringing frequently as a common block to their rest time and stated how helpful it was to use an answering machine."

—Lamp, 1992, page 85

Learners who had previous experience with childbirth supported the other group members and shared solutions. Formal evaluations confirmed that this creative technique was an effective teaching tool, stimulating interaction and enhancing retention of information. One week after the presentation, all the learners that were called remembered Fredricka and were able to mention at least two concerns she predicted that they experienced.

Another Example of a Way to Teach Groups

Sometimes there is a good deal of content that learners need before they can practice skills. In these cases, the instructor needs to present information before the learners can actively participate. Here's an example of how such a group teaching, combining lecture with practice, might work.

As part of a hospital outreach education program, I co-taught a series of classes entitled, "Childhood Emergency Workshops." Participants attended a series of classes that involved use of slides, lecture, and a handbook about common childhood accidents and appropriate home care and infant/child CPR.

Following the lecture, participants were divided into groups of three around infant or child mannequins and given a list of written scenarios designed to reinforce application of the lecture and handbook material. One participant was designated as the responder, one designated the scenario reader, and one designated the observer. The observer was to assess the rescuer's response without comment during the response. The rescuer was to talk through and demonstrate their response to the situation.

At the end of the response, the group discussed and identified other response alternatives. Evaluations for this teaching format were consistently positive. People had fun participating in this activity. It seemed to be a very effective means of promoting learning about childhood safety and CPR.

—An RN

A learning task doesn't have to be complicated or super-creative to be good. Simple, true-to-life scenarios that give the learners practical experience are quite effective.

Did They Learn Anything?

"Check for understanding."
—Ancheta, 1996, page 26

Activities that engage everyone in the group should help you evaluate understanding throughout the group session or at least identify learners who are having difficulty keeping up.

Sometimes the most important learning in a group is not a skill, but an attitude and increased self-efficacy. This is still important learning. Do not underestimate its value.

"Group teaching sessions lessen the feelings of alienation and being different that many people experience with acute and chronic conditions. Patients frequently remark after attending a group teaching that it was helpful to hear that others share the same problems and feelings."
—Rankin & Stallings, 1996, page 326

True evaluation of learning should be done by members of the health care team who follow up with the learners. They will be able to evaluate learning, reinforce key information, and document to share progress with others on the health care team.

Don't Stop There

"Help students transfer their new knowledge to their future . . . experiences."
—Ancheta, 1996, page 26

Think about ways the material learned in your group is repeated, reinforced, and used. Involve all the members of the health care team in this process. Following are possible methods:

- The written teaching materials you provide should include activities your learners can engage in on their own, such as explaining to a family member what was learned.
- Give each learner an opportunity to roll a die.

"The number on the die that is rolled represents the number of minutes the participant commits to taking as a health break back on the job."
—Backer et al., 1995, page 113

- Have learners write on a piece of paper or postcard a goal they want to accomplish related to the group's topic. Have them address these to themselves and give them to you, the group leader. After an appropriate time (weeks to months), send these goals back to the learners with an encouraging comment.
- Videos or posters used in the session should be repeated in clinic waiting rooms or other places learners will go to reinforce the message.
- Follow up with telephone calls to all who participated in the group to find out how they have applied the information they learned and if any questions have come up.
- Send follow up postcards or e-mails to learners with reminders of goals and to encourage new behaviors.
- Offer a review of the content in another format on a website. Consider an on-line multiple-choice or true-false quiz that provides immediate feedback.
- Provide a list of community resources for independent follow-up.

Give the participants in your group handouts: a written summary of the skills and behaviors covered and resources for additional learning. This will help them review and continue learning, as needed.

Don't stop there. There are more things you can do to help your learners integrate this new information and apply it in their lives.

"Suggest further practice to help them store what they learned in long-term memory."
—Ancheta, 1996, page 27

The written materials you send home with your learners should include homework assignments. For example, the participants in the asthma class may be given a chart to document the results of their peak flow meter readings. Ask them to share this chart with their primary care physicians at the next office visit. (Peak flow meters are one of the methods to help prevent future asthma attacks.)

"Provide an application assignment immediately following the program."
—Bader & Bloom, 1994, page 67

You're not alone. Access the rest of the health care team to repeat and reinforce the group's message. If the learner is a patient in the hospital, communicate with that learner's nurse what was taught and what needs to be practiced. If the learner is not a hospital patient, communicate with the primary care provider, the home health nurse, or the school nurse what was taught and what needs to be practiced.

"By using this repetitive process, patients' understanding of key points of therapy have improved."
—Ramsdell & Annisrove, 1996

Communicate your plan for follow through with other members of the health care team. Give them the tools to monitor and measure the progress. Give them lists of the key content taught and suggestions on how they might evaluate learning and continue the process.

"Plan time for follow-through practice and feedback activities to reinforce new or changed behaviors."
—Bader & Bloom, 1994, page 98

Evaluate the Group

"Complete a thorough course evaluation."
—Bader & Bloom, 1994, page 104

Ask your learners for written, anonymous feedback from the participants on satisfaction with the group session. You can also ask, "What is the most important thing you learned in this session?" "What was the least important information covered in this session?" Include questions that will help you determine if the group achieved its intended purposes.

Responses to these questions will help you plan future sessions.

Collect similar data from the learners and health care providers who are providing follow-up reinforcement and evaluation of learning.

Compile data from the group and follow-up evaluations:

- Did the group teaching change anything?
- What are the outcomes? (Evaluate against your objectives in the "for what" planning step.)
- Was the amount of change achieved worth the effort?
- Calculate the level of activity: number of learners, hours of group teaching done, costs.
- Calculate the costs compared to outcomes based on your "for what" objectives, such as decrease in number of admissions for asthma, reduced length of stay, increased independence in self-care, decreased use of pain medication.

The financial benefit from the patient education programs may not be cost savings (money you could put in the bank and save), but cost avoidance (money not spent). Both are valuable, but be clear when you report the results (Haggard, 1989).

If the group did not show an improvement in outcome or a financial benefit, what can you change to improve the intervention?

Several problems may occur:

- Unclear objectives
- Unrealistic objectives
- Inappropriate tasks
- Unclear tasks
- Tasks that are too difficult
- Tasks that did not fit in time allowed

Look at the problems honestly, and with adjustments, these problems can readily be repaired.

Groups can reach adult learners in effective ways that one-on-one teaching by a nurse cannot. Teaching groups takes time and preparation but is well worth the effort when you respect your learners as adults and actively involve them in the learning process.

If you want to learn more:

(1996). Assessing your target population to build the most effective programs. *Patient Education Management, 3*(3), 25–28.

(1998). Teach through a variety of education methods. *Patient Education Management, May,* 65.

Ancheta, R. (1996). How to teach a how-to: Helping your clients learn for themselves. *Childbirth Instructor Magazine, 4,* 24–27.

Backer, L., Deck, M., & McCallum, D. (1995). *The presenter's survival kit: It's a jungle out there!* St. Louis, MO: Mosby Year-Book, Inc.

Bader, G.E., & Bloom, A.E. (1994). *Make your training results last: A practical guide to successful training follow-through.* Irvine, CA: Richard Chang Associates.

Benner, P. (1984). *From novice to expert: Excellence and power in clinical nursing practice.* Menlo Park, CA: Addison-Wesley.

Berk, R.A. (1998). *Professors are from Mars, students are from Snickers: How to write and deliver humor in the classroom and in presentations.* Madison, WI: Mendota Press.

Charney, C., & Conway, K. (1998). *The trainer's tool kit.* New York: AMACOM, American Management Association.

Droz, M., & Ellis, L. (1996). *Laughing while learning: Using humor in the classroom.* Longmont, CO: Sopris West.

Haggard, A. (1989). *Handbook of patient education.* Rockville, MD: Aspen Publishers.

Hill, D.J. (1988). *Humor in the classroom: A handbook for teachers (and other entertainers!).* Springfield, IL: Charles C. Thomas.

Hopkins, K.R. (1997). Choosing the right presentation platform. *AV Video and Multimedia Producer, October,* 109.

Lamp, J.M. (1992). Humor in postpartum education: Depicting a new mother's worst nightmare. *The American Journal of Maternal/Child Nursing, 17*(March/April), 83–85.

Lawlor, M., & Handley, P. (1996). *The creative trainer: Holistic facilitation skills for accelerated learning.* London: McGraw-Hill.

Loomans, D., & Kolberg, K.J. (1993). *The laughing classroom: Everyone's guide to teaching with humor and play.* Tiburon, CA: H.J. Kramer.

Lorig, K. (1996). *Patient education: A practical approach.* Thousand Oaks, CA: Sage Publications.

Morgan, D.L., & Krueger, R.A. (Eds.). (1998). *The focus group kit.* Thousand Oaks, CA: Sage Publications.

Nasmith, L., & Daigle, N. (1996). Small-group teaching in patient education. *Medical Teacher, 18*(3), 209–211. [On-line]. Available: EBSCO.

Ramsdell, R., & Annisrove, C. (1996). Patient education: A continuing repetitive process. *ANNA Journal, 23*(2), 217–221. [On-line]. Available: EBSCO.

Rankin, S.H., & Stallings, K.D. (1996). *Patient education: Issues, principles, practices* (3rd ed.). Philadelphia: Lippincott-Raven.

Senge, P.M., Kleiner, A., Roberts, C., Ross, R.B., & Smith, B.J. (1994). *The fifth discipline fieldbook: Strategies and tools for building a learning organization.* New York: Currency.

Theis, S.L., & Johnson, J.H. (1995). Strategies for teaching patients: A meta-analysis. *Clinical Nurse Specialist, 9*(2), 100–104.

Vella, J. (1994). *Learning to listen, learning to teach: The power of dialogue in educating adults.* San Francisco: Jossey-Bass.

Yingling, L., & Trocino, L. (1997). Strategies to integrate patient and family education into patient care redesign. *AACN Clinical Issues, 8*(2), 246–252.

Frequently Asked
Questions

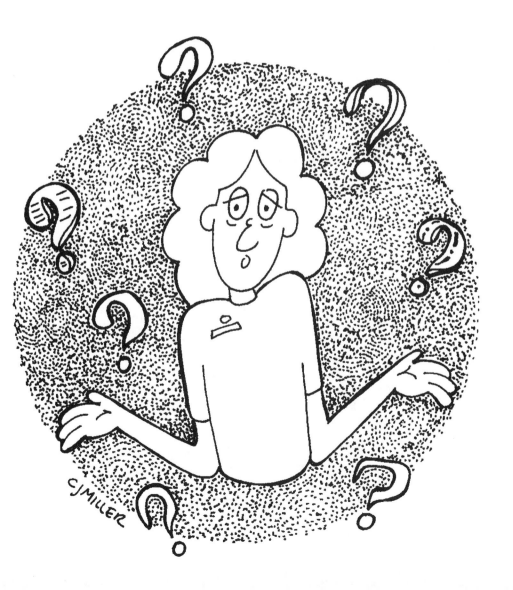

T here are times when I feel like I need to scream because I can't accomplish eveything I am asked to do."
—Rita Becchetti, MHS, RNC, FHCE (1998, *Patient Education Management*, p. 3)

"With all that's going on, how can I find the time to teach?"
—an RN

....

Some questions come up over and over again. Perhaps yours are in this collection.

"How do I get staff to document their teaching?"

An extensive literature review reveals no answer to this question. However, I can offer an observation and hope some nurse researcher is inspired to test my hypothesis.

I believe this universal problem of getting staff to document their teaching is the result of our unwillingness to look at this question honestly. The answer is clear, but we ignore it, because it is a painful reality.

Patient and family education is not documented because we are ambivalent about it.

This is the rationale:

- If we agreed documentation of patient and family education was a professional obligation, we would hold one another accountable for it. Nurses would confront their colleagues when it was not done. Nurse managers would weigh it seriously when doing performance evaluations. The problem would disappear overnight.
- If we agreed documentation of patient and family education was not necessary, we would form a consensus, produce studies that substantiated our view, and inform the Joint Commission on the Accreditation of Healthcare Organizations (JCAHO) that their requirements are outdated and inappropriate.
- We do neither. We respond to this issue with feelings instead of rational problem solving.
  - Nurses feel it's more important to do teaching than write about it.
  - Nursing management and administration also feel it's more important to do teaching than write about it.
  - As pressure increases to cut staffing, we do not calculate in and advocate for enough nursing time to complete professional nursing activities, such as documentation. Nurse managers and administrators feel guilty because

they have been unable to staff adequately to support quality care.

- Nurses work within their limits and do as much teaching as possible in the time available. However, they feel angry that their professional nursing care is not supported adequately by management and administration, and they rebel. They prioritize, and documentation of patient and family education falls to the bottom of the list.
- Consequently, staff nurses and nurse managers have come to a tacit agreement. Staff members do not hold management and administration accountable for supporting professional practice fully. Management and administration do not hold staff accountable for documentation of patient and family education.

When we prepare for a JCAHO review, we realize we fall short on documentation, so nurse managers ask, "How do I get staff to document their teaching?" Staff and management then play a little need-to-document-teaching game until the crisis passes. The real issue is not addressed.

We have trouble holding other people accountable for things we're not so invested in ourselves. We will find the answer to this question when we honestly face our ambivalence.

"Documentation is a cross to bear!"

—An RN

To be fair, there are other possible explanations for nurses not documenting their teaching. Some believe nurses don't document because they don't know how to teach and don't want anyone to find out.

"I think the problem is nurses focus on themselves, not on the patient. They feel it looks bad if they don't know the answers to questions. They feel it looks bad if they don't teach everything, so they don't document at all, so no one will know."

—An RN

"Part of this reluctance, I believe, is because they don't know the 'language of education' and need to learn how to describe patient response to teaching . . . . Also, they don't value it in quite the same way as other components of care, unless they are held accountable by managers and managers value patient teaching. They won't admit that and they say education is extremely important, but when push comes to shove, it's education that doesn't get done when they are strapped. Part of that is what is valued and expected by the leadership, and where they put their priorities."

—An RN

These nurses think teaching isn't documented because nurses lack skills and don't think teaching is important. They don't think highly of teaching; they don't value it. Their proposed solutions are reaching nurses effectively to help them appreciate the usefulness of teaching:

"Teaching is episodic. We need to show the effects of this on the patient. Maybe we need to interview a patient and family on video to show nurses how this impacts care. Nurses need teaching skills, passion for teaching, and time."

—An RN

Perhaps instructors in nursing schools don't communicate to their students that patient teaching is a professional activity. We need to teach nurses the skills they need to teach well and not be afraid to document:

"They learn how to describe an infiltrated IV in their charting because they have been taught that, and they need to be taught how to describe the educational process."

—An RN

A third viewpoint came out of a meeting of one hospital's Patient and Family Education Committee. Attendees of that meeting proposed that formal teaching is documented, but informal teaching is either not recognized as teaching or not recognized as significant enough to document.

If this is the true reason nurses don't document their teaching, then perhaps nursing schools emphasize formal teaching skills but not informal teaching skills. Perhaps informal teaching skills are more sophisticated than formal, because it takes experience to get comfortable doing tasks and listening to the learner simultaneously. Perhaps informal teaching skills should be introduced in undergraduate nursing programs but taught in graduate school.

In any case, this view of the problem indicates we need to teach nurses that informal teaching is still patient and family education. When nurses learn how to recognize that they are teaching within conversations, it could correct the documentation problem.

What's your theory? Why don't nurses, and most other health care providers, document their teaching?

"How do I assess someone's learning style quickly?"

To assess someone's learning style quickly, ask him or her, "Think back to the last time you wanted to learn something. How did you go about it?"

"How do I evaluate the effectiveness of teaching quickly?"

To evaluate effectiveness of teaching quickly, ask the learner to show you or repeat the information in his or her own words.

"Ask the patient to repeat some of what you've explained. Avoid asking questions that require a Yes or No answer."
—Platt, Tippy, Dennis, & Turk, 1994

"How do I assess for learning readiness, and if they are not ready, how do I help them become ready to learn? What else can I do?"

"All we have to do is listen—really listen."
—Dass & Gorman, 1985, page 69

The learner is ready for information at teachable moments. The learner makes a provocative statement ("I'll never remember to take all these pills") or asks a question ("What if the pain comes back?"). The better you learn to recognize teachable moments, the more you will realize learners are often ready to learn. It just may not be the same stuff you want to teach. Present information in the order determined by their needs. Then ask questions to get them to realize they'll also need the information you want to teach.

For example, a family member may express feeling guilty, because he or she didn't recognize the signs of a stroke and did not act quickly to help the patient. In response, you can provide emotional support and suggest a number of things the learner can do to help the patient in the future. List a few, like feeding and ambulation, and say you will teach the learner how to do these when he or she is ready.

Patients and family members who are not ready to learn are preoccupied with other issues. Have you and the other members of the health care team addressed those distracting issues?

You can help patients and family members get ready to learn by coaching them. Help them identify their needs for information. Patients and families need information for the following reasons:

- To make informed decisions
- To develop basic self-care skills to survive
- To recognize problems and know what to do in response
- To get questions answered and find resources for answers

Ask the learner to explain his or her understanding of the treatment options. Correct misperceptions, and fill in missing information.

Ask the learner how he or she will handle certain self-care needs, like hygiene, cooking, or getting the prescription medicine.

Offer a scenario that could occur at home, and ask how the learner will manage the situation. For example, what would the learner do if in 3 days, the surgical site became red, hard, and painful?

"How do I involve the patient and family in their own learning?"

You can involve the patient and family in their own learning by having conversations. Find out what they know, what they need to know, and what they want to know. Find out what worries them and what bothers them. Set mutual goals.

When you teach, don't lecture. Teach with methods that use active involvement. Refer learners to resources they can access on their own, when ready.

"Patients are informed about access to additional resources in the community."

—JCAHO, 1998, page 106

"How do I come up with answers to questions that I, as a nurse, cannot answer?"

If you, as a nurse, cannot answer a learner's question because it is in a physician's scope of practice (such as, "how long do I have to live?") and not yours, then do the following:

- Tell the learner that is a very good question, but he or she needs to ask the physician.
- Give the learner a pencil and paper to write down the question so he or she doesn't forget.
- If there is some urgency to the question, offer to call the physician for the learner.

If you, as a nurse, cannot answer a learner's question because it is out of your scope of practice but within that of a clergy person's, social worker's, or any other member of the health care team's scope of practice, offer to call the team member for the learner, or give the learner the name and telephone number to call. You can also offer the paper and pencil so the question isn't forgotten.

If you don't know the answer the question, but it is within your scope of practice, then do the following:

- Tell the learner you don't know the answer, but will find out and get back to him or her.
- Find out.
- Get back to him or her.

If you don't know the answer and neither will anyone else (such as, "will I lose my leg?"), tell the learner no one on the health care team can predict the future, and invite the learner to discuss his or her fears, worries, or feelings.

Always respond to the question in some helpful way. Do not ignore or make light of a learner's concerns.

"How do I know if I'm overloading the patient with too much information?"

Don't lecture. Pay attention to the response you're getting. Is the learner continuing to interact? Is the learner not responding very well? Is your learner yawning, staring into space, fidgeting, or ignoring you? You may be talking too much or too long. You may be offering more detail than the learner wants. If you teach in two-way conversation, you are less likely to overload the learner. You will hear or see the learner telling you it's time to stop.

Evaluate understanding frequently enough to know if your learner is keeping up with you. This will also help you determine when it's time to stop.

Teachable moments are opportunities for teaching, when the learner is ready. Teachable moments may only last for moments and be gone once the question is answered. That's fine. There will be another moment. Just pay attention so you can take advantage of it when it arrives.

"What is the best tool for providing education for patients that do not speak English?"

The best tool for providing education to patients that do not speak English is a language interpreter.

If you do not have access to professional interpreters, ask your organization to subscribe to a telephone translation service, such as the AT&T Language Line. With this, you can access professional interpreters for almost any language from any telephone.

It is also good to have written materials in the learner's language for backup if the learner or family members can read. Make sure the learner has appropriate resources for follow-up.

"We use interpreters when a patient doesn't speak English. Often, patients don't want to impose and they tell us not to bother getting an interpreter. But what if they have questions later?"

Look at your behavior. If your patients often tell you not to bother, your feelings may be showing. Are you frustrated by this extra step in the teaching process? Do you resent having to use interpreters? Does your manager imply your department is spending too much money on interpretation, so you're uncomfortable using interpreters?

Learners' refusal of an interpreter may not mean they do not want teaching or have no questions. They may just see your hesitation and are trying to make your job easier.

Do your job. Get an interpreter. Teach.

"Do you think that an educator should know the beliefs and practices of a particular ethnic group to do education appropriately?"

No. To do education appropriately, the educator should know the beliefs and practices of the specific learner.

Even if you know the beliefs and practices of a particular ethnic group, unless you assess your learner directly, you will not know where your learner is right now. When cultures mix, as they do in the United States, they mix dynamically and on a continuum. Learners are in a mixed culture, which may be anywhere on the continuum, such as 20%/80%, 40%/60%, or 90%/10%. They may speak their native language at home but English when they're out. They may see both traditional healers and allopathic health care providers (that is, you). This bicultural state can, at times, cause internal stress and conflict. The two cultures may have opposing viewpoints, such as emphasis on independence in the United States and, in their native culture, on interdependence of family members. This interplay between two cultures is dynamic, not static. Internal and external pressures create changes.

In addition, there is a danger that if you focus on learning about a culture, you will stereotype your learners. This can interfere with development of a therapeutic relationship. Instead, if you focus on understanding the specific learner, you will hone right in on the issues you need to consider when individualizing teaching.

"All we have to do is listen—really listen."
                                    —Dass & Gorman, 1985, page 69

If you stay aware when you teach enough people from the same ethnic community, you will, in time, understand their range of beliefs and practices. Then you may develop specific questions about the culture, and you may turn to literature and your resources in that community to get answers. As you gain understanding, you will learn to assess a specific learner faster and more accurately. This process is going on in the background, as part of your professional growth and development. When you are teaching, your focus is listening to the specific learner and understanding his or her story.

"I am often confused on how much information about side effects of medications to give patients so not to confuse them but at least keep them informed. Do you have any tips?"

How do you teach enough but not too much? Use conversation, interaction, and assessment.

For example, prepare a tool for teaching about side effects. Print a double-spaced list of common side effects of medications in general, glue the sheet onto cardboard, and cut to make a little card for each side effect. Put the cards into a box. Keep the box in the medication room.

When it's time to teach, give your learner the box, and ask him or her to go through the cards and pull out all the possible side effects of his or her medication. Return in a while, and review the learner's work. Make sure your learner pulled out all the significant side effects. If not, add those that were missing, and explain. Then ask your learner how he or she will respond if those side effects occur. Which can be self-treated? Which need medical follow-up? Which are emergencies?

> *"Patients are educated about the safe and effective use of medication, according to law and their needs."*
> —JCAHO, 1998, page 106

> *"Patients are educated about potential drug-food interactions, and provided counseling on nutrition and modified diets."*
> —JCAHO, 1998, page 106

By involving the learner, you will know if he or she remembers every little side effect or only a few big ones. Because the learner needs to recognize problems and know what to do in response, make sure the significant side effects are discussed. Because your learner needs to give informed consent, make sure he or she understands the purpose of the medication and the risks involved. Tailor your teaching to the learner's focus.

"How do we get physicians to participate in our patient education efforts? They do not like it when we tell patients too much."

This question on multidisciplinary team building suggests you want to interact with other disciplines. However, it also sounds like you started without them. You want physicians to participate in your patient education efforts. That may be part of your problem; an interdisciplinary approach would be more collaborative.

Instead of starting patient education efforts and inviting physicians to participate, meet with the whole health care team, and develop the patient education efforts together. If they're part of the process, they'll participate. Discuss with them the benefits of educating patients and families.

> *"The better the patient understands the medical situation, the better the treatment compliance and follow-up cooperation will be. The synchronization of patient, family and physician fosters an atmosphere of continuing trust which can contribute to greater satisfaction for both the patient and physician, while improving quality of life."*
> —Oberst, page 1

Now the second part of your question: Physicians do not like it when you tell patients too much. If any members of the health care team do not want something taught, find out what part of the goals of patient and family education they do not want the learner to meet.

Do they not want the learner to make informed decisions?
Do they not want the learner to develop basic self-care skills?
Do they not want the learner to learn to recognize problems and know what to do in response?
Do they not want the learner to have answers to questions?

If the health care provider says yes to one of the above questions, show that person the Patient's Bill of Rights. Patients have a right to the information defined in the goals.

Sometimes a physician may want specific information shared only after test results are in or a specialist is consulted. This is not a concern about telling patients too much but too soon. It may make sense not to discuss treatment options until the diagnosis is clear. If the learner is asking questions, it is not too soon to discuss the topic, but present information as tentative. If the learner is not asking questions about this topic and the physician wants you to wait, why do you want to teach it now?

If you still disagree about what to teach, talk to the physician. You don't need a doctor's order to do patient and family education, but you do need to nourish good relationships between team members to have an effective health care team. Ask what his or her concerns are. What could happen if the learner got "too much" information? Is the learner asking for this information? Could the learner also get this information from a library, the internet, or a second opinion? Is it not best to respond to the learner's needs and control the accuracy of the information the learner gets?

What is best for the patient?

"It may be necessary to have the patient himself request patient teaching and put pressure on the doctor to provide it."
—Rankin & Stallings, 1996, page 308

"Why don't we have nursing assistants do some teaching? They could teach simple things, like cough, turn, and deep breathe."

"Patient teaching requires the depth of information that only nurses have. It is one of the truly independent functions of nursing practice that springs from our ability to synthesize our broad base of knowledge; its loss would be devastating to the profession."
—Freda, 1997, page 330

Theoretically, a nursing assistant could teach a patient to cough, turn, and deep breathe, but would he or she know why this is done? If asked, would he or she be able to explain it to the patient?

Patient and family education should be multidisciplinary. On the other hand, the most accurate and thorough teaching will be done by health care professionals who know the subject and resources for additional information.

If you want health care team members who are not professionally trained to augment teaching, check their scope of practice and job descriptions. Then check yours. Do not allow anyone to practice nursing or medicine without a license.

Use your nursing assistants well, and don't abdicate your responsibility to teach. Nursing assistants can best support patient and family education in the following ways:

- Identifying teachable moments
- Alerting an appropriate professional health care team member (nurse, nutritionist, physician) to the nature of the teachable moment
- Promoting an environment that supports patient and family education, such as maintaining and stocking teaching tools

"How do we get the organization's top leadership to see the value of patient education (other than when a JCAHO visit is upcoming) and provide the necessary financial resources?"

Your organization's top leadership probably knows the value of patient and family education. One of the highest correlates with patient satisfaction is education.

On the other hand, top leadership may not understand what is taught and when and how it is taught. They may not understand that to be most cost-effective, we need to take advantage of teachable moments. This means we need to maintain an environment that supports readiness to teach and flexibility of professionals' time to be able to take advantage when opportunities arise. If the organization is too tightly staffed with no room for spontaneity, teaching opportunities will be missed. Teaching done at the wrong times will be more time consuming and less effective.

Your top leadership may not know that people provide most of their own health care through maintenance activities and self-treatments. It is possible your top leadership does not know that teaching is one of the biggest responsibilities of health care providers to ensure safe and effective self-care.

To help top leadership value patient and family education, educate them year round about its importance in terms that are meaningful to them. Use their criteria for significance. Keep top leadership informed of the latest research findings. For example, cite studies that correlate excellence in patient and family education with cost effectiveness, patient satisfaction, and low readmissions.

Suggest they use patient and family education as a tool for promotion of the organization, a customer service. It is a low-tech, high-touch balance to the cold, impersonal side of health care. It is a way to reach out into the community.

If that doesn't work, remind them JCAHO says,

> *"The hospital identifies and provides the educational resources required to achieve its educational objectives."*
>
> —JCAHO, 1998, page 10

Remind them it's their responsibility.

"How do we have nurses do patient education on the units and not dump on the nurse educator?"

"How does a nurse educator ensure core-competency for staff nurses to do patient teaching?"

"How do we train staff to be patient educators?"

Train staff to be patient educators the same way you train them in other skills. Identify their learning needs, and teach those skills.

> *"One- or 2-day workshops offered to all health professionals are an effective means of imparting teaching and learning principles and securing interest in patient education."*
>
> —Rankin & Stallings, 1996, page 302

If you are looking for structure for a program to teach health professionals how to teach, see Barber, Belton, and Simpson's *Teach to Teach: Teach Staff to Plan and Implement Effective Patient Education* (1993). It includes content to present, pages to make into overhead transparencies, and bibliographies.

> *"Many nurses remark that they do not know what to teach. Although we believe that most nurses do have the pertinent information stored away, we feel that anxiety can be decreased by helping the staff to organize and review the information that patients need."*
>
> —Rankin & Stallings, 1996, page 302

Another effective tool in teaching patient and family education is the use of exemplars. Exemplars are anecdotes, examples of excellence in our care of patients and families. Several are included in this book and in Benner's *From Novice to Expert* (1984). Exemplars are useful because they help us understand nursing activities that are interpersonal skills, not delegable tasks. They put nursing care in context.

Exemplars may be expressed in writing, audiotape, or videotape. You can use exemplars in the following ways:

- By sharing them in groups
- By making them available to colleagues in a notebook or display
- By publishing them in internal publications
- To teach skills to preceptors, orientees, and students
- In the performance evaluation or clinical ladder process

See Box 12-1 for details on how to create exemplars.

"The patient only needs one injection a day. When I teach, should I make the patient do it that day, or have him practice that first day then watch him do it the next day?"

Every learner is different. Remember the top time-saving teaching tips from Chapter 2. Two of the tips answer this question:

- Partner with the learner to establish learning objectives.
- Individualize your teaching.

Present the two options to the patient, and ask which he or she prefers.

"How do we really show evidence of an interdisciplinary approach to patient education?"

If you're having trouble showing evidence, make sure you do have an interdisciplinary approach to patient education. If you do talk to one another about the progress and outcomes of patient and family education, then demonstrate it.

You can really show evidence of an interdisciplinary approach to patient education through documentation:

- Notes from multidisciplinary care conferences, signed by the team members who participated
- Documentation on education records by representatives of all disciplines
- Evidence in progress notes

BOX 12-1   Share Your Success With Exemplars

If we don't make an effort to notice and celebrate our successes, we may never notice them at all. Exemplars are ways to document examples of excellence in our care of patients and families.   .

They are useful:

- They increase our awareness of what we do and how we do it.
- They are powerful ways to communicate the impact we have on the lives of our patients and families.
- They increase our ability to define our professional practice.

Here's how to write an exemplar:

1. Notice when you feel like you've made an impact in the life of a patient or family. Write notes about it right away, before you forget.
2. When you have a moment, read your notes, and let them trigger your memory of the experience. Think about the details. Then, as if you were telling a friend, write, audiotape, or videotape the story. To protect confidentiality, do not use real names. Include the following:
   - What happened
   - What people said, with quotes if possible
   - What you thought at the time; what you were trying to accomplish
   - What you learned
   - Why you remembered this experience; what was important
3. Review your exemplar. Did you leave anything out? How could you make the story clearer? Rework it if necessary.
4. If you wrote the exemplar rather than recorded it, check for grammer, punctuation, and spelling.
5. Share your exemplar with others. Listen to their exemplars.
6. Collect your exemplars over time, and watch your professional practice grow.

For samples of exemplars, see Benner, P. (1984). *From novice to expert: Excellence and power in clinical nursing practice.* Menlo Park, CA: Addison-Wesley.

"When a child is terminal and will pass on soon, what and how do you teach the parents?"

Individualize teaching to the needs of the learner. What do they want to know? What are their concerns? What do they need to know to make informed decisions? What skills do they need to care for their child through this transition? What do they know about grief and how it feels to lose a child? They may feel like they are going crazy and not understand the power of the grief. Conflicts may arise within the family. Listen to them. They may need anticipatory guidance and emotional support.

"We don't teach patients that are dying, right?"
Let's think this one through. Why do we teach?

We teach to meet the goals of patient and family education. Do dying patients have the same goals? Do they still need to make informed decisions? Do they still need to take care of themselves, as their physical condition deteriorates? Do they still need to recognize problems and know what to do in response? Do they still have questions?

The need for information does not disappear when a person is proclaimed terminal. It just changes. The content of what we teach is individualized to the learner's needs. When a patient has 6 months or less to live, he or she may have a greater need for information about pain management and may need anticipatory guidance about the dying process.

"He not busy being born is busy dying."
                                        —Dylan, 1995, page 176

Do patient's rights end when there is no hope for cure, or do we provide care throughout the lifespan?

Professional nurses do teach patients who are dying. It's the compassionate thing to do.

"I work in a nursing home. I don't have to do any teaching, do I?"
Just because a patient cannot care for himself or herself, does that mean he or she cannot or should not participate? Does the patient still need to make informed decisions? Does the patient still need to recognize problems and know what to do in response? Does the patient still have questions? If the patient can hear you, explain what you are doing and why. Do this even if you are not able to evaluate understanding. An aware patient who knows his or her medications can help prevent mistakes.

If the patient is in a coma or is mentally incompetent, would you avoid teaching the family members? Teach them how to help with the patient's hygiene, or feeding, or exercise. It will help them feel involved and give them an opportunity to show they care. This is especially important if the patient cannot recognize them or respond.

Does everyone who checks in to your nursing home die there, or occasionally does someone return home? Certainly, anyone who is discharged, or a family member, needs to understand self-care and how to recognize problems and what to do in response.

"How can you do teaching if the family is not there?"

Did this ever happen to you? You know your patient cannot care for himself or herself and will need complex home care. You're ready to start teaching, but the family members and significant others never come into the hospital to be taught!

They may not come in because they have children to care for, a great distance to travel (a subjective factor, but can be a real barrier), transportation problems, jobs or responsibilities that take up their time, or a combination of these. Maybe they can't agree on who will care for your patient. You may never know why they don't come in.

Are you frustrated?

Here are a few tips on effectively teaching the absent care provider:

- Do the family members know you expect them to be part of the patient's health care team? Do they know that part of the treatment includes teaching them how to care for the patient at home? How do you know they know?
- Call the significant other or family members. What are their expectations of hospitalization and home care? What are their concerns? Are there other care providers involved? Is the person you're trying to meet with the right person to teach?
- Think mutuality. Identify shared goals, and use those goals to plan your teaching.
- When your teaching plan is established, communicate it to everyone on the health care team. Include details. Make sure your documentation is clear enough so everyone on the team can participate.
- Collaborate. Involve all the disciplines on the health care team in the teaching plan. Does the family member call the attending physician for medical updates? Does the social worker or case manager contact the family? Perhaps a nurse on another shift sees the family members more often than you do and needs to take primary teaching responsibility. Identify who is responsible for what.
- Take advantage of even brief teachable moments. Assess understanding, teach, or evaluate some bit of knowledge every time you walk into the room.
- If teachable moments are few and far between, everyone on the health care team needs to be primed to take advantage of them. Clear verbal communications and documentation are essential.
- Do you need an interpreter to facilitate communication? Perhaps the family members speak English but would learn better in their native language.
- Does the family have transportation problems? Consult social services or the member of your health care team who knows those resources.

- Be creative. If the care provider is unable to come in, can you mail or fax teaching materials and discuss them by telephone?
- If the family member can only visit the hospital occasionally, make an appointment for teaching. Follow up with a written reminder or phone call. Obtain backup support so you are free at appointment time to teach.
- If you meet with much resistance, go back to the step on mutuality. Are you trying to meet their learning goals or your teaching goals? Do family members believe they are capable of caring for this patient at home? Should other team members, such as the primary care physician, social worker, home care nurse, or school nurse, take a bigger role?
- Communicate. Document each of your planning efforts and the teaching you accomplish.

"Are patient satisfaction surveys a good measure of the effectiveness of teaching or an educational program?"

"Research links patient satisfaction with economic survival of healthcare organizations."

—Bonheur, 1995, page 36

Satisfaction is important.

"Did the patient learn everything if he or she was satisfied with teaching?"

No. If the patient was satisfied with teaching, that does not mean he or she learned the information. It might mean the teaching was individualized and tailored to the learner's needs. When teaching is not individualized, learners get frustrated and dissatisfied, because they feel they are not being heard, and their concerns are not being addressed.

Patient satisfaction is a general barometer, but it does not tell you which team member taught or didn't teach; what, if anything, was learned; or if any of the new information will be applied. Health outcomes are not addressed by questions of satisfaction with teaching.

"What factors contribute to patient satisfaction? Is the patient always objective? Could the score be low if the patient doesn't like the instructor?"

Is the patient always objective? If you want an objective answer, don't ask a subjective question. You're asking the learner's opinion: did he or she feel satisfied? Satisfaction is a subjective quality, not objective. If you want to know objectively what the patient and family learned, that's another question.

Of course dislike for an instructor contributes to a negative opinion. That is one of the factors contributing to patient satisfaction—relationships. When patients feel they are not heard, therapeutic relationships suffer and satisfaction decreases. That is one of the reasons individualization of teaching is so important.

If you want to learn more:

(1998). Accomplishing too many tasks in too little time. *Patient Education Management,* 5(1), 3–4.

AT&T Language Line. Telephone interpretation in 140 languages. Services include critical interpretation assistance, Personal Interpretation service, Membership Interpretation, and Subscribed Interpretation. For information about services, call 1-800-752-0093, ext. 196.

Personal Interpretation service, single use with credit card, 1-800-528-5888. http://www.att.com/languageline.

Barber, L., Belton, A., & Simpson, N. (1993). *Teach to teach: Teach staff to plan and implement effective patient education.* Toronto, Ontario, Canada: Medical Audio Visual Communications, P.O. Box 84548, 2336 Bloor Street West, Toronto, Ontario M6S 1T0, Canada, 1-800-757-4868.

Benner, P. (1984). *From novice to expert: Excellence and power in clinical nursing practice.* Menlo Park, CA: Addison-Wesley.

Bonheur, B.B. (1995). Measuring satisfaction with patient education. *Journal of Nursing Staff Development, 11*(1), 35.

Dass, R., & Gorman, P. (1985). *How Can I Help? Stories and reflections on service.* New York: Alfred A. Knopf.

Dylan, B. (1985). *It's alright, ma (I'm only bleeding).* In Lyrics, 1962–1985. New York: Alfred A. Knopf.

Freda, M.C. (1997). Don't give it away. *The American Journal of Maternal/Child Nursing, 22*(December), 330.

Joint Commission on Accreditation of Healthcare Organizations. (1998). *1998 Hospital Accreditation Standards.* Oakbrook Terrace, IL: Author.

Oberst, B.B. (no year). *Patient and parent education: Why? What? How?* Gerber Medical Services.

Platt, F.W., Tippy, P.K., Dennis C., & Turk, D.C. (1994). Helping patients adhere to the regimen. *Patient Care, 28*(17), 43–53. [On-Line] Available: EBSCO.

Rankin, S.H., & Stallings, K.D. (1996). *Patient education: Issues, principles, practices* (3rd ed.). Philadelphia: Lippincott-Raven.

Measuring Outcomes

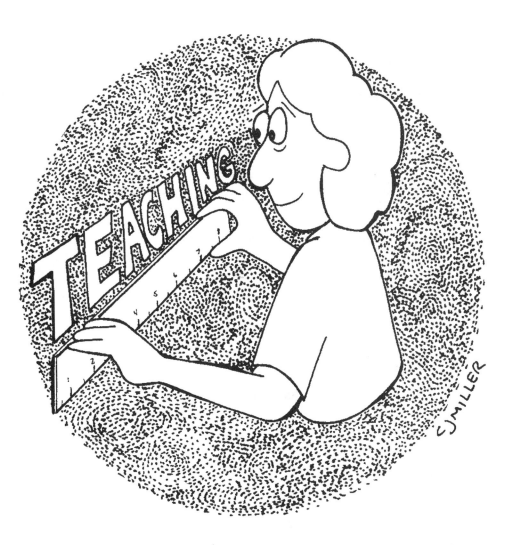

As it is, we don't have enough time to teach. Why bother measuring teaching outcomes? We could use that time to take care of patients!"

—An RN

•••••••••••••••••••••••••

Measuring outcomes is not just for the Joint Commission on Accreditation of Healthcare Organizations (JCAHO), accountants, or third-party payers. It's the evaluation part of nursing process. You know, the nursing process, A PIE: Assessment, Plan, Intervention, and Evaluation. It tells us if our intervention worked as we intended. It's part of our professional practice. It helps us continually make improvements. Measuring outcomes is part of taking care of patients.

In addition, if we want more time to teach, we have to convince the people with the money that it's a good investment. We have to show them it works. Evaluation serves that purpose, too.

What Were We Teaching for Again?

As a result of education, we expect the learner to be able to do the following:

- Make informed decisions
- Have skills for basic self-care to survive
- Recognize problems and know what to do in response
- Get questions answered; find resources for answers

These are short-term goals to be accomplished during our time with the learner. We reach them primarily by using conversation in informal teaching. Sometimes we teach more intentionally, with planned content and tangible tools. Through these short-term goals, we help learners take care of themselves and their families better. These contribute toward the ultimate long-term goal: improved health outcomes.

Many of our nursing interventions have only short-term impact. Medications relieve pain, but when they wear off, we have to give more. Treatments can manage symptoms of chronic illnesses, but they last only so long and need to be repeated.

Patient and family education is different. Conversation is as low-tech as you get and only costs as much as a nurse's salary. However, patient and family education has the potential for life-changing, long-term effects. Effective teaching is inexpensive, needs no special equipment, improves quality of life, and saves lives.

More Than Filling a Knowledge Deficit

Patient and family education is more than teaching medical facts. Yes, we do teach information, but the nursing diagnosis of "knowledge deficit" can be misleading. Providing a learner with knowledge is only the first step. Knowledge alone will not necessarily have an impact on outcomes. When we teach, our intention is to impact not only knowledge, but also the following:

- Attitudes
- Skills
- Ability to apply skills
- Behavior changes
- Health outcomes

Every time you interact with a learner, you engage in some teaching activity. Test this. After your next conversation with a patient or family member, ask yourself, "Based on my observations of that interaction, what knowledge or skills can I say I assessed, taught, or evaluated?"

You thought you had no time to teach! You're doing it all the time.

You're Part of the Big Picture

"Informed patients are more satisfied with the care they receive and more likely to comply with treatment and medication regimens. As a result, they generally enjoy better outcomes."

—Deye et al., 1997

Patient and family education is not limited to your interaction with the learner. All members of the health care team, across the continuum of care and across time, teach. Learners also obtain information on their own, through television, radio, books, magazines, friends, and family members. All these contribute to the learner's knowledge and skills.

This collection of knowledge and skills can be demonstrated as outcomes on many different levels. Rankin and Stallings (1996) identified four levels of learning outcomes:

1. Patient's participation during interventions.
2. Patient's performance immediately after the learning experience.
3. Patient's performance at home.
4. Patient's overall self-care and health management.

"All levels of evaluation provide important evidence. . . . Every nurse who teaches a patient can document an outcome at some level, and learning outcomes can be reflected in documentation in the patient's record on a daily basis."

—Rankin & Stallings, 1996, page 224

That means every day, on every patient, whether you see him or her in a clinic, in a hospital, in an office, or in a home, you have something to document about patient and family education.

Obviously, interventions of health care providers are not the only variables that impact outcomes of patient and family education. There are other variables:

- Timing of teaching
- Patient characteristics
- Socioeconomic status
- Education
- Family involvement

We can't control everything. Patient and family education is complex and dynamic. Consequently, we may sometimes have an overwhelming sense that there's no time to teach, we're not adequately prepared to teach, and we have no idea what to document.

How can we measure outcomes of teaching when there are so many variables? How can we say we made a difference?

Take a deep breath. Look at your piece of the big picture. At what level do you work, and at what level are you evaluating outcomes of teaching?

- During interventions?
- Immediately after the learning experience?
- During learner's performance at home?
- During patient's overall self-care and health management?
- On effectiveness of programs in patient and family education?

Steps for Evaluating Outcomes

Let's go through this step by step.

Did the Learner Get it?

Nurse: Do you understand?
Learner: Yes.
Nurse: Do you have any questions?
Learner: No.
Nurse: Are you ready to go home?
Learner: Yes.

Is this a familiar conversation? We know this offers no evidence that the teaching was effective. The poorest measures of evaluating teaching are the most popular. One is to ask the learner, "Did you understand that?" and the other, to ask, "Do you have any questions?"

These are ineffective measures, because their implied messages discourage an honest response. If you ask, "Did you understand that?" and the learner admits to not understanding, he or she may feel that he or she is admitting to being slow or stupid. It's safer for the learner to say he or she understands everything and not create an anxiety-producing situation. Similarly, if you ask, "Do you have any questions?" and the learner responds with a dumb question, he or she could be demonstrating a lack of intelligence.

Another drawback to these evaluation methods is that even if the learner says he or she understands, you are not evaluating whether that understanding is accurate.

Here are some specific ways to find out if the learner understands. Ask the following:

- **"Tell me what you know about . . . "**
  amoxicillin, bipolar disorder, prostate cancer
- **"How you would know if . . . "**
  the lice were gone, the incision was infected, you were getting side effects from the medication
- **"Show me how you would . . . "**
  take your temperature, change the dressing, pick an appropriate meal from this menu
- **"What would you do if . . . ?"**
  pus started oozing from the wound, she had another seizure, you had a bad pain in your chest
- **"Who would you call if . . . ?"**
  he says he wants to kill himself, the line clots off, you thought you were having a stroke

Ask the learner, "What have I forgotten to explain?" or, "What could the video have explained better?" instead of, "Do you have any other questions?"

These methods also reinforce learning and enhance later recall by actively involving the learner in the process.

Develop Games

Games can also measure learning:

- Create flash cards with questions on one side and answers on the other. Test the learner with them.
- Show a medical supply or piece of equipment, and ask the learner how it relates to the skill or what can go wrong with it. Create "what if" scenarios out of the responses.
- Adapt a commercial game, such as Trivial Pursuit, to evaluate knowledge. Encourage the whole family to play and learn.

Create Puzzles

Puzzles can help you evaluate understanding if you use them as tools to facilitate conversations.

- Create crossword puzzles that review and measure learning on the topic.
- Have the learner fill in missing key words in a paragraph on the topic taught and then find those words hidden in a word search puzzle.

Consider Written Tests: Quizzes, Questionnaires, Pretests, Post-tests

Adult learners may not respond well to written tests. Tests are reminiscent of school days; they make the learner and teacher less equal. A learner can fail a written test. Tests do not contribute to a sense of safety. Conversations are far less threatening, take less preparation and scoring time, and are more easily individualized.

On the other hand, self-learning modules may include tests that are self-scored. These are safer, because they are private. In addition, the learner is testing himself or herself and not being tested by an authority figure. The learner can look up the answer. The learner can decide how much time to take to process the material.

One study looked at whether learners would be interested in self-learning modules. In their study population, the answer was yes.

"Most (81%) patients in this group were willing to spend some of their own time learning information that they thought was important. The results may allow for patient education program designs that put more responsibility for learning with the patient."

—Piccininni & Vernon, 1997, page 41

Keep in mind the written questions in self-learning modules are part of the learning process. To know if the teaching method was effective in transferring knowledge, health care providers still have to evaluate the learner's understanding and ability to apply this information.

If you want to evaluate a teaching program, you can use quizzes to see if your methods work. To measure the effectiveness of teaching, use these same questions as a pretest and post-test. Let the learners know you are evaluating the program, and they may not be as concerned about the focus on their performance.

Written pretests and post-tests are the identical test given before and after teaching to determine how much learning has taken place. They are most appropriate when you are formally studying the effectiveness of teaching, and learners know they are part of this study. Written tests are generic, including information everyone in the same circumstance needs to know. They are also limited, because content is not individualized, and only literate learners can participate. Prepare questions on information the learner needs to know. You can present them as a written quiz or an oral challenge.

Another way to evaluate teaching is to send a questionnaire to patients at home. This reinforces teaching and gives you an opportunity to identify misunderstandings. You can send questionnaires 2 to 3 days after you see the patient to evaluate learning and retention.

Introduce the questionnaire with your purpose, such as, "Our job is to help you best take care of yourself. We taught you many things when you were with us. We want to know what you remembered and what was important to you. Please answer these questions and send us your answers. This will help us teach you, and other people, better."

In most patient and family education, evaluation of learning is verbal, not written, and individualized to the learner's needs. Knowledge is assessed before teaching (comparable to the pretest) and evaluated after teaching (comparable to the post-test).

Document Extent of the Learner's Understanding

When a nurse documents, "Patient verbalized understanding of teaching," what does that mean?

Did the patient say, "Yeah, I understand. Can I go back to sleep now?"

You wouldn't write on a flow sheet, under "temperature," the word "fever," right? You would write something like, "102.6."

When you evaluate understanding, describe how you know the learner understands, just like you would describe how you know the patient has a fever. For example, write, "Teaching was done re: infections. Patient accurately defined the signs and symptoms of infection, and reported if any one of them developed, he would call his PCP."

It is more important to define the extent of the learner's understanding than it is to define the content of your teaching. You can save time if you don't double document.

How Do I Know You Can Apply it?

"Did you hear about the newly diagnosed diabetic who came back with a high blood sugar? She didn't understand why. Every time her insulin was due, she drew up the right amount and injected it into her orange with good technique . . ."

—An RN

The most important evaluation of patient education is health outcome. If the learner understood, internalized, and applied the new information and consequently had a positive outcome, we assume learning occurred.

However, most nursing roles don't have the luxury of continuity to measure the outcome of patient education. All we can do is make sure the learner understands the information, set the stage for its internalization and application, communicate with members of the health care team who will provide continuing care, and hope progress will continue and a change in outcome will follow.

How can the short-term effectiveness of patient education be evaluated? Only your creativity limits the list. Here are a few options:

Ask the Learner to Explain it

Before you start to teach intentionally, tell the learner you will ask him or her to explain the information, skill, or behavior to a family member or significant other. This will help the learner pay attention better.

After teaching, either observe the learner teaching the information to another, or have the learner practice by teaching you, in his or her own words. When the learner is done, compliment the learner on information conveyed correctly, and discuss the parts the learner did not explain or demonstrate so well. Correct misperceptions and misunderstandings.

Through this process, the learner has reviewed and reinforced the information. It has also given you the opportunity to evaluate and document evidence of understanding.

Offer "What If" Scenarios

"What if" scenarios evaluate the learner's understanding and problem-solving skills. The learner's personality, social situation, lifestyle, and resources will alert you to potential problems. Ask open-ended questions about a situation the learner is likely to experience. Ask what the learner's behavioral response would be to specific challenges that might occur.

If the learner expresses concern about a specific potential problem, ask how the learner might respond. Teach from there. Then try other related "what if" scenarios to help the learner integrate the new responses.

This is especially helpful when guiding learners through behavior changes. For example, your learner is in the hospital for emphysema, has been off cigarettes since he was admitted, and swears he will never smoke again. Compliment the learner on this health-promoting decision, and reinforce that this is especially important, because he is going home on oxygen. Then offer "what if" scenarios for the learner to problem solve. What if his friend comes over to watch the game, takes out his cigarettes, and offers the learner one? What will the learner say? What if the learner is at his daughter's house, and the lingering odor of cigarettes in the family room makes him yearn for one? What will the learner do? If he meets these situations with a plan, he is more likely to succeed.

Have the Learner Show You

I used to think it was condescending to ask patients for a return demonstration.

I should have asked my daughter to show me how she took her medicine! Now I understand why we ran out of it so fast! She took too much.

—An RN

You are probably familiar with return demonstrations, because many nursing schools teach this evaluation technique. Return demonstrations show you clearly whether or not the learner can apply the information correctly. They are especially effective when working with learners with low literacy skills or learning disabilities. Performing a skill teaches and demonstrates whether instructions can be carried out.

Document the learner's progress every step of the way so other health care providers on the team can readily pick up where you left off. Here's a summary of the process:

1. Prepare your learner. Tell him or her why you're teaching this skill and what you expect from the learner.
2. Show the learner how you do it. Perform the skill with the learner watching, describe what you are doing, and explain why you are doing it.
3. Have the learner practice the steps in the skill. In this stage of learning, he or she may ask for clarification of details and express feelings about the process. Provide encouragement, give tips, and guide the learner into correct performance. Provide rationales as needed.
4. Have the learner repeat the skill, with your feedback, until the learner expresses comfort with the skill, and you are confident that the learner can perform the skill correctly.
5. When the learner feels ready, have him or her perform an independent return demonstration.
6. If there is time, have the learner complete at least three unassisted, accurate return demonstrations (over time; not one after the other). Of course, you do not have to observe each of these. Others on the health care team can share in this evaluation of learning.

- The first return demonstration shows the learner can do the skills.
- The second demonstrates the learner can recall the skills over time.
- By the third, something may go wrong (break in sterile technique, wrong size gauze). This will let you evaluate the learner's understanding of each step and problem-solving skills.

Create Steps-in-the-Skill Checklist

If the skills you are teaching are complex, you may want to make sure all the steps are understood and performed correctly in return demonstration. A steps-in-the-skill checklist can help you follow along, evaluate the accuracy of the return demonstration, and focus your teaching where it is needed most.

There may be several ways to perform the skill or behavior correctly. However, if you hone them all down, there are basic steps they share. These are the steps on your steps-in-the-skill checklist.

Each step should be clear, simple, and have one measurable action. Use the checklist when you teach. Give the learner a copy of this checklist to follow to walk through the skill. Encourage the learner to evaluate himself or herself on the skill, and identify problem areas.

Make sure the learner masters each step before going on to teach the next. Use the checklist's objective criteria to evaluate and document the learner's ability to perform the skill steps.

We were having a difficult time trying to determine the best way to have families demonstrate that they knew how to mix formula for their babies. We needed a new system for ensuring families were taught correctly and had a record that they actually demonstrated that they knew how to mix formula.

One of the formula companies donated what we have come to call discharge formula teaching kits. They include measuring cups, measuring spoons, the actual bottles they will use to mix the formula, syringes for liquid additives, and a can of formula filled with sugar to be used for practice. We used sugar because so many hands were in the practice can. It was stored in the formula room, and we wanted to prevent accidentally giving contaminated formula to babies. One of the nurses worked to revise a new skills checklist. This form is signed off by the RN, showing that the family can do each step to mix the formula correctly.

Once, when we taught a Spanish-speaking family, the instruction was done using the discharge teaching kit and a Spanish interpreter. The mother was able to measure out all the liquid and powder appropriately, using the correct utensils, and did a perfect demonstration. Because it was practice, we were using the sugar in the formula can to represent the powder. The interpreter was convinced the mother understood exactly what she was doing.

When the mother was all finished and was asked if there were any questions, she asked, through the interpreter, when should she add the sugar?! Even though we very carefully explained to her that the sugar was used only to demonstrate, she was still confused. The mother even asked whether the powdered formula looked the same as the sugar.

Then another case occurred, when an English-speaking mom asked us about the sugar, too. It certainly caused us to rethink what seemed like a sure way to teach. We needed to put actual formula powder in our teaching kits and reuse the powder for demonstration. Since we have done this, we have not had any further questions about mixing.

—An RD

If possible, when having learners practice skills, avoid symbolism and substitutions. Have the learner do it for real: Actually make the formula and then feed the child, or fill the syringe and give the shot. Don't assume understanding, and don't take anything for granted.

Always Evaluate Understanding

Some evaluation techniques should be applied after every formal teaching session and whenever a handout, pamphlet, or video is used. Never assume learning occurred unless you have measurable evidence. Choose the evaluation technique that is most appropriate to the material and the learner. If the learner cannot read, use oral questioning or return demonstration. If the learner is anxious, consider offering appropriate games and puzzles to ease the tension. If the learner is uncomfortable speaking to you, an authority figure, evaluate learning with nonverbal, demonstration methods.

Have you put your written teaching materials through patient and family review to be sure they are understood and can be applied? One company that produces written teaching materials includes in its advertisements the results of independent research resources looking at the effectiveness of their booklets. They looked at successful transfer of information, relevancy of content to the reader's circumstances, and the reader's intent to act. More than 1,000 adults participated. Their booklets for low-literacy and average adult readers were studied separately. Among participants expressing little or no intention to take a specific action before reading the booklet, there was a 38% to 56% increase in reported intention to act (Channing L. Bete Company, 1997).

Read what others on the health care team have documented about where they left off on teaching. Evaluate for understanding, acceptance, and application before you teach more. Evaluate and address your learner's affective responses. This will guide you in enhancing the learner's alliance with the mutually identified goals and promote a positive outcome. Put learning in the context of expected outcome. Document the results of your evaluation so others on the health care team can build on your findings.

As your evaluation skills improve, you may be surprised by how much of your teaching is not understood. You may be surprised at how little your learner knows of basic body processes and self-care. This may upset you, but it is good information. Use this new knowledge to improve your teaching skills. This is the continuous loop of nursing process in action.

Remember to Focus on Goals

"Consumers self-treat four times more health problems than doctors treat."
                                                    —Farley, 1997

Most interventions involve the participation of the learner to succeed. We can't change many outcomes directly and solely with our interventions. Other than surgery, little we do to patients makes them healthier. To change health outcomes, learners need to participate. We can bring them medicine, but they have to take it. They need to follow up after our interventions. We can recommend adjustments in behaviors related to exercise, work, nutrition, drugs, alcohol, tobacco, safety, hygiene, and risk taking, but they have to make those changes. We can help them when things go wrong, but they need to call us.

Our interventions depend on our learners' abilities to understand our instructions and ability and willingness to follow through. This is best accomplished through individualizing our teaching.

"Measuring outcomes is accountability in its truest form, and with the changing climate in healthcare, is more important than ever."
                                                    —Considine, 1996, page 488

As good as our interventions are, they may only work some of the time. We can offer interventions, but they must also be received. For example, patients with tuberculosis or high blood pressure need to take their medications for a very long time. The medications we have may work well, but when they are not taken, they don't work at all.

Our responsibility includes giving the medication and partnering with the learner to optimize the medication's opportunities to work. We need to help learners apply skills and behavior changes we prescribe. We need to teach.

"Achieving worthwhile gains in compliance, recall and satisfaction should be possible if clinicians use techniques to enhance the comprehension of health messages."
                                                    —Doak, Doak, Friedell, & Meade, 1998

Focus on shared goals. Information that does not relate to the learner's goal will probably not be applied. The family who brings sweets to the patient with diabetes is probably not homicidal. They may just want to improve the patient's quality of life and don't know how else to accomplish this goal.

Does Teaching Change Anything?

It's important to make sure the learner understands our teaching and is able perform the skills. The next step is determining if the learner can apply the skills within the context of his or her life.

"Testing can certainly help educators measure gains in knowledge levels, but unfortunately they prove nothing about whether patients will apply their knowledge to self-care."
—Haggard, 1989, page 168

Within the hospital setting, we can prepare the learner to apply the information, but nurses and other health care providers in the community can best determine if the learner is succeeding. Nurses in home care, clinics, doctors offices, and schools are especially well positioned to assess and facilitate application of knowledge.

Did our teaching of information, skills, and behaviors do anything? Is the learner less anxious? Is the learner better able to function? And ultimately,

"What objective proof do we have that what we have done has made an impact in the patient's overall quality of life?"
—Considine, 1996, page 488

Measure Short-Term Outcomes

The first step is to measure our success in short-term outcomes. Health care providers who deal with learners in inpatient settings generally see them over a short span of time and tend to focus on the present. Short-term outcomes to be evaluated include the following:

- Increases in knowledge (comparison of pretest and post-test scores or assessment and evaluation of knowledge)
- Demonstrates understanding
- Performs specific technical skills
- Demonstrates ability to problem solve
- Applies coping skills
- Shows self-efficacy (does the learner believe he or she can do it?)
- Is satisfied
- Has enhanced sense of well-being

One of the most commonly used of these short-term outcomes is patient satisfaction. It is common in part because satisfaction is easy to measure with a survey. However, it also is an important factor, and teaching is important to overall patient satisfaction.

"Patients who reported having discussed any health education topics with a health care provider were more likely to be satisfied with their physician than patients who reported that they did not."

—Schauffler, Rodriguez, & Milstein, 1996

Research has shown that understanding of health teaching correlates well with patient satisfaction, recall of information, and compliance (Doak, et al., 1998).

Short-term teaching outcomes are often documented on a patient education form. The VNA Community Care Services (1998) actually named one of their patient education documentation tools "Patient Outcome Tool: Heart Failure." Like similar tools, it includes spaces for documenting understanding and application of knowledge about medications, disease management, how to recognize problems, and what to do in response. The outcomes they measure include both knowledge and level of functioning. The form includes evaluation of level of functioning, including bathing, mobility, dressing, toileting, and eating. These are evaluated at the first visit, visit 12, and at discharge.

Measure Long-Term and Big Picture Outcomes

This leads us toward long-term outcomes. Health care providers who interact with learners in outpatient settings are in a better position to assess and facilitate application of knowledge.

"Measure the long-term effect of education on patients' knowledge, behaviors, attitudes, and skills required to maintain or improve their health. Such factors often determine a patient's willingness and ability to comply with a treatment regimen and self-manage his or her condition."

—Spath, 1997, page 51

Not that long ago, our measures of health outcomes focused primarily on the traditional five D's: death, disability, dissatisfaction, disease, and discomfort (Mitchell, Ferketich, & Jennings, 1998). These are still very important. However, we began to ask more questions, such as, "Is a long life necessarily a good life?" "Is this intervention worth it?" "What? We spend most of our health care money on the last few weeks of life?" Consequently, what we measure has evolved.

"Steadily, the criteria for determining a client's health outcome have changed from extending the duration of life to assessing the quality of life."

—Hoeman, 1995, page 106

We now look at other outcomes:

- Retention of knowledge
- Changes in attitudes and beliefs
- Application of the information (alliance with plan of care)
- Early recognition of problems and appropriate response
- Health-promoting behaviors
- Health-related quality of life (such as, "What bothers you most?" "What worries you most?")
- Health status
- Satisfaction with patient and family education
- Satisfaction with clinical outcome; perception of being well cared for
- Demonstration of competence in symptom management
- Use of services (number and appropriateness of visits, telephone contacts, hospitalizations, use of ancillary health care services)
- Health care costs

There are many outcomes we can evaluate to determine if our interventions worked, but how do we measure them?

Ways to Measure Outcomes

To find out if your intervention was followed by improvements, you need to compare data:

- Before and after the intervention (such as pretest, post-test)
- Measuring changes over time
- Comparing two matched, randomly selected groups

This comparison lets you measure the extent of improvement.

Do you want to measure effectiveness of patient and family education? Then look at the outcomes for which you are reaching. Define your objectives in ways that can be measured, such as decrease in blood levels of cholesterol or ability to ambulate independently with prosthesis. Then decide which method is appropriate for gathering data on that variable. Here are some possible methods.

Physical Evidence

Examine the learner for presence or absence of desired health outcomes. Did the learner lose weight? Is the blood pressure within normal limits? Are laboratory values within normal limits?

Interviews

Interviews can be done in person or by telephone. Call the learner at intervals, weeks or months after the teaching. Review and reinforce teaching, answer questions, and inquire about compliance. Data gathered this way may or may not be meaningful, because accuracy depends on honesty. However, accurate learner feedback can be very valuable.

Another way to measure your progress toward goals is to ask for personal anecdotes.

> *"You may also ask patients to write a letter describing the birth experience or a surgical experience and explaining how prepared they felt for it. They can offer suggestions for how to best prepare others on their experiences."*
> —Rankin & Stallings, 1996, page 228

Self-Report Diary

This is a written record kept by the learner and shared with the health care team in follow-up. The learner can record any data that are appropriate for the plan of care, such as a record of food intake, blood sugar readings, or hours of sleep.

Again, accuracy depends on honesty, but if nothing else, a self-report diary would regularly remind the learner of the mutual goals. Self-report diaries collect data but also help learners gain awareness of health-related variables.

> *"Patients can be taught to be good reporters if they are given specific directions about collecting and recording significant information and if they are told how they are expected to contribute to the evaluation process."*
> —Rankin & Stallings, 1996, page 227

Review of Medical Records

Review medical records for evidence of presence or absence of desired health outcomes.

Quality Assurance Programs

> *"Quality assurance programs are an effective vehicle for evaluating the effectiveness of patient education programs."*
> —Rankin & Stallings, 1996, page 336

Another way to measure quality of teaching is to compare performance against JCAHO standards (1998). Variables you can look at include critical incidents, length of stay, and readmissions.

Program Evaluation

Some nurses work in positions where they develop programs that teach populations of learners. How can you tell if the program is working? Again, compare data. Look at knowledge, skills, or behaviors before and after the intervention; measure changes over time; or compare two matched, randomly selected groups (if ethically appropriate).

It is important to evaluate the effectiveness of educational programs to improve them, to demonstrate their usefulness, and to justify continued or additional funding. Ideally, when you design a program, you build in the evaluation parameters, so you collect data before the intervention begins.

In the past, much money was needed for salaries for skilled staff to collect and process data for program evaluation. Technology is making that easier, cheaper, and faster. For example, one program collects information on quality of life from breast cancer patients on every clinic visit. The computer operator hands the patient a pen-based, hand-held computer, and the learner fills out the questionnaire, using the pen on the screen. The patient returns the computer to the computer operator. The computer operator uploads the patient's responses on to the desktop computer through a wireless infrared connection. Push, zap, and data are in. The program makes some identification checks, then calculates the results, using the patient's responses. The system updates the database with the new entry, and the patient's responses are printed out for the physician to view before seeing the patient (Le et al., 1998). All sorts of data can be collected and managed using a system like this.

If you want or need to evaluate the effectiveness of a patient and family education program, don't begin until you read Lorig et al. (1996), *Outcome Measures for Health Education and Other Health Care Interventions*. In it, the authors detail study instruments, how they determine which outcomes to measure, and coding in a chronic disease self-management study. They measure behaviors, self-efficacy, and outcomes from the patient's perspective.

Research: An Organized Way to Get Answers

"I love bedside nursing! You won't find me getting get stuck in that theoretical stuff that has nothing to do with real clinical issues. I'm not interested in research. I'm a real nurse."

—An RN

If you're a real nurse, you care about patient outcomes. You want your patient to be as pain free as possible, as functional as possible, and as healthy as possible. How do you know what to do to accomplish this? You look at the data. You notice your patients on morphine are more comfortable than those on meperidine, with fewer side effects. You notice decubiti heal faster on this bed than that one. You notice that patients on this cardiac medication often have strokes. That's evaluation of outcomes. That's the start of research.

"Research, a tool of science, facilitates the development of a knowledge base for practice. Nursing research endeavors to describe, explain, and predict outcomes of nursing interventions with one of the most important interventions being the practice of patient education."

—Rankin & Stallings, 1996, page 332

Don't be intimidated by the jargon, charts, and math of research. Underneath the language of research are important findings that can help you improve your clinical care. Like anything else, if you practice reading research, in time you will get better at understanding and applying it.

How do you start? You start with a problem, something you want to learn more about. When you decide to look up studies relating to a problem, you need to locate them. Ask your librarian for help. She or he may be able to show you resources that didn't exist when you were writing papers in nursing school.

Then, when you find studies, you need to be able to tell if the writers' conclusions were true and whether the conclusions are worth anything to you in your practice. Much has been written on how to evaluate research studies. Box 13-1 is a summary of some of the key questions you can ask. For more detail, check your library (or the carton in your attic or basement) for a nursing research text.

BOX 13-1   How to Review the Literature

Why?

Health care is science and research based. Over time, our understanding of physiology, illnesses, treatments, and patient and family education evolve. Therefore, it is important for health care providers to keep current on information to ensure our practice is state-of-the-art. Reviewing the literature is one way to keep up.

What Is "the Literature?"

"The literature" is written by professionals for professionals. It consists of journals, books, conference proceedings, and other media.

The most reliable literature is research that is peer reviewed. This means that a group of experts in the field agreed it was worthy of publication.

Literature that is not peer reviewed is considered less reliable. Information based on research results is preferred. When deciding practice issues, opinion pieces are of lowest value.

How do I Find "the Literature" on a Specific Topic?

Write down the questions you want answered. What are the key words in your topic? How big is your scope, such as population or timeframe? What is your viewpoint, such as nursing, medicine, or psychology? This will help you decide which databases are appropriate to use.

Use only research from the last 3 years. When 6 to 10 research studies have the same results, you can be confident that the findings are ready to be instituted into practice. Reviews of the literature and meta-analyses may summarize some of this for you.

Searches are now generally done on a computer database, such as CINAHL, MEDLINE, or Grateful Med. If you want to learn how to do the search yourself, make an appointment with a librarian. You could also ask a librarian to conduct an on-line search for you.

Some articles or books identified in your search may not be available locally. Ask if you can get them through your library's interlibrary loan department.

What Do I Do With These Articles and Books?

Read them. Take notes or highlight the important points. Look at their reference lists for additional resources.

It may help to use note cards or a computer to organize information into the categories of your outline.

Box 13-1 *(Continued)*

Use your clinical experience to evaluate the information critically. Decide what information belongs and what doesn't. To evaluate a research article, get out your old nursing statistics textbook (What? You sold it?) and review it, piece by piece.

- What problem does the research study? Is it similar to your problem?
- What does it say about other research on the topic?
- What does it say about the nonresearch information on the topic?
- Is the review of the literature complete and balanced?
- Is the setting of the study sample similar to the setting in which you are interested?

Are they similar enough to make comparisons?

- Is the population of the study sample similar to the population in which you are interested? Are they similar enough to make comparisons?
- What is the study's sample size?
- Is the sample representative of the population?
- Do the author(s) identify limitations or factors that influenced the study results?
- How were the study's findings measured?
- How were the data collected?
- How appropriate were the statistical methods used? (I told you you'd need that old textbook.)
- Are the findings significant?
- Were appropriate statistical methods used to analyze the data?
- Does the study discuss clinical implications?
- What do you think of the study? Do you believe the results, based on your clinical experience?
- Based on your answers to the above questions, are the findings of the study appropriate for your needs?

You may be considering applying the findings in practice:

- Have you looked at six independent studies that recommend the same changes and believe they are good studies?
- How much potential risk would you take by implementing the findings?
- How many resources would you need to implement the findings?
- Who in your organization would need to be involved in implementing the findings?
- How ready are these others for change?

Box 13-1 (*Continued*)

- If you want to move ahead to make the change, what is your plan?
- How would you evaluate effectiveness of the change?

Also, look for articles that are meta-analyses or reviews of the literature on your topic. Meta-analyses actually apply statistics to summarize, mathematically, the collective findings of a set of studies. Reviews of the literature critically discuss, compare, and contrast studies on a topic. Both can be very useful in giving you a sense of where results are leaning.

However, meta-analyses and reviews of the literature, like research studies, may be flawed. Their selection criteria or limitations on access to materials may have left out studies that would have swayed their conclusions in another direction.

Read all research critically. Don't believe everything you read. Trust your clinical experiences. If the research contradicts what you've experienced, try to figure out why. Is it a different population, location, or culture? What, in the structure of the study, may have contributed to the researchers getting that result?

Many conclusions from research are presented in this book. They are presented in the context of your practice, illustrated by anecdotes that describe situations similar to those you might have experienced. The intent is to help you see the connections between research and practice. The objective is to help you apply this information so you can teach faster and better. Research may seem nerdy, but it's really very cool. Perhaps it might even inspire you to apply quality patient and family education skills in your practice.

Current Answers From the Literature

Most of our learners are adults. Even if we work in pediatrics, we teach the parents (although, admittedly, many parents are not adults yet). Consequently, we apply adult education research in patient and family education. It makes sense. We need to learn how to teach adults quickly and effectively, and this research holds the answers.

What Teaching Methods Work Best?

"Given the large volume of articles about patient education found in the literature, proportionately few report systematic evaluation of patient education interventions."

—Falvo, 1995, page 229

Most patient and family education is informal, occurring in casual conversations. It is difficult to design a research study that depends on evaluating the use of teachable moments.

Theis and Johnson (1995), through meta-analysis, found the four most effective teaching methods to be structured teaching, reinforcement, independent study, and the use of multiple strategies. Structured teaching includes planned teaching.

However, this study got its results by looking at all the research studies that met criteria, including randomization into treatment and control groups. Only 73 studies done between 1960 and 1992 met these criteria. Teaching methods that were not studied, like informal, individualized teaching using teachable moments, were not included.

A different study with a small sample of 24 patients came to the following conclusion:

"Perhaps the best type of patient-education program would be one in which the clinician offers and directs one or two small group sessions per week while still encouraging individually directed learning from a resource library."

—Piccininni & Vernon, 1997, page 43

This needs to be tested with other populations and other topics to be validated. However, it does agree with the many studies that indicate the most effective way to teach is to combine methods.

"In summarizing findings from review articles . . . one-on-one, group, audiovisual and psychoeducational strategies have proved useful. The combination of strategies to reinforce learning is probably more effective than any single strategy."

—Rankin & Stallings, 1996, page 341

Another review article also discussed the need for a variety of teaching methods:

"Clinicians should develop strategies and media that can be introduced in the acute care setting and then taken home for reinforcement, as many homes now have videotape recorders and/or computers. Verbal instructions should only be used with some form of media support."

—Theis & Johnson, 1995, page 104

Using a variety of methods may work well because you deliver the same message in several different ways. Different methods help you repeat a message without being boring. Using a variety of methods also delivers the message through many senses, enhancing learning. Also, when using a variety of methods, the same message is repeated over time, so the learner is reminded of it.

"In summarizing findings from review articles . . . patient education must be repetitive and reinforced at different time periods."
                                    —Rankin & Stallings, 1996, page 341

Evidence on effective methods of patient and family education is so consistent that when you see a study that claims something other than what you would expect, look carefully at the variables. Compare the teaching practices described in the study with the principles of teaching well (such as mutually establishing goals with the learner, using the teachable moment, and individualizing instruction).

For example, Goldstein, Snyder, Edin, Lindgren, and Finkelstein (1996) compare the effectiveness of teaching lung and lung–heart transplant patients in two different environments: in the clinic setting, referred to as an integrated approach, and in a patient learning center (PLC), referred to as a separate approach. The authors concluded that "the PLC-instructed group was more adherent than the clinic-instructed group in following the home monitoring protocol" (Goldstein et al., 1996).

Why would teaching at a separate site, rather than integrating teaching into the clinic visit, improve outcomes?

In both sites, nurses taught learners one-to-one. Upon reading the article, it becomes clear that the differences in teaching methods between the two settings were probably more responsible for this result than the separate location of the teaching.

"Education received in a PLC, which allows hands-on learning in an unhurried, relaxed, and quiet environment, is a more effective way of teaching patients to use an electronic spirometer/diary instrument at home than is teaching conducted in a clinic setting. . . . There is no feeling of being rushed in the PLC; patients know they can return for a review session at no extra charge. . . . Because there is more time available for teaching in the PLC (90 minutes in the PLC, as opposed to 30 minutes in the clinic), patients' individual learning needs and style can be accommodated, and additional time can be spent helping patients determine how to fit home monitoring into their daily schedule and reviewing what to do if problems should occur."
                                    —Goldstein et al., 1996

The authors concluded that "findings from this study support a structured approach that takes place in a separate setting" (Goldstein et al., 1996), but do they, really?

Too many variables were unequal. The learners in the clinic were given one third of the teaching time of those in the PLC! This study merely demonstrated that you get better results by spending more time doing individualized teaching in a learning environment.

Why did the authors think the separate setting was significant? The authors did not attempt to create a learning environment in the clinic. The differences between the integrated (clinic) and separate (PLC) settings were not well controlled.

If given that same quiet 90 minutes to teach, would clinic nurses have the same or better results than PLC nurses? The clinic nurses already have an ongoing relationship with the learners and can mutually arrive at goals and assess learning needs within the context of their interactions. The nurses in the PLC probably spent some of their teaching time building a relationship with the learners, establishing mutual goals, and assessing needs.

How much more did it cost to establish and run a separate PLC, compared to giving clinic nurses enough time to teach their patients?

See, looking at research can be fun.

Does Patient and Family Education Change Behaviors and Outcomes?

Yes. Many studies in the literature demonstrate the effectiveness of patient and family education in changing both behaviors and outcomes.

For example, many studies have looked at educating people with arthritis about their disease and teaching them skills for living with it. A meta-analysis of these studies indicated that education increased functional ability and reduced tender joint counts.

> *"Based on this meta-analysis, patient education interventions provide additional benefits that are 20%–30% as great as the effects of NSAID treatment for pain relief in OA and RA, 40% as great as NSAID treatment for improvement in functional ability in RA, and 60%–80% as great as NSAID treatment in reduction in tender joint counts in RA."*
> —Superio-Cabuslay, Ward, & Lorig, 1996, page 292

Did you notice the use of acronyms in this quote? These terms were defined at the beginning of the article, as they should always be (NSAID = nonsteroidal anti-inflammatory drug, OA = osteoarthritis, RA = rheumatoid arthritis). Definition of terms is one of the factors you consider when evaluating a research study. Definitions should be there. Look for them.

There were a lot of acronyms and percentages in this quote and many commas. Don't let that intimidate you. Break each sentence down into manageable parts, take some time with it, and you should be able to understand what the author is saying.

Here's another example of how patient and family education measurably impacts outcomes:

> *"Education and counseling can help patients understand heart failure, recognize the need for medical attention, and adapt psychologically to their condition. . . . Counseling and education can improve patient outcomes and decrease unnecessary hospitalizations."*

—Dracup et al., 1994

Education also works to help learners get early screenings, which, by finding cancer earlier, often improves survival.

> *"Women who received the education program exhibited a greater knowledge about cervical cancer prevention and were more likely to have reported having a Pap smear within the past year than women who did not receive the program."*

—Dignan et al., 1996

Many studies address effectiveness of teaching, and the number of articles is growing all the time. Very little published research indicates patient and family education is ineffective or offers too few benefits for the expense. Those that have been published often are unclear about the teaching methods used, use teaching methods that are not the most effective, or use teaching inappropriately.

For example, one study looked at the value of purely educational approaches in treating back pain. It concluded the following:

> *"Although back pain patients like the educational interventions and may have benefited from them in some ways, the interventions had no impact on symptoms, function, disability or health care use. . . . Because of limited benefits, there is little justification for implementing this type of nurse education program in primary care. Although patients feel a need for more and better information about back problems, it is not clear how this can be accomplished cost-effectively."*
> —Cherkin, Dayo, Street, Hunt, & Barlow, 1996, page 353

The investigators hypothesized that if teaching changed the subjects' perceptions, the teaching, as compared with usual care, would lead to:

> *"1) greater use of recommended exercise, 2) better physical and social function, 3) less disability, and 4) less use of health care services for back pain."*
> —Cherkin et al., 1996, page 348

Their results showed teaching clearly didn't achieve these goals.

However, they expected to accomplish these impressive goals with a minimum of effort. One group had the usual care. A second group received an educational booklet. The third group received a teaching session with a clinic nurse, an educational booklet, and one follow-up telephone call 1 week after the teaching session.

The nurses in that third group spent an average of 17.0 minutes teaching each subject, with a range of 8 to 30 minutes. The average time spent on the follow-up phone call was 6 minutes. Outcomes were assessed 1, 3, 7, and 52 weeks after the intervention. Other than the follow-up phone call, no evaluation, continuation, or reinforcement of teaching was done.

By the last assessment, 1 year after the intervention, the three groups showed no difference in expected outcomes. Given the interventions, are you surprised? Fortunately, the study ends with,

"Future efforts to promote self-care for back pain should first identify the underlying needs of persons with recurrent episodes of care and then develop intensive interventions that directly address those needs."
—Cherkin et al., 1996, page 348

They concluded individualized teaching might work better. If you're going to teach, save time and money, and do it right.

Is Teaching Cost Effective?

"How do we show that patient education is cost effective to justify spending money?"
—An RN

To show that patient education is cost effective, we need to demonstrate that teaching is a good investment. This can be done in several ways.

We can look at the research that's been done on this topic. Indeed, it's true:

"A growing body of research supports the idea that improved patient and family education produces positive health outcomes for patients and decreases the overall costs of care."
—Kantz et al., 1998, page 12

A review of research that looked at the cost benefits of patient education concluded:

"On the average, for every dollar invested in patient education, $3-4 were saved."
—Bartlett, 1995, page 89

That puts it in tangible dollar terms. It makes sense. If learners know how to take care of themselves, recognize problems, and know how to respond, fewer complications will occur, and problems that do occur will be identified and corrected early. Because the cost of teaching learners is less than the cost of treating the complications that could arise, money will be saved.

Another way to demonstrate that teaching is a good investment is to show how the teaching you do works. Before you make changes in your patient and family education program, note the status of key indicators you hope to impact, such as length of stay or readmissions. Remember, you need to compare data to be able to show there is an improvement.

Data you collect can then be applied to a cost-benefit analysis, where the benefits (disease prevention) are compared with the costs of the program. A cost-benefit analysis puts a price on health outcome. This sort of calculation makes some people uncomfortable.

An alternative calculation is cost-effectiveness analysis (CEA). CEA measures health outcome in terms of health units (such as years of life saved) compared to the cost of the treatment, which is measured in dollars. This does not give you an absolute decision about benefits outweighing costs, but it does give a measure that can be used to compare programs, to determine which is most cost-effective.

One nurse researcher (Stone, 1998) describes CEA in some detail. This process takes into account many variables. Her article ends with,

> "In most cases, the education of nurses, physicians, and others has ill prepared them to make decisions regarding cost-effectiveness. But in years to come, conducting CEAs or using information from multiple CEAs to make an informed decision will become important for clinicians, particularly those who practice in price and quality competitive environments. Nurses who understand CEA and how to use it to solve problems will not only be highly valued by organizations and policy makers, but will enrich their capacity to make contributions that advance the profession and increase nurses' influence on people's care."
>
> —Stone, 1998, page 233

Cost-effectiveness analysis has been applied to variables like pneumo-coccal vaccines, Pap smears, and cholesterol-modifying agents (Buerhaus, 1998). Could we see CEAs of patient and family education programs in the future?

Make Your Point With Research

Remember one thing about research: Study results do not prove anything, but significant results from several studies that all support the same conclusion provide really good evidence for that side of the argument. Research can be a powerful tool. There is already a strong body of evidence that can help you advocate for support of patient and family education.

> "In summarizing findings from review articles . . . patient education is positively related to knowledge accrual and a number of beneficial psychosocial and physical health outcomes."
> —Rankin & Stallings, 1996, page 341

Practice reading the research so you can gain critical evaluation skills. Whether you agree or disagree with an article, critically evaluate it. The more insight you have into the research process, the better you can meet challenges to your stance.

Look at how patient and family education fits into your nursing role, and become familiar with relevant research studies. What works for you? Do you want to learn how to teach groups best? Which methods are effective in diabetes teaching? How do you reach underserved populations?

Use the information you learn from that research in your practice. Apply methods that have been demonstrated to be effective. When you advocate for more teaching time or supplies, use research results to support your requests. Cite relevant research when you apply for grants, and keep your focus on what's best for the patient and family.

Make your point with research. It's a powerful tool.

How You Can Contribute

Even if you are not a nurse researcher with a PhD, there is still much you can contribute to the measuring of outcomes of patient and family education. (If you are a nurse researcher with a PhD, you know how you can contribute to the measuring of outcomes. Have you looked at outcomes of patient and family education lately?)

Check your patient's chart for details on what other health care providers have taught, evaluate understanding, and teach from there. Make sure your learner understands your teaching, and demonstrates the ability to apply it. Share your evaluation of understanding with your colleagues on the health care team through discussions and documentation. This will help continuity and save teaching time for all.

You can also role model your skills in evaluation of understanding to teach your colleagues, students, and orientees. If your patients have been in the hospital for 3 days and no one's documented on the education record yet, be the first. Someone's got to begin the process.

Notice when your learner meets the goals of patient and family education. Notice when your teaching has an impact on outcome. Enjoy it! Record a description of the situation as an exemplar, described in Figure 12-1, on page 372. Collect these success stories, and encourage your colleagues to do the same.

Take some time to look at your collection of exemplars. Do you see themes? What observation jumps out at you? How can you use this information?

These anecdotes may help you feel good about the care you are providing. Your discoveries may help you advocate for more resources for teaching or more time to teach. You may find themes that you want to explore further, either through informal reading or designing a little study.

You may be asked to participate in gathering data to evaluate the effectiveness of a patient and family education program. You may be asked to participate in a research study, where the outcomes of your teaching are followed. Get involved.

If inspired, you may become a nurse researcher in patient and family education. You know which teaching methods work and which don't work. Now demonstrate it in statistical terms administrators and third-party payers can understand. Let's do what's best for patients and families.

Historical Note on Measuring Outcomes

Are you still not convinced this measuring stuff is really nursing?

Did you know that Florence Nightingale got so frustrated with not being listened to by the military authorities, Parliament, and Queen Victoria that she invented a new kind of statistical graph that convinced them to carry out her proposed improvements?

During the Crimean War, Florence kept records of the incidence of needless deaths caused by unsanitary conditions. She presented her data to the appropriate government powers and was ignored, so she invented polar-area charts (she called them Coxcombs). These clearly showed that far more deaths were attributable to nonbattle than battle-related causes.

The graph she used to display her data is at the website http://www.math.yorku.ca/SCS/Gallery/.

These polar-area charts are like pie charts but more complex. They're sort of circular histograms. Equal-angle sections represent data sets (such as time periods), and the area represents volume. Unlike pie charts, polar-area charts keep angles constant and vary the radius.

Florence's charts made her point graphically. She was listened to, and the changes she wanted were put into place. Her calculations demonstrated that an improvement of sanitary methods would decrease deaths. She was right.

Florence Nightingale didn't just invent this chart. She innovated the collection, tabulation, graphical display, and interpretation of descriptive statistics. In 1858, she became a Fellow of the Royal Statistical Society and in 1874, an honorary member of the American Statistical Association.

What's the moral?

When the system gets you down, collect data and advocate for what's best for the patient.

 If you want to learn more:

Bartlett, E.E. (1995). Cost-benefit analysis of patient education. *Patient Education and Counseling, 26,* 87–91.

Buerhaus, P.I. (1998). Milton Weinstein's insights on the development, use, and methodologic problems in cost-effectiveness analysis. *Image: Journal of Nursing Scholarship, 30*(3), 223–227.

Bonheur, B.B. (1995). Measuring satisfaction with patient education. *Journal of Nursing Staff Development, 11*(1), 35.

Channing L. Bete Co., Inc., 200 State Road, South Deerfield, MA 01373-0200; 1-800-628-7733. Source of written materials for patient and family education. 1997 pamphlet titled, "Our educational materials have been proven effective in a nationwide study conducted by independent experts."

Cherkin, D.C., Dayo, R.A., Street, J.H., Hunt, M., & Barlow, W. (1996). Pitfalls of patient education: Limited success of a program for back pain in primary care. *SPINE, 21*(3), 345–355.

Considine, C.J. (1996). Measurement of outcomes: What does it really mean? *Home Healthcare Nurse, 14*(6), 488.

Deye, D.L., Kahn, G., Jimison, H.B., Renner, J.H., Wenner, A.R., & Gabello, W.J. (1997). How computers enrich patient education. *Patient Care, 31*(3), 88–100. [On-line]. Available: EBSCO.

Dignan, M., Michielutte, R., Blinson, K., Wells, H.B., Case, L.D., Sharp, P., Davis, S., Konen, J., & McQuellon, R.P. (1996). Effectiveness of health education to increase screening for cervical cancer among Eastern-Band Cherokee Indian women in North Carolina. *Journal of the National Cancer Institute, 88*(22), 160–167. [On-line] Available: EBSCO.

Doak, C.C., Doak, L.G., Friedell, G.H., & Meade, C.D. (1998). Improving comprehension for cancer patients with low literacy skills: Strategies for clinicians. *CA: Cancer Journal Clinics, 48,* 151–162. [On-line]. Available: http://www.ca-journal.org/frames/articles/articles_1998/48_151-162_frame.htm.

Dracup, K., Baker, D.W., Dunbar, S.B., Dacey, R.A., Brooks, N.H., Johnson, J. C., Oken, C., & Massie, B.M. (1994). Counseling, education, and lifestyle modifications. *Journal of the American Medical Association, 272*(18), 1442–1447. [On-line]. Available: EBSCO.

Einhorn, C. (1998). *Steps of patient education.* [On-line]. Available: http://nisc8a.upenn.edu/psychosocial/pat_educ.html.

Farley, D. (1997). Label literacy for OTC drugs. *FDA Consumer, May-June,* [On-line]. Available: http://www.fda.gov/dfac/features/1997/497_otc.html.

Falvo, D.R. (1995). Educational evaluation: What are the outcomes? *Advances in Renal Replacement Therapy, 2*(3), 227–233.

Goldstein, N.L., Snyder, M., Edin, C., Lindgren, B., & Finkelstein, S.M. (1996). Comparison of two teaching strategies: Adherence to a home monitoring program. *Clinical Nursing Research, 5*(2), 150–177. [On-line]. Available: InfoTrac.

Haggard, A. (1989). *Handbook of patient education.* Rockville, MD: Aspen Publishers.

Hoeman, S.P. (1995). Nursing's expected and unexpected outcomes. *Clinical Nurse Specialist, 9*(2), 106.

Joint Commission on Accreditation of Healthcare Organizations. (1998). *1998 Hospital Accreditation Standards.* Oakbrook Terrace, IL: Author.

Kantz, B., Wandel, J., Fladger, A., Folcarelli, P., Burger, S., & Clifford, J.C. (1998). Developing patient and family education services. *The Journal of Nursing Administration, 28*(2), 11–18.

Le, P.P., Kohane, I.S., & Weeks, J.C. (1998). Collection of health related quality of life information using a pen-based computer. [On-line]. http:// www.chip.org/chip/projects/pdaquality/pdaquality.html

Lorig, K., Stewart, A., Ritter, P., González, V., Laurent, D., & Lynch, J. (1996). *Outcome measures for health education and other health care interventions.* Thousand Oaks, CA: SAGE Publications.

Lorig, K. (1996). *Patient education: A practical approach.* Thousand Oaks, CA: Sage Publications.

Mitchell, P.H., Ferketich, S., & Jennings, B.M. (1998). Quality health outcomes model. *Image: Journal of Nursing Scholarship, 30*(1), 43–46.

Mullen, P.D., Simons-Morton, D.G., Ramírez, G., Frankowski, R.F.L., Green, W., & Mains, D. A. (1997). A meta-analysis of trials evaluating patient education and counseling for three groups of preventive health behaviors. *Patient Education and Counseling, 32*, 157–173.

Piccininni, J.J., & Vernon, H.T. (1997). Self-directed patient education in soft-tissue rehabilitation: Rationale and analysis of a pilot project. *Journal of Manipulative and Physiological Therapeutics, 20*(1), 41–46.

Rankin, S.H., & Stallings, K.D. (1996). *Patient education: Issues, principles, practices* (3rd ed.). Philadelphia: Lippincott-Raven.

Schauffler, H.H., Rodriguez, T., & Milstein, A. (1996). Health education and patient satisfaction. *Journal of Family Practice, 42*(1), 62–69. [On-line]. Available: EBSCO.

Sidani, S., & Braden, C.J. (1998). *Evaluating nursing interventions: A theory driven approach.* Thousand Oaks, CA: Sage Publications.

Spath, P. (1997). Do your patient education programs pull their weight? *Hospital Case Management, March,* 51–54.

Stone, P.W. (1998). Methods for conducting and reporting cost-effectiveness analysis in nursing. *Image: Journal of Nursing Scholarship, 30*(3), 229–234.

Superio-Cabuslay, E., Ward, M.M., & Lorig, K.R. (1996). Patient education interventions in osteoarthritis and rheumatoid arthritis: A meta-analytic comparison with nonsteroidal antiinflammatory drug treatment. *Arthritis Care Research, 9*(4), 292–301.

Theis, S.L., & Johnson, J.H. (1995). Strategies for teaching patients: A meta-analysis. *Clinical Nurse Specialist, 9*(2), 100–104.

VNA Community Care Services (1998). Patient outcome tool: Heart failure. *Home Healthcare Nurse, 16*(1), 17.

If you want to learn more about Florence Nightingale's statistical prowess, here are four websites:

Lipsey, S. (1993). Mathematical education in the life of Florence Nightingale. *Newsletter of the Association for Women in Mathematics, 23*(4), 11–12. [On-line]. Available: http://www.scottlan.edu/lriddle/women/night_educ.htm http://www.scottlan.edu/lriddle/women/nitegale.htm http://www.math.yorku.ca/SCS/Gallery/ http://daisy.co.uk/daisy003.html

Only the Beginning

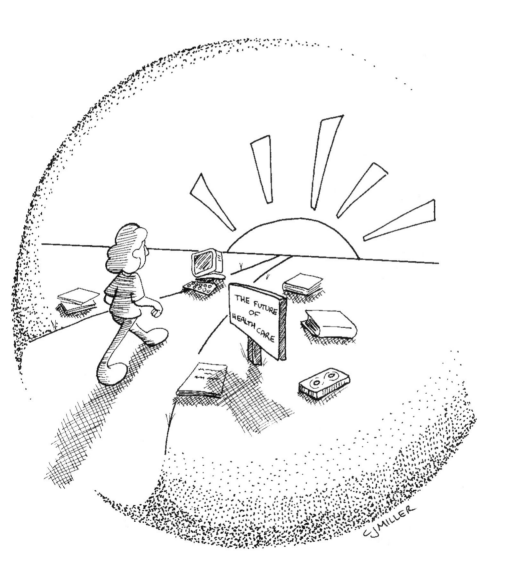

A t a time when hospital LOS is becoming shorter and staff have too many duties and not enough time, patient education managers must find a way to work smarter, not longer. The solution is to review the process and determine ways to streamline and re-engineer patient education."

—Joyce Dittmer, MSN, RN

(1998, *Patient Education Management,* 5(1), p. 2)

....

On the Road

As you travel the road of your career in nursing, look at your opportunities for teaching patients and families. Listen to their needs, look at how and when you teach, and see what works or doesn't work. Stay focused on the goals of patient and family education, and keep your care centered on your learner's needs. Use the most effective teaching methods, as defined by research.

As you increase awareness of your role as educator of patients and families, watch your expertise develop. Benner (1984) defines the competencies of the teaching-coaching function of nursing as follows:

- Timing: capturing a patient's readiness to learn
- Assisting patients to integrate the implications of illness and recovery into their lifestyles
- Eliciting and understanding the patient's interpretation of his or her illness
- Providing an interpretation of the patient's condition and giving a rationale for procedures
- The coaching function: making culturally avoided aspects of an illness approachable and understandable

These are some of the ways nurses treat the human response. Expertise in these skills can be very rewarding, both professionally and personally.

No Time to Teach? has shown how you can save time teaching by teaching well. Teach only what is necessary and appropriate. Use methods that are demonstrated to work effectively. Individualize teaching to your learner. If you didn't learn much about these techniques in nursing school, they may not make much sense until you apply them.

Research in patient and family education is growing quickly, so don't stop your education here. Periodically review the current literature for updates. Attend inservices and conferences. Make your learners into your teachers.

If you have internet access and e-mail, use them to keep in touch with colleagues and share knowledge. Also use them to keep up on the literature. If you want to learn about professional and lay patient education books in your clinical area, sign up with Amazon.com's Amazon Eyes service (http://www.amazon.com). If you belong to Sigma Theta Tau, ask for information about their book service. When a book in one of the topics you define is published, these services will send you an e-mail to let you know. They also offer you the opportunity to order the book, with a credit card, over the internet.

As you learn, gain experience, and grow in your patient and family education skills, consider sharing your challenges and successes with others in the profession. Share your exemplars. If you develop a teaching tool or program or build a successful team out of chaos, tell others about it at conferences, or write about it. Choose a nursing journal in which you can imagine your story appearing, and format your article in the style they publish. Submit it for publication.

We will all save teaching time if we stop simultaneously solving problems independently and share our knowledge and build the base together.

Who Empowered Dorothy?

Have you noticed this book did not once say that patient and family education empowers learners?

Do you know why?

It doesn't.

> "Teachers do not empower adult learners; they encourage the use of the power that learners were born with."
>
> —Vella, 1994, page 8

In *The Wizard of Oz*, Dorothy always had the power to go home. She just didn't realize it. She just needed someone to tell her how.

It's the same for your learners. They've been taking care of themselves their whole lives. They just need some encouragement and guidance to meet the newest challenges in their journeys.

It's the same for you.

You've always had the power to get the time you need to teach patients and families.

Where are your ruby red shoes? They're in the form of a little card. The one that licenses you to introduce yourself as a professional registered nurse.

You, and all other RNs, have had the power all along.

If we discharge patients before they are ready and able to care for themselves, we would be practicing unsafely. Our patients and families want to understand what is happening to them and what they have to do to take care of themselves. Our nurse practice acts tell us we are licensed and obligated to teach. The Joint Commission on Accreditation of Healthcare Organizations (JCAHO) insists that teaching be done and done well. JCAHO also wants us to make teaching an integral part of our business, by collaborating on it in our multidisciplinary teams and across the continuum of care.

The mission statement of the organization you work for probably mentions something about striving for excellence, quality of care, or patient satisfaction. Because patient satisfaction is strongly correlated with the effectiveness of patient and family education, that means your mission includes teaching.

What sort of power are you waiting to get?

Who are you struggling against to gain power? Is it the system? Who's that?

What profession has the greatest numbers in the system?

Nurses. We're in the community, all the health care facilities, and academia. We're even in managed care. We've infiltrated the system from the trenches, to quality improvement, to middle management, to the boardrooms.

Nurses are in position, have the support of learners and license, and have the skills to do it. We've had the power to teach all along. Now with the system's emphasis on cost-effectiveness and movement to increase self-care, timing is on our side too.

Continuous Learning

Unlike clicking our heels to get home, we're on our journey to the future of health care. We need to identify our challenges and deal with them, one by one.

The health care environment contains many structures that are inconsistent with our stated objectives. We say we want to cut costs but still emphasize development of high-tech, expensive interventions. We need to increase awareness about these inconsistencies and better align our resources with our objectives.

Do you need a tangible example?

"Most acuity systems ignore the importance of nursing interventions as patients get closer to discharge, reflected in decreased acuity levels at this time. However, the identification of activities relating to teaching interventions provides nurses with evidence that these interventions take as much nursing time and effort as frequent monitoring or assistance with self-care needs."

—Rakel, 1992, page 403

The system's intention is to decrease cost of care while maintaining quality. Patient and family education is demonstrated to be cost-effective and health promoting. If we don't document our teaching, don't document what's left undone, and don't advocate for quality care, we are undermining ourselves and our profession and cheating our patients and families.

It's similar to what happens if just to get your job done, you work unpaid overtime too often. In time, administration believes the time they're paying you for is all the time you need to accomplish your work. You've set yourself up by not communicating your needs.

We've had the power to teach all along. The external forces are on our side: patients, families, JCAHO, quality, cost-effectiveness, re-search, and timing. Now we have to document better the need for teaching, demonstrate its effectiveness to those controlling our bud-gets, and advocate better for our patients' rights to know, understand, and care for themselves.

The Essence of Nursing

"We, and only we, have the knowledge, skill, and ability to teach patients about their health. No one else can do it as well as we can."
—Freda, 1997, page 330

Quality patient and family education reflects the essence of profes-sional nursing.

"Nurses . . . through their education and experience, develop ways to observe and understand many ways of experiencing and coping with illness, suffering, pain, death, or birth and to offer patients avenues of understanding, increased control, acceptance and even triumph in the midst of these foreign, uncharted happenings. Experience in addition to formal educational preparation is required for the development of this competency, since it is impossible to learn these ways of being and coping with an illness solely by precept. A deep understanding of the situation is required, and often the ways of being and coping are transmitted without words but by demonstration, attitudes, and reactions."
—Benner, 1984, pages 89–90

Still No Time to Teach?

An expert on time management stood in front of a group of business students (high-powered overachievers) and said, "Okay, time for a quiz."

Then he pulled out a one-gallon, wide-mouthed mason jar and set it on a table in front of him. Then he produced about a dozen fist-sized rocks and carefully placed them, one at a time, into the jar.

When the jar was filled to the top and no more rocks would fit inside, he asked, "Is this jar full?"

Everyone in the class said, "Yes."

Then he said, "Really?" He reached under the table and pulled out a bucket of gravel. Then he dumped some gravel in and shook the jar causing pieces of gravel to work themselves down into the spaces between the big rocks.

Then he asked the group once more, "Is the jar full?"

By this time the class was onto him. "Probably not," one of them answered.

"Good!" the speaker replied.

He reached under the table and brought out a bucket of sand. He started dumping the sand in and it went into all the spaces left between the rocks and the gravel.

Once more he asked the question, "Is this jar full?"

"No!" the class shouted.

Once again the speaker said, "Good!" Then he grabbed a pitcher of water and poured it in until the jar was filled to the brim. Then he looked up at the class and asked, "What is the point of this demonstration?"

One eager beaver raised his hand and said, "The point is, no matter how full your schedule is, if you try really hard, you can always fit some more things into it!"

"No," the speaker replied. "Good guess, but wrong. What does this demonstration really show us? If you don't put the big rocks in first, you'll never get them in at all."

What's the moral of the story? If you have no time to teach, maybe you're treating patient and family education like gravel, sand, or water. Maybe you're squeezing it into the empty spaces of your day.

If you have no time to teach and teaching is one of your big rocks, maybe it's a big rock you didn't get in the jar.

Put your big rocks in first.

If you want to learn more about providing high quality patient and family education, here are key resources for the journey:

(1998). Process improvement teams revamp teaching programs to fit busy schedules. *Patient Education Management,* 5(1), 1–3.

Baker, C. (1992). *Just say it! How to write for readers who don't read well: A training manual for writers.* Washington, D.C.: Plan, Inc.

Bartlett, E.E. (1995). Cost-benefit analysis of patient education. *Patient Education and Counseling, 26,* 87–91.

Benner, P. (1984). *From novice to expert: Excellence and power in clinical nursing practice.* Menlo Park, CA: Addison-Wesley.

Dass, R., & Gorman, P. (1985). *How can I help? Stories and reflections on service.* New York: Alfred A. Knopf.

Doak, C.C., Doak, L.G., & Root, J.H. (1996). Teaching patients with low literacy skills (2nd ed.). Philadelphia: Lippincott-Raven.

Fink, A. (Ed.). (1995). *The survey kit.* Thousand Oaks, CA: Sage Publications.

Freda, M.C. (1997). Don't give it away. *The American Journal of Maternal/Child Nursing, 22*(December), 330.

Lawlor, M., & Handley, P. (1996). *The creative trainer: Holistic facilitation skills for accelerated learning.* London: McGraw-Hill.

Literacy Volunteers of America. (1992). *Secret survivors: The plight of functionally illiterate adults in the health care environment.* [Video.] Syracuse, NY: Author.

Lorig, K., Stewart, A., Ritter, P., González, V., Laurent, D., & John, L.J. (1996). *Outcome measures for health education and other health care interventions.* Thousand Oaks, CA: Sage Publications.

Lorig, K. (1996). *Patient education: A practical approach.* Thousand Oaks, CA: Sage Publications.

Morgan, D.L., & Krueger, R.A. (Eds.). (1998). *The focus group kit.* Thousand Oaks, CA: Sage Publications.

Pirsig, R.M. (1974). *Zen and the art of motorcycle maintenance.* New York: Bantam Books.

Rakel, B.A. (1992). Interventions related to patient teaching. *Nursing Clinics of North America, 27*(2), 397–423.

Rankin, S.H., & Stallings, K.D. (1996). *Patient education: Issues, principles, practices* (3rd ed.). Philadelphia: Lippincott-Raven.

Stallings, K.D. (1996). *Integrating patient education in your nursing practice.* [Video] Durham, NC: Horizon Video Productions.

Vella, J. (1994). *Learning to listen, learning to teach: The power of dialogue in educating adults.* San Francisco: Jossey-Bass.

A Summary for Those Too Busy to Read This Book

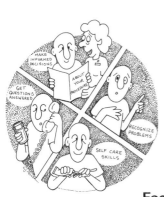

Focus on behaviors and skills

Be ready

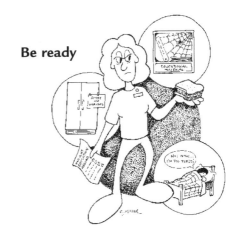

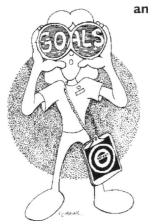

Frustration

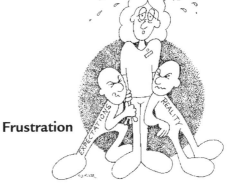

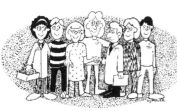

Partnerships

Listen, listen, listen

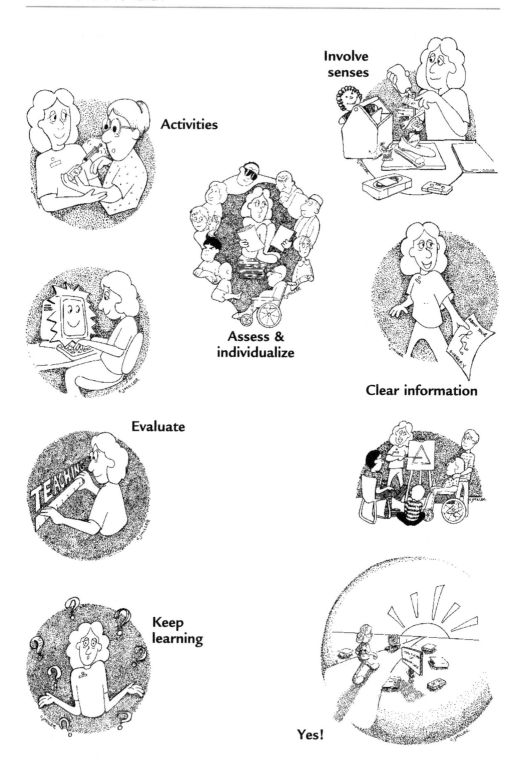

Activities

Involve senses

Assess & individualize

Clear information

Evaluate

Keep learning

Yes!

Appendix: The Goals of Patient and Family Education From the View of the Health Care Team

We teach to optimize health outcomes.

As a result of the education we provide, the learner can do the following:

- Make informed decisions
- Develop basic self-care skills to survive
- Recognize problems and know what to do in response
- Get questions answered; find resources for answers

Theory to Practice

Adult learning principles provide the structure for the contents of this book. Similarly, the cover of this book binds it and gives it structure. In this book, this metaphor has been made concrete. The guidelines for how adults learn appear on the inside covers of this book. They provide the theoretical framework.

How do you get from theory to practice? Here are some ways to apply the principles of adult education in the health care setting. The guideline is in bold, and the application below it.

- **Collaborate with the learner on goals, content, methods, and evaluation of teaching.**

    "You will be going home with a cast. Have you ever had a cast before?"

    "This is a big decision. What sort of information would help you decide which treatment to choose?"
- **Encourage learners to identify their own learning needs.**

    "What concerns you about this?"

    "What bothers you about this?"

    "What sorts of things might make it difficult for you to do this at home?"
- **Teach with active involvement, activity, and reflection.**
    - **Involvement:** "There are lots of ways people remind themselves to take their medicine. How do you remind yourself?"

- **Activity:** "Here's a form that can help you keep track of your medicine. Write the names of the medicines in this column, and the times you take them here . . ."
- **Reflection:** "What do you think about this system of keeping track of your medicine?"
   "If you used this at home, how would it work?"
   "What would make it work better?"
- **Encourage learners to identify resources and to create strategies for using such resources.**
   "If you had that question at home, where might you find the answer?"
   "When would you call the doctor?"
   "When would you go to the emergency room?"
   "When you're home, who can help you with this?"
- **Help learners carry out their learning plans.**
   "Here's a list of good diabetes cookbooks."
   "Here's the phone number of a consumer health library."
   "Here's a list of support group meetings."
- **Involve learners in evaluating their learnng.**
   "How are you going to explain this to your husband? Pretend I'm your husband. Tell me what you have to do."
   "What's the best way for us to be sure you can do this at home?"

The following are examples of ways to obtain information:

- **Assessing learning needs:**
   "Why are you here?"
   "Why do you think you have [this illness, this problem]?"
   "What have you done already to treat [this illness, this problem]?"
   "What would help you now?"
   "If you went home now, what would be your biggest concern?"
- **Identifying learning style:**
   "The last time you wanted to learn something on your own, how did you do it?"
   "How would you like to learn that? Would you use a fact sheet or a video? Do you want me to show you? Do you want to meet someone like you who learned how to do it?"
- **Evaluating understanding:**
   "Show me how you do that."

"Put [these pictures, these steps] in order. Now, tell me about each one."

"How would you explain [this medicine, this self-care skill] to your family?"

"If [describe a situation] happened, what would you do?"

"When you get home, what will you do differently?"

- **Establish learning priorities:**
  - Identification of needs by patient or family member
  - Sources of anxiety for patient or family member
  - Data to make informed decisions
  - Preparation for treatments and procedures, in terms of sensory experiences to expect
  - Basic self-care survival skills; importance of continuing therapy
  - Recognition of problems and what to do in response

Teaching Pitfalls

- The least effective question is, "Do you have any questions?" because a "no" response shuts off discussion.
  - Instead, ask "Is there anything I didn't say clearly enough?"
  - With this question, you take responsibility for individualizing teaching.
- The least effective method is not allowing the learner to interrupt your presentation of information.
  - This does not incorporate the learner in the process.
  - Teaching is most effective and takes less time when it involves dialogue.
- The least effective attitude is treating medical information as dogma, based on belief rather than science.
  - Political and religious idealogues believe they have universal and divinely ordained truth. They do not feel they need to learn from others and see criticism as irrelevant.
  - Medical information changes as we gain new information. Health information is not dogma. There is not one right way for the learner to behave. Learners have choices.
  - In effective teaching–learning interactions, all participants learn.
  - If teaching is taking too long, are you trying to convince learners you are right and they are wrong?

- The answer is not always education.
  - Sometimes people know what to do but choose not to do it. This is not corrected by providing the same information again.
  - This is corrected by determining why they are choosing not to change behaviors and dealing with the relevant issues.
- Assess knowledge before you teach.
- Save teaching time by teaching only when teaching is appropriate.

If you want to learn more, here are some classic resources:

Brookfield, S.D. (1986). *Understanding and facilitating adult learning: A comprehensive analysis of principles and effective practices.* San Francisco, CA: Jossey-Bass.

Smith, R.M. (1982). *Learning how to learn: Applied theory for adults.* Chicago, IL: Follett Publishing Company.

Knowles, M. (1984). *The adult learner: The neglected species.* Houston, TX: Gulf Publishing.

Knowles, M.S., Holton, E.F., & Swanson, R.A. (1998). *The Adult Learner.* Houston, TX: Gulf Publishing.

Wise, P.S.Y. (1980). Adult teaching strategies. *Journal of Continuing Education in Nursing, 2*(6), 15–17.

Index